THE PANDEMIC IN BRITAIN

This book offers a political analysis and sociological critique of the UK government's response to the novel coronavirus outbreak, interpreting the inadequacies of government policy with regard to COVID-19 as the results of neoliberal ideology, the protection of corporate interests, Brexit nationalism, and the peculiarities of a British model of capitalism based on international trade and labour market precarity.

Arguing that institutionalized corporate-capitalist control of state and science generates new and growing public health risks, and that consumer-driven individualism has eroded community life and the protections this might offer against pandemics, the author contends that the UK government's catastrophic response to the COVID-19 pandemic was the result of peculiarly British socioeconomic and political phenomena.

The Pandemic in Britain will appeal to scholars of sociology, philosophy and politics with interests in the COVID-19 pandemic as well as neoliberal ideology and its manifestation in political life.

Sean Creaven is Senior Lecturer in Sociology and Criminology at the University of the West of England, UK. His research interests include the sociology of modernity and postmodernity, sociological theory, critical theory, Marxism and Post-Marxism, critical realism and criminological theory. He is the author of *Against the Spiritual Turn: Marxism, Realism, and Critical Theory* (Routledge, 2010), *Emergentist Marxism: Dialectical Philosophy and Social Theory* (Routledge, 2007), and *Marxism and Realism: A Materialistic Application of Realism in the Social Sciences* (Routledge, 2000).

The COVID-19 Pandemic Series

Series Editor: J. Michael Ryan

This series examines the impact of the COVID-19 pandemic on individuals, communities, countries, and the larger global society from a social scientific perspective. It represents a timely and critical advance in knowledge related to what many believe to be the greatest threat to global ways of being in more than a century. It is imperative that academics take their rightful place alongside medical professionals as the world attempts to figure out how to deal with the current global pandemic, and how society might move forward in the future. This series represents a response to that imperative.

Titles in this Series:

COVID 19: Surviving a Pandemic
Edited by J. Michael Ryan

Pandemic Pedagogies
Teaching and Learning during the COVID-19 Pandemic
Edited by J. Michael Ryan

COVID-19 in Brooklyn
Everyday Life During a Pandemic
Jerome Krase and Judith DeSena

The Pandemic in Britain
COVID-19, British Exceptionalism and Neoliberalism
Sean Creaven

For more information about this series, please visit: www.routledge.com

THE PANDEMIC IN BRITAIN

COVID-19, British Exceptionalism and Neoliberalism

Sean Creaven

Routledge
Taylor & Francis Group

LONDON AND NEW YORK

Designed cover image: 'M5 in Lockdown. MMXX' © Maria Stadnicka 2020

First published 2023
by Routledge
4 Park Square, Milton Park, Abingdon, Oxon OX14 4RN

and by Routledge
605 Third Avenue, New York, NY 10158

Routledge is an imprint of the Taylor & Francis Group, an informa business

British Library Cataloguing-in-Publication Data
A catalogue record for this book is available from the British Library

ISBN: 978-1-032-19168-3 (hbk)
ISBN: 978-1-032-22985-0 (pbk)
ISBN: 978-1-003-27503-9 (ebk)

DOI: 10.4324/9781003275039

Typeset in Bembo
by Apex CoVantage, LLC

This book is dedicated to workers in social care and the NHS – heroes of the British pandemic, our saviours from British exceptionalism

CONTENTS

FOREWORD

The UK is exceptional in many ways, some of them good, some of them not so good. The Government's response to the pandemic has been equally as nuanced. Thus, while the UK was the first country in the world to administer a post-clinical-trial COVID-19 vaccine, they are also one of the countries with the highest infection, and death, rates per capita, and one where some arguably very bad decisions (at least from the perspective of public health) have made global headlines. Headlines, in fact, that helped lead to the ousting of a prime minister and a rejuvenated debate about the National Health Service.

The history of UK exceptionalism also includes being a pioneer in neoliberalism, spearheaded most notably by former prime minister Margaret Thatcher and her government. From a social science perspective, the impact of neoliberalism on issues like public health has been well documented, and very rarely with findings that indicate it is a life-saving approach to societal organization. Indeed, the neoliberal focus on profits over people has continued to rear its ugly head even as the world has experienced its most exceptional global health crisis in more than a century.

One of the strengths of this volume is that it was written as events unfolded. Indeed, as the reader will note, Creaven makes a number of predictions that, in the end, did not come to pass (although many of them did, unfortunately for public health and individual wellbeing). From a social and political perspective, this style only adds strength to the arguments as it shows how events unfolded in real time and gives insights into the "thinking of the times" that helped shape future decisions. One of the challenges of scholarship related to the *ongoing* COVID-19 pandemic is that it is often outdated by the time it comes to print. By framing the analysis in terms of a specific point in time, Creaven has overcome this challenge and, with little doubt, created a work that will be not only of social and political interest, but of historical interest as well.

Readers of this volume will not find it difficult to keep turning the page as Creaven's writing style is as engaging as it is informative. Indeed, this book is well poised to become *the* historical narrative of how the COVID-19 pandemic unfolded in the UK.

J. Michael Ryan
Series Editor, *The COVID-19 Pandemic Series*
September 2022

PREFACE

This book is to a large degree an attempt to examine the reasons for the UK government's internationally suboptimal performance in addressing the novel coronavirus pandemic. As such, this is conceived as a work of political *and* social critique. The two aspects of critique are interlinked. The political dimension of critique is of the gross inadequacies of UK government policy with regard to COVID-19 as this response has been framed by neoliberal ideology, the protection of corporate interests, the constraints of austerity politics, Brexit nationalism, and the peculiarities of a British model of capitalism that is more internationalized or export-based than those of the other developed countries. The social (or socio-economic) dimension of critique is of a type of society in which corporate-capitalist control of economy and state and science is institutionalized. British exceptionalism is a concept that is deployed in this book to account for these national policy failings.

The bulk of this book was written in draft before 19 July 2021's "Freedom Day". Indeed, the earliest draft was a polemical work titled *The Peculiarities of the British: Coronavirus UK – A Critical Analysis of the Government's Response*. This was written for students of Sociology at UWE in the spring of 2020 in the midst of lockdown and posted on the programme Blackboard pages. Thereafter, the present volume was set aside as I embarked on the task of analysing the pandemic in the global framework of political economy, scientism, consumerism, and the crisis of ecological sustainability of our civilization within which local pandemic events and policy responses to address them need (in my view) to be grasped.

This means that this book often refers to past events as present or upcoming events and offers forecasts of scenarios to come that either did or did not happen. This conveys a sense of the ongoing immediacy of the pandemic and of the way the UK state authorities responded to it, of the experience of these things as they unfolded in time, and of the concerns they raised. This also allows self-reflection by this author on the degree to which predicted happenings happened and the reasons why they did or did not. The reader will notice that I have dated the chapters to convey when they were completed in draft in the midst of the unfolding crisis. I have also indicated when they were finalized. The finalization in each case was mostly the addition of new references to support the earlier analysis. The concluding chapter updates the account and the timeline of events that supports the earlier analysis up until the summer of 2022.

ACKNOWLEDGEMENTS

My previous published work has all been situated on the terrain of social theory (much of it in the interface between Critical Realist philosophy and Marxian social science) and was informed by the work of a number of theoretically minded academics to which it was heavily indebted. This is not the case this time. This is a straightforward current affairs and politics book.

It would not have got started unless I (in common with everyone else) had been placed in hermit-like isolation during the first lockdown and if students of sociology of mine at the University of the West of England were not asking questions about the Government's handling of the crisis that were hardly acknowledged let alone answered in the corporate media – not until the first lockdown was upon us.

I would like to thank my students for asking those questions and for sharing their own critical ideas, focusing me on this project. Thanks as well as always to certain colleague-comrades at UWE (especially Andy, Ian, and Jack, but also Lita, Finn, and Maria) for tolerating my musings on the events and arguments this book addresses and the reasons for them. In the case of Jack, Andy, and Ian, these voicings were perhaps rather rambling and repetitive! For me, articulating ideas in conversation (or was it in monologue!) is a way of clarifying them. Do they *sound* right?

Maria Stadnicka warrants a special mention. This is for kindly allowing me to select an image from her wonderful photo exhibition on the pandemic for the front cover of this book. Jack Spicer too merits a special mention, for two reasons. Firstly, for reminding me in his own exemplary professional academic practice of delivering outstanding teaching and support for students as well as producing research outputs of the highest quality that I can once again (as I once did and doubted I would again) be an active researcher and published author, despite my heavy investments in students and the academic programmes I run. Secondly, for convincing me that being as such is of equal importance to these other commitments. Thanks, Jack!

INTRODUCTION

Anatomy of the UK pandemic

This undertaking is to a large degree intended as a critical analysis of the UK government's response to the novel coronavirus pandemic in this country. In that respect, it is conceived as a work of political critique, albeit informed by the analytical tools of social science. This may be of interest to those who have struggled to understand why we (here in the UK) have twice become (i.e. by the end of the first and second and perhaps third waves of the pandemic) the worst-hit European country for COVID-19 deaths, and among the world leaders internationally for mortality from the new disease.

At the time of writing this introduction (15 July 2021), the official UK death count from the virus stands at 128,609.[1] This places the UK in 19th place out of 222 countries internationally for mortality rate per head of the population and in second place in Europe (behind Russia) for absolute number of fatalities. The UK is presently the second worst performer for minimizing COVID-19 mortalities among all of the developed countries of the Global North, topped only by the USA.[2] Indeed, the Government's performance in containing the negative impacts of the pandemic on public health is much less impressive than in a large majority of developing countries of the Global South. These are countries that fared better in managing their own crises despite a level of per capita income considerably less than is enjoyed by the UK – the world's fifth or sixth largest economy – and despite in most cases having far less developed public health infrastructure and medicare resources at their disposal.

This undertaking is to a large degree intended as an attempt to examine the reasons for the internationally and regionally suboptimal performance of the UK in addressing the pandemic.

As such, this book is conceived as a work of political *and* social critique. The two aspects of critique are interlinked. The political dimension of critique is of the gross inadequacies of UK government policy with regard to COVID-19 as

DOI: 10.4324/9781003275039-1

this response has been framed by neoliberal ideology, the protection of corporate interests, and the peculiarities of a British model of capitalism that is more internationalized or export-based than those of the other developed countries, and which is focused especially on retail, hospitalities, tourism, and finance – with a substantial low-pay sector of the labour market characterized by precarity. The social (or socio-economic) dimension of critique is of a type of society in which corporate-capitalist control of economy and state and science is institutionalized. The ill-effects of the latter are manifold. Some of these will be addressed in this book.

Of particular interest has been the subordination of political and scientific judgements of what would be appropriate public health protections against the pandemic to those which are concerned with protecting corporate enterprise from the economic deficits of physical distancing. As this book will argue, British exceptionalism with regard to COVID-19 – which in practice consisted of eschewing a range of community protection measures on the grounds that each and every one of these was not "proven" to generate major advantages – was not simply an artifice of politicians, but also of scientists close to government. Ministers and establishment scientists alike were reluctant to cause economic harm to capitalist enterprise through speedy and proactive physical distancing measures unless there was incontrovertible evidence that these would, on a case-by-case basis, function almost as a magic bullet in controlling the virus.

Government scientists, as did the politicians, recognized that such protective measures would yield positive results, but these were deemed likely to be insufficient to warrant the economic price (slower growth, reduced profits, perhaps even a recession) that would need to be paid. This was especially if they were brought in "prematurely", that is, before the crisis spiralled out of control and threatened to overwhelm healthcare services. This mindset ensured that, right up to the first community lockdown towards the end of March 2020, there was in practice no policy of community protection or prevention against COVID-19. Rather, policy goals were restricted to the far more tepid reactive ones of slowing or delaying the spread of the virus and managing its impact on the National Health Service (NHS), with the result that the outbreak was much more intense and harmful to public health (and to the economy) than it would have been if a "safety first" approach had been taken from the outset.

This book is informed by media stories and reports as they unfolded over the course of the pandemic in Britain up until the present, illuminating some of the key issues surrounding the crisis. This is up to mid-July 2021, as the UK was engulfed by what is commonly represented as its third pandemic wave, but which with equal justice may be conceived of as its fourth wave. The narrative draws on these empirical materials to chart the development of the UK crisis and the unfolding government response to it since the start. This aspect of the work is a thematic critical-reflective analysis of the crisis, in the spirit of bearing witness, which may be as difficult for some to read as it was for me to write. Difficult because this is an account of a human tragedy in the making that was certainly avoidable.

The British first wave and its aftermath

In the period from 14 March until 15 May 2020, it has been estimated by the Office for National Statistics (ONS) that there were 54,032 excess deaths in England and Wales, or 76 percent more than would be typical based on comparisons with the equivalent timeframe in previous years.[3]

At the peak of the first wave of the pandemic in England and Wales (the weeks ending 17 and 24 April), the total number of deaths per week was more than twice normal levels. This was largely because more than 8,000 people died with COVID-19 in both weeks.

Of the four home nations, England suffered the most during the peak infection period. Moreover, the UK experienced over this period the longest uninterrupted period of excess mortality and the highest numbers of excess deaths in Europe.[4] At the peak of the first wave, on four consecutive days, from 7 to 10 April, the number of deaths was in excess of 1,000, hitting a daily peak of 1,168 on 21 April.[5]

The ONS reported 51,935 deaths from COVID-19 in England and Wales based on information on death certificates from the first one recorded up until 7 August (compared to the Government's official count of 38,266) and calculated 58,000 excess deaths since the start of March up until 7 August based on comparison with the equivalent timeframe for the years 2015–2019.[6] By contrast, according to the official GOV.UK statistics, the UK death toll from COVID-19 up to and including 14 May, when the curve of infection began to dip and the numbers of transmissions began to slow, was 33,614, with 233,151 cases of infection.[7] But this was a major under-estimate of the real scale of human harm and suffering that had been perpetrated especially up to that point, despite the Government's belated decision to add deaths outside hospital to the official count. That was because the number of deaths at home, in hospices, in care institutions and elsewhere must have been much higher than those which were officially recorded. The *Independent* reported on 9 May 2020:

> NHS England said earlier that the number of registered deaths involving COVID-19 had increased to 33,021, but new figures show that a further 3,610 hospital patients who had tested positive for COVID-19 died up to yesterday. Added together, they suggest the overall death toll for the UK has now passed 36,600.[8]

On 12 May 2020, *The Independent* re-calculated that the number of COVID-19-related deaths across the whole of the UK up to and including 9 May had risen to almost 51,000. COVID-19 was directly responsible for 33,257 of these deaths, or 71 percent of the total. The others were the results of the "collateral" damage caused by the disease. They were

> connected with wider changes in England and Wales since the lockdown began: a reluctance on the part of some people to visit a doctor or a hospital, for instance, or the result of long-term health conditions being made worse by having to remain at home.

The figure was arrived at by combining statistics on mortality rates from the Office for National Statistics (for England and Wales), the National Records of Scotland, and the Northern Ireland Statistics and Research Agency; and then comparing the number of deaths counted with the typical or average number that have previously occurred over the same timeframe.[9]

The Government's failure for several crucial months following the arrival of the novel coronavirus on these shores to embark on the kind of systematic community testing and track-tracing programme that was operationalized from the beginning in other European (including Italy) and South Asian countries ensured that the UK figures for infection and mortality in the run-up to and over the course of the first wave, irrespective of ambiguities in data collection, were likely to be much more in the way of under-estimates than in these other countries. Initially, there was not even routine testing of patients in hospital before community release or indeed testing of medical front-liners unless they displayed symptoms. In the early months, even testing of hospital patients who manifested obvious symptoms of infection was rate, whereas testing of poorly residents in care homes was negligible.[10]

Outside the hospitals and care homes, in the wider community, deaths were scarcely registered at all in the period from the start of the pandemic up until after the curve of the first wave began to flatten. This was simply due to the paucity of contact tracing and mass population testing.[11] There was also, according to a whistle-blower heavily involved in the registration of deaths, the problem of over-pressed GPs simply not citing COVID-19 on death certificates as an actual or suspected cause of a mortality where this was medically warranted, for various reasons.[12] This was the case even where such suspicions were plausible, and such deaths probable, owing to a reluctance of GPs to cite the new disease as the cause of death in the absence of a positive test result. All of this would have led to a substantial undercounting of fatalities.[13]

Fatalities in care homes were not even included in the official government statistics until 29 April 2020.[14] Statistical measures indicate that between 42 percent and 57 percent of COVID-19 deaths in European countries (Italy, Spain, France, Belgium, and Ireland) up to that point had taken place in care homes.[15] By contrast, the UK government estimated that, up to and including 10 April, only 16 percent of COVID-19 deaths in this country were in care homes,[16] whereas only 25 percent had been up to and including 1 May.[17] According to the Health Care Foundation, in the week ending 24 April, a total of 7,911 deaths were recorded in

UK care homes compared with 2,471 in the week ending 13 March when at a relatively early stage of the first wave. That was an increase of 220 percent that may be explained only by the intervention of an unprecedentedly calamitous event. This is suggestive that 5,440 deaths related to COVID-19 infection in UK care homes were likely to have occurred between 14 March and 24 April 2020 – far higher than the official government record of 3,096. Many others that were not attributed to COVID-19 infection would have occurred before the week starting 6 March, dating back to the start of the outbreak on 29 January.[18]

The ONS, whose statistics for deaths in care homes have since 29 April 2020 been counted by ministers as part of the "official" count, recorded 8,310 deaths from COVID-19 in care homes from 13 March to 1 May of that year. But a study conducted by London School of Economics (LSE) researchers concluded that the probable actual death toll in care homes over that same period was 19,938, since that was the number of excess deaths compared to the number recorded over the same period for the previous five years.[19] More recently, based on a study of excess deaths, between 13 March and 26 June 2020, it is estimated that 21,775 fatalities were of care home residents, or 40 percent of the total of the UK pandemic up to that point.[20] The reasons for this woeful performance will be discussed later in this book.

The second wave and after

Even before the first wave of the virus had receded, the UK had become the European leader and an outlier internationally for COVID-19 fatalities. This remained the case deep into autumn of that calamitous first year. By mid-October 2020, of the developed countries, with advanced healthcare systems, and relatively low household densities, the UK was in fourth place internationally for the total number of people who have contracted COVID-19. This was on the official count (i.e. statistics generated by Public Health England and the equivalent authorities for Scotland, Northern Ireland, and Wales). As of 14 October 2020, there were 654,644 officially acknowledged UK cases of the virus. By then, the UK was in seventh place internationally among the advanced countries in terms of relative infection rates, with 9,629 cases per million of the population. This was more than double the international average of 4,978 cases per million.[21]

In terms of fatalities, as the second wave of the virus began to gather pace from the latter part of September 2020 onwards, the UK had established itself as a world leader of the wrong kind in another way. Based on the official government (GOV. UK) statistics, 43,155 people in the UK died from COVID-19 up to and including 14 October. This situated the country in fifth place internationally for the total number of COVID-19 deaths. Moreover, of the developed OECD countries, the UK was in second place for the total number of officially recognized COVID-19 fatalities, trailing only the USA. By then, the UK also occupied fifth place among the advanced countries in terms of relative fatality rates adjusted for population densities (deaths per million of the population) and was in ninth place internationally under this same metric.[22]

The relative situation has since been improved, however. This is owing to major outbreaks of the virus in a number of less developed countries (Brazil, India, Mexico, etc.) alongside weak or negligent government responses to these outbreaks in those countries. But, in terms of international comparisons, the UK's situation has not been substantially improved by these events. By mid-July 2021, the UK remained in the top quintile of countries for death rate per million of the population (19 out of 222), and in second place in Europe (behind Russia) on total number of deaths. The UK, with 0.87 percent of the world's population, recorded 4,096,239 cases of infection by mid-July 2021, almost 3 percent of the world's then-total caseload (of 177,327,697).[23] Moreover, the UK remained by then the second worst performer of the developed world (behind the USA) in terms of COVID-19 mortalities.[24] Simultaneously, the absolute situation in Britain dramatically deteriorated especially since December 2020, owing to the impact of the second (or second and third) waves. Thus, up to and including 15 July 2021, 128,609 people in Britain have died from the virus, on the official counts. This was 3.1 percent of the world's total recorded fatalities. This was also a death rate per million almost three-and-a-half times higher than the international average.[25]

The cost of the new waves of infection on human life has been far greater than was caused by the first wave. The second wave (or second and third waves) was ascending from September 24 (2020) and receding by 24 March (2021). During this period, the number of people killed by the virus had, according to government statistics, increased by more than threefold, from 42,115 to 126,328. The first wave from its March 2020 beginnings to its 21 April peak (i.e. its peak in terms of the highest number of deaths on a single day) brought about 22,888 mortalities. The second wave from 28 September 2020 through to its peak (i.e. in terms of the highest daily number of fatalities) on 23 December added a further 28,813 to the number killed by the virus.[26] At this point, the four-week "circuit-breaker" lockdown that the Government brought in from 5 November to 2 December of that first year had at last begun to lower the number of daily mortalities (albeit briefly). This was more than three weeks after it was terminated. The circuit breaker also reduced transmission rates from their second wave peak of 33,407 new cases recorded on 12 November to 12,130 new cases recorded on 12 December 2020.[27]

Yet there were almost 101,000 new cases of infection during the week prior to the ending of the circuit-breaker, according to the official daily counts. This was a rate of community transmission that was more than three times higher than it was in the seven-day period before the start of the gradual unlocking of the first lockdown in the spring.[28] So, the ending of the second lockdown not only repeated the error of prematurity of the first one but also radicalized it. Infection rates were still almost 60 percent of the second wave weekly peak (of 170,686 new cases) when the total lockdown was abandoned in favour of a return to the failed tier system. This was manifestly insufficient to defuse the second wave or prevent its rapid metamorphoses into a bigger third wave. The third wave (or second upsurge of the second wave) then increased, on the Government's statistics, the number killed by a further 55,736, before it gradually receded. This was from 27 December 2020 through to 20 January 2021 when a record number of deaths on a single day (of 1,823 persons) was officially acknowledged.

The scale of the second and third waves seemingly dwarfed that of the first. The peak number of infections of the second wave (33,407 on 12 November 2020) was more than four times higher than it was on the first wave (7,646 on 10 April). The peak number of infections of the third wave (67,803 on 8 January 2021) was more than eight-and-a-half times higher than it was on the first wave. This is purely at the level of statistics, however. Of course, the real number of cases during the first wave would have been several times higher than those captured by the data, since in the absence of general testing (or even much specific or targeted testing) only a small minority of infected people (those serious enough to require hospitalization) were enumerated. Nonetheless, the increase of the death rate on the second spike (albeit over a much longer period than the first) and its doubling on the third was strongly suggestive of a major upsizing of the caseload volume. This was nothing less than a human calamity. The start of 2021 was disastrous. Between 6 January and 30 January, the daily death toll was in excess of 1,000 people on 19 days out of 25.[29]

As previously observed, during the first wave, official UK data on mortalities were undoubtedly considerable underestimates of the real magnitude of the human costs of the crisis, and these statistical inaccuracies that depressed the volumes were likely to be more pronounced in the UK than in comparable countries. Statistics on excess death rates revealed a much higher count. Excess deaths were "most pronounced in the first wave in early 2020, with 48% more deaths than usual in the three months to mid-June". But, during the summer of that year, the excess death rate dropped to a level that paralleled the statistical counts for COVID-19 fatalities, before rising to 24 percent above the norm owing to the second wave that was building towards the end of the year and the third wave which let rip in January 2021. These had climbed above 100,000 by the start of February of that year.[30]

However, the variation between calculations of COVID-19 deaths based on excess mortality and the actual counts collated by the Government on its daily dashboard narrowed if not disappeared over the course of the spring and summer of 2021. There are several reasons for this.

> As the pandemic has progressed, changes in coding have closed the gap between deaths from COVID-19 and excess deaths, and from December non-COVID deaths were below the five-year average. The understanding of how the disease affects different groups of patients has increased, and clinicians have much more experience in identifying and treating the disease. There is also more capacity to test patients for COVID-19, so it is likely to be identified at an earlier stage of their illness.

The Nuffield Trust estimates "the overall impact of the pandemic by comparing the number of deaths each week with those we would expect to see based on the average for the same week over the last five years". Based on this:

> For the weeks ending 13 March 2020 to 12 March 2021, there were 651,327 deaths registered in England and Wales which is 112,244 above the expected number of 539,083 – indicating there were 21% more deaths registered over this period. Two-thirds of these excess deaths occurred within the first two months, and at the height of the first wave there were more than double the expected number of deaths in a week. The second wave occurred over winter, when the expected number of deaths each week is at its peak, and hence the difference between this year and the average is smaller.[31]

This was not particularly out of step with government daily estimates based on counts of those who had died within 28 days of receiving a positive diagnosis. Yet the Government's decision in June 2020 to recalculate the number of COVID-19 dead based on the "28-day cut-off rule" is estimated to have resulted in an undercount of 20 percent on all mortalities before mid-February 2021.[32] This translated into potentially as many as 23,000 lost lives effectively chalked off the ledger. Previously, all those who died following a positive test were counted among the COVID-19 dead, whereas most medical-scientific experts opined that counting all those who died within 60 days of a positive test would arrive at more reliable and accurate figures.[33]

Counting all deaths following a positive diagnosis would undoubtedly inflate the figures. This was the stated rationale of ministers for bringing in the 28-day rule – along with the need to generate speedy data that would inform policy decisions in the teeth and claw of the crisis and to bring the collection of statistics in England into line with those in the devolved countries. However, the previous counting method was unlikely to have significantly inflated the death count, whereas the 28-day limit on counting deaths would radically deflate it. This, indeed, was bound to be the intention of a government with vested interests in finding a reason to drag the mortality rate closer to those European Union (EU) countries (Spain, Italy, and France) that were also hard hit by the first wave in order to evade or disguise its own outlier status among nations.

For sure, it is possible to recover from an attack of the virus, only to step under a bus a few weeks later, but that mischance is rather improbable.[34] Virtually all people who died after falling ill from COVID-19 would have done so either because the virus caused them to die or because it was a major contributor to their death, whether that was within 28 days or two or three months later. As reported in the *Guardian* newspaper, research at Leicester University tracked 40,000 COVID-19 patients for 140 days after their discharge from hospital. This study revealed that almost one-third of them were back in hospital within five months owing to health problems caused by the virus whereas 23 percent were re-hospitalized within 60 days. Not only that, the study also found that 12.5 percent of them died from

COVID-19 "complications" or from other conditions exacerbated by these complications whereas 9 percent died within 60 days but after 28 days.[35]

Calculations based on excess death statistics are also likely to underestimate mortalities. One reason for this is that there has been a long-run tendency for mortality rates to fall, which has continued in recent years. This means that estimating current death rates based on rates in the five preceding years loses sight of the fact that the size of the former would be greater if the expected continued progress in mortality performance had continued in the COVID-19-ravaged years rather than being thrown into sharp reverse. However, this is a relatively minor matter. A second, more significant, reason for regarding excess death statistics as underestimating COVID-19 fatalities is that the lockdowns and other physical distancing and public health precautions offered the population much greater protection from the typical seasonal illnesses (especially influenza) that normally cause thousands of winter deaths among the elderly and vulnerable.[36]

By contrast, if we instead base our estimate of COVID-19 mortality on the number of death certificates issued that present the disease as the cause of death or as a major contributor to the cause of death, the number of fatalities has been even more calamitous. This, according to ONS data, had reached 150,000 towards the end of March 2021,[37] and by 15 July had climbed to 154,000.[38] Death certificate data collated by the ONS confirms the basic patterns revealed by the Government's statistics, but at much higher scales:

> The death toll of the second wave was higher, with 56,735 fatalities 30 days either side of the peak, compared with 44,235 in the same timeframe during the first wave, according to UK death certificate figures from the Office for National Statistics. Coronavirus deaths also hit a fresh peak in early January when 1,465 deaths were registered across the UK on 19 January, similar to the previous record daily death toll of 1,459 just over nine months earlier, on 8 April 2020.[39]

But, again, even these figures were an underestimate. During the first wave, as we have seen, it is likely as well that many COVID-19-caused deaths (especially of the old and those with other major illnesses or frailties) were not acknowledged on death certificates by over-pressed medics. Rather, unfamiliar with the disease, or in denial about it, doctors often attributed deaths to underlying conditions (such as dementia) or to events (such as coronaries) that may have been triggered by an attack by the virus, or who confused its symptoms with those of other respiratory illnesses.

There is also the negative impact of Post-COVID-19 Syndrome or "Long Covid" that manifests as a wide range of symptoms. These, according to the NHS website, include: fatigue; shortness of breath; chest pain or tightness; problems with memory and concentration; insomnia; heat palpitations; dizziness; pins and needles; joint pain; depression and anxiety; tinnitus and ear ache; nausea, diarrhoea and stomach aches; loss of appetite; high temperature, sore throat, and cough; loss of sense of smell or taste; and rashes.[40]

British exceptionalism

As I write this introduction (15 July 2021), the UK is caught in the grip of a third (or even fourth) wave of the novel coronavirus.[41] The origins of this latest wave can be traced to the back end of May as infection rates renewed their upwards climb and as this trend accelerated from 23 June onwards. This was after a period of static infection rates for most of May at the lower scales following on from a dramatic decline from the astronomical peak of the preceding wave (of 60,407 new cases on 2 January) through to the end of April. On 30 May, 4,240 new cases were recorded. By 11 June, this had climbed to 11,625 new cases. By 1 July, 27,704 new cases were recorded – the highest daily increase since 28 January. By 15 July, 60,680 new cases were recorded – the highest tally ever. During the period from 30 May to 15 July (2021), there were on average 19,305 cases per day.

Unlike the earlier waves, however, this latest one has not been accompanied so far by big increases in hospitalizations or deaths. During the period from 30 May up to and including 3 July, as the present wave began to build and accelerate, there was an average of 12,779 new cases of infection per day. Over this same period, however, there were 444 new deaths – an average of 12.68 per day. By contrast, during the longer gestation period of the second wave (from 16 September 2020 until the second lockdown of 5 November that year), the total death tally was 6,460. This was an average of 126.7 per day, with 25,128 new cases reported on the day before the second lockdown began, and with an average caseload over the whole period of 14,470 per day.[42]

This turnaround of performance in terms of minimizing casualties is due to the impact of the vaccination programme. This is estimated by Public Health England to have prevented between 6.4 million and 7.9 million infections and between 26,000 and 28,000 deaths in England alone since it was rolled out from mid-December 2020 up until June 2021.[43] This is a striking success story, but one which also points immediately to the bigger shortcomings. This is the failure (for reasons explored in this book) of other government pandemic-management policies to protect the public from disease and save lives that preceded the vaccination programme and that have continued alongside it.

The chief failures in question are those of mishandled lockdowns and unlockings, insufficiently robust physical distancing and other precautionary public protection policies, inconsistent and unclear public health information (which watered down public compliance with lockdown and physical distancing restrictions), and delayed and dysfunctional test-and-trace systems. The UK's vaccination programme was initially much more advanced than those in the EU countries (though the EU is now vaccinating at a faster rate than in Britain and the USA and is fast catching up).[44] However, at the time of writing, the UK is still an international leader in the race to inoculate.[45] Yet the official death toll in the UK (which was 128,103 on the day that the PHE report was released)[46] remains higher than everywhere on the continent except Russia, and is now set for more sharp increases as physical distancing recedes in the aftermath of 19 July's "Freedom Day".

Given these circumstances, if the Government had not placed the UK in the international vanguard for mass vaccination, the magnitude of the public health disaster would have been considerably, catastrophically, worse. Pre-vaccination, the UK was a poorer performer for COVID-19 deaths than every one of the EU states, and already the second worst performer for deaths among all of the developed countries. And so, were it not for pharmaceutical technoscience's "sending in the cavalry" (so to speak), the outlier status of the UK for pandemic management failures would have been even more starkly exposed. Instead of 128,000-plus official deaths, there would probably have been 155,000.

To put it starkly, there were not many countries that needed the vaccine solution more urgently than the UK. The gap between this country's pandemic performance and that of all other comparable countries except the USA would have been so great that denial of British exceptionalism could invite only incredulity. That the UK has evaded this new disaster cannot be considered as anything less than fortuitous. For all of its flaws, "big" corporate science delivered its bio-technical fix far quicker than could reasonably be aspired. Set alongside this get-out-of-gaol card, the Government's early contract signings (compared to the EU) for vaccine procurements and fast-tracking (compared to everywhere else) of regulatory clearance for the vaccines was a secondary matter.[47]

Basically, the success of the vaccination programme has licensed ministers to dilute its gains in favour of other benefits and indeed to risk these gains altogether in a breathless dash for virtually full economic and social normalcy. Such risky premature unlockings of physical distancing protections are an aspect of British exceptionalism. British exceptionalism refers to the particularity or peculiarity of the UK government's policy response (and non-response) to the pandemic. The phenomenon includes delayed or tardy (but also piecemeal and unthorough) lockdowns, in comparison to those in many other countries. This is deferral in the sense that these are enacted in response to crises that have escaped controllability rather than as a means of averting crises or preventing these from spilling out of control. British exceptionalism also manifests as ambivalent or even inconsistent public health and safety messaging, so that public compliance with physical distancing rules is potentially compromised. A further aspect of the phenomenon is foot-dragging over the full spectrum of health and safety protection measures (including mask-wearing, border controls and travel restrictions), motivated seemingly by either scepticism or fatalism. Moreover, there was as well the lack of advance preparedness for pandemic events, seemingly rooted in complacency.

British exceptionalism is a somewhat inexact term, however. This is inasmuch as it denotes more the policies of the Westminster government than those of the devolved authorities – especially those of Scotland and Wales. (In this undertaking, the focus of critique has been on decision-making and decision-non-making by the British or UK government.) *English* exceptionalism may, therefore, be a better fit, with regard to the political events addressed in this book. Yet the term *British* exceptionalism nonetheless retains efficacy owing to the predominance of England in the union and the overall political authority exercised from Whitehall over the

UK. This is also because, in practice, the degree of policy variance in the UK with regard to the pandemic has been fairly narrow (though the devolved governments of Scotland and Wales have on occasions exercised a somewhat greater degree of caution than Johnson's with regard to unlockings and a somewhat greater willingness to impose restrictions in response to escalating caseloads).

British exceptionalism is intended not simply to describe the multiple failings of the UK government's response to the pandemic that made it calamitous but also to get started on the task of explaining these failings – how and why they occurred. A full explanation of British exceptionalism and its effects is not possible without attention being paid to sociological context. This is especially of how British exceptionalism was made by the politics of neoliberalism (as a mode of state and governance and its ideological legitimations) and is very much expressive of these politics.

At the economic level, policy failure is attributable to pressures exerted on capitalism-supportive governments by the law of value (the dynamic of inter-capitalist rivalries). This is the pressure of constraint to speedily restore profitability faced with the threat of comparative competitive disadvantage in the global marketplace. At the political level, this is a story of the international dominance of neoliberalism, since neoliberalism is no prisoner of corporate capitalism, but is its active and willing accomplice. Neoliberalism is a form of governmentality that sees its role as building a business state, a consumer society, and a fully commodified culture, since all of this is regarded as indispensable to economic success under conditions where capitalism is internationalized. Finally, at the ideological level, this is the success of neoliberalism in promulgating myths of "globalization" (i.e. of capitalism as irresistible juggernaut, unbound by national borders, compelling state-actors to bend-the-knee to market forces, and seeing in this master–servant relationship only virtue).

To be clear, the concept of British exceptionalism does not mean that the UK government response has been unique among all nation-states in manifesting any one or more of these specific failings, or even all of them collectively. On the contrary, there have been strikingly similar policy failings to greater or lesser degrees in most countries, as well as some striking national success stories. Moreover, where there have been these failings, they are attributable to the same political, ideological, and economic factors that account for British exceptionalism. So, in that sense, British exceptionalism cannot be seen as unprecedented. Rather, the exceptionality of the exceptionalism consists in the fact that this has been characterized by *each and every one* of the policy failings or "errors" found elsewhere, and on a bigger scale than in most other places. This is especially among governments of the developed world (with the possible exception of the USA), but also among those of a large swathe of those of developing countries, especially in Southeast Asia.

Many other states other than the UK have not coped well with the pandemic. This is owing to a considerable degree to the kinds of constraints (as well as imperatives) that are exerted on policymaking by global political economy. That is, by the near-hegemonic status of neoliberalism in some shape and to some degree among the leading state actors, and the system of untrammelled corporate-capitalist power in world economy that neoliberalism was designed to unleash and empower. Yet none of the governments of the G7 (and few of those of the G20) have handled the pandemic worse than the British government. The UK response has been especially compromised (or more compromised than elsewhere) in terms of offering effective public health protection because state and governance in the UK has been far more absorbed by neoliberalism and by the imperatives of corporate enterprise than in most other countries. Most pertinently, the impact of neoliberalism in undermining vital public services in the UK, especially those of healthcare and social care, and to a greater degree than in other developed countries, this has actually posed a considerable risk of undermining the effectiveness of public health protections when faced with the peculiar challenges of the pandemic. This was by sustaining an almost perpetual austerity or retrenchment of the non-commercial sector, as this book will set out.

Themes

This book will explore the following themes. (1) British exceptionalism in its many aspects. These are basically policy aspects as these unfolded over the course of the pandemic. (2) The nature of neoliberalism as a mode of politics and ideology as this has developed in the UK in the run-up to the pandemic and in relation to British capitalism. (3) The impact of this neoliberal governance in corporate Britain on those social and welfare services (the NHS and social care) that were to bear the brunt of managing the pandemic and which owing to chronic under-funding under years of neoliberal hyper-austerity were placed under intolerable strain. (4) The political mobilization of science and expertise as modes of legitimation for government policies that compromised public health in the service of the interests of economic powerholders.

Timeline

The period of coverage of the analysis is divided into five phases. First: *Phase 1*. This was from the start of the crisis, as this originated overseas, in Wuhan City and Hubei province, China, through to the first wave of community transmissions in the UK that eventually triggered the first general lockdown of the country. This is the period from the start of 2020 until 24 March of that year. This was characterized by government inactivity and complacency, a policy of "wait and see", as the pandemic headed towards these shores, as evidence accumulated overseas of the scale of the crisis to come, and as community outbreaks in the UK began to spiral.

During this period, a lack of advance government preparations was followed by a reticent, tardy, and wholly reactive policy response, for reasons that will be diagnosed. This was at odds with the World Health Organization (WHO) guidance and with the policy approach taken by most other governments. Not only that, it was seemingly blind to the lessons to be learned from the devastating effects of the virus in neighbouring EU states which were experiencing major community outbreaks (with heavy death tolls and overwhelmed healthcare systems) several weeks in advance of this country. The UK lockdown when it arrived was indeed at least two weeks too late. This was even though the Government had the opportunity to learn from the devastating consequences of delayed lockdowns in Italy and Spain (whose governments were less well placed to enact border-defence policies and did not have, as the UK government did, the advantage of hindsight in appreciating the immediate necessity of radical physical distancing policies).

Second: *Phase 2*. This was the period of de-escalation or un-locking of the first UK lockdown, commencing in the middle part of May 2020, and increasing rapidly through June, July, and August of that year. This is the period when the Government attempted to fast-track the country back towards "business as usual", following the devastation wreaked on families, communities, health and care services and the economy by the pandemic's first wave. Compared to the other European countries that introduced full community lockdowns, not only was the UK's long deferred but it was also curtailed much sooner. A reactive, tardy approach to radical physical distancing was followed by its contrary: an aggressively proactive approach to scaling it down. The reasons for both, I will argue, were identical.

Third: *Phase 3*. This was the period since the start of September 2020 up until the start of the second lockdown starting in November of that year. This witnessed the dramatic resurgence of COVID-19 transmissions, with rapid upsurges in community infections in most parts of the country, alongside the steady ramping-up of the fatality rate nationally. During this period, the rate of community transmission was higher than it was when the Prime Minister (PM) announced the first national lockdown in his belated response to the first wave of community transmission towards the end of March. This period elicited a disjointed and reactive policy approach by government – as physical distancing measures were strengthened (albeit only in certain ways and up to a point) in areas where transmission rates spiked radically but were elsewhere avoided until further notice, even as caseloads inexorably ascended. Such resembled a repetition of the earlier *ad hoc* "wait and see" and "hope for the best" strategy in the runup to the first wave. The key objective of government policy during this phase, it would appear, was *avoidance* – not so much of community spread of the virus but of a second lockdown.

Yet the timing of the second wave – in autumn and on the cusp of winter – was always likely to necessitate exactly a repeat of the earlier shutdown, unless the virus was to be allowed free reign. Allowing it free reign, however, would almost certainly have overwhelmed an NHS that had suffered decades of austerity-motivated underfunding and which had barely coped during the first wave. The reluctance of the Government to countenance a nationwide radicalization of physical distancing measures, on the grounds that piecemeal tightening of restrictions here and there under the newly introduced three-tier alert system would be sufficient to bring the second wave under control, was never a remotely feasible strategy. This sowed the seeds for a bigger health crisis than would otherwise have transpired if earlier more decisive nationwide action had been taken.

Far too late, several weeks after government scientists and the political opposition in parliament had begun calling for tightening of restrictions, the Government acquiesced to a four-week "circuit-breaker" lockdown, from 5 November to 2 December 2020. This was necessary, in the words of PM Boris Johnson, to "prevent a medical and moral disaster for the NHS".[48] This succeeded in lowering transmission rates and easing the pressures on the NHS as this was faced with fast-rising hospitalizations. But, given the abbreviated timeframe of the second lockdown and the lack of intent to extend this if warranted, this was sufficient only to dampen rather than defuse the second wave. Or, perhaps it was insufficient to prevent the rapid transition from a second to a third wave, once the restrictions were lifted. As was planned from the start, the lockdown was abandoned in favour of a return to a modified multi-tiered system of local alert-based controls – basically the same policy approach that had failed to flatten the second wave. This led ultimately to thousands more unnecessary deaths and a more protracted third lockdown.

Next: *Phase 4*. This includes the period after the late-autumn early-winter circuit-breaker of 2020 ended, the run-up to Christmas that year, and the Christmas holiday period thereafter. The latter was especially notable for the Government's remarkable decision to majorly suspend its own physical distancing rules by permitting gatherings of extended family in indoor gatherings in all tiers except the red-flagged ones on Christmas Day. Initially, the suspension of this aspect of physical distancing was to be applied nationwide irrespective of tier and for several days over the seasonable holiday. But, under the pressure of critique from oppositionists, this was scaled down, but not until the cusp of the holiday season, by which time millions had made their travel plans – with predictable results.

This period also covers the third and longest of the nationwide lockdowns starting on 5 January 2021. This the Government could defer but not avoid owing to the tardiness and insufficiency (in terms of duration) of the late-autumn early-winter circuit-breaker plus the ill-fated (and disadvised by government scientists and other non-aligned scientists and public health professionals) suspension of physical distancing norms on family mixing over Christmas. The third national lockdown (like the second) was thereafter notable for being less stringent or thoroughgoing than the first, owing to more exemptions. This was despite the fact that transmission rates, hospitalizations and mortalities exceeded the first wave.

Finally: *Phase 5*. Included in this period are the key events of the step-by-step unlocking of the third lockdown, starting from 8 March 2021 with school returns, along with the roll-out of the vaccine programmes (which were started on 8 December the year before) that accompanied this process. This unlocking of lockdown was, like the first one, a phased one, on the basis of a roadmap to normalcy. But, unsurprisingly, this second de-escalation was rather more cautious and tentative and hence more protracted than its predecessor. Government ministers with their eyes on the polls simply could not afford a third public health mauling having fast-tracked de-escalation before. Moreover, it would have been prohibitively unpopular in the court of public opinion to unlock lockdown ahead of progress in the vaccination programme, given the scale of death in the second wave (or second and third waves combined). Nonetheless, Johnson's "roadmap" of 22 February 2021 was confident enough to commit to the abolition of physical distancing by 21 June. Moreover, there were missteps and calamities along the de-locking road (as will be set out in the next chapter). These mirrored the bigger ones of the first unlocking, and for the same basic reason – a willingness to minimize business harm at the cost of taking more risks with public safety.

By contrast, the vaccination programme may be counted as the only highlight of the Johnson government's handling of the pandemic, since this proceeded rela-tively smoothly and efficiently, delivering impressive rates of vaccination. These exceeded the ambitious schedules set out by the Government just as they steadily and radically drove down hospitalizations and mortalities from April 2021 onwards. This success may be attributed to three main factors.

Firstly, this was incentivized by all of the previous failures – including especially by the inadequacies of the track-and-trace systems that were supposed to prevent new lockdowns and allow an earlier release from them. This meant that the only prospect of escaping the cycle of the upscaling and downscaling of physical dis-tancing rules was by fast-tracking vaccination. Secondly, the vaccination project chimed with neoliberal agendas whereas the public health protection measures that came beforehand and ran adjacently did not. Vaccination was not about pub-lic health protection (the minimization of death or permanent disability in the vulnerable population). Rather, this was about rendering the caseload of hospital admissions manageable for the NHS, so that the lockdown could be lifted as soon as possible, enabling people to be returned to work. So, it was driven by the usual prioritization of the economic over the social that was characteristic from the start. Finally, owing to the necessity of avoiding yet another misstep that would place the ruling party beyond the electoral last-chance saloon, ministers for once resisted the lure of their own neoliberal fetish of appointing VIPs ("dynamic" entrepreneurs, i.e. corporate businesspersons) to oversee and organize the rollout. Instead, this was placed in the hands of public health administrators and experts and the NHS, to be delivered mostly by GP practices, hospitals, pharmacies, and care homes.

Freedom Day?

As I write this introduction, however, new storm clouds are gathering – or rather a repetition of earlier ones are. These are those posed by the prospect of another reckless dash for complete normalcy. Ministers have been emboldened by the success of the vaccination programme in extending double-dose protection to the 60-plus age groups and those with underlying health vulnerabilities and in extend-ing the scope of vaccine coverage to all but the under-thirties demographic. But a government with this one's track record of aversion to decisive action in defence of public health becomes more dangerous as it becomes more confident. Conse-quently, the unlocking of the third lockdown, already well advanced by the end of May, was due to be completed by 21 June 2021.

However, the third (or fourth wave) of the pandemic was then beginning. Cases were rising, fuelled by rapid community infection rates among the unvaccinated younger demographic groups. This was owing to the history of unlocking up to that point and the way the steady easing of restrictions (and the way these were presented by the Government as irreversible steps towards freedom and liberty) emboldened young people to take liberties with the watered-down controls on physical distancing that remained. Not only that, escalating transmissions were being driven by potentially more dangerous variants of earlier strains of the virus (i.e. in terms of their greater infectiousness and perhaps enhanced vaccine resistance). Consequently, Health Minister Matt Hancock along with Chancellor Rishi Sunak and Michael Gove were persuaded to bow to the advice of government scientists (and the lobbying of independent scientists) who urged caution on the final unlocking that would end controls on all indoor settings and gatherings. These three subsequently secured Johnson's "approval" (or rather forced it on him) for a delay on ending all restrictions by a further month – until 19 July 2021. This was to give scientists close to the Government time to study the latest data on the impact of vaccination on the new variants in relation to hospitalization rates.[49]

This decision was unpopular in the governing party (just as Johnson's acceptance of the delay was grudgingly conceded): unpopular among the grassroots constituency members; and unpopular for a growing number of MPs and government ministers, perhaps even a majority of both.[50] Disquiet on the backbenches over pandemic restrictions existed from the start. This had grown into a vociferous and organized campaign of opposition to physical distancing within the parliamentary party under the misnamed Covid Recovery Group in the run-up to the second lockdown as the tier restrictions were phased in.[51] So, following Johnson's decision to delay the final unlocking, press reports circulated alleging that, driven by overcaution, Hancock had helped secure cabinet approval for the delay by suppressing the most recent scientific study data that showed that this was unwarranted.[52] This data reputedly showed that, despite the rapid spread of infection owing to the new variants, this was not significantly upscaling hospital admissions or mortalities.

Two weeks later, Hancock was no longer in post, owing to either resignation or dismissal – which is not clear. This was after a video recording of him in a compromising embrace with one of his aids whom he was accused of having an extra-marital affair with was leaked to the *Sun* newspaper.[53] The scandal rendered Hancock's tenure as Health Secretary untenable, since he was exposed not only as disregarding physical distancing rules imposed by his own ministry but as an adulterer to boot. Perplexingly, the incriminating video images were captured by a CCTV camera that had been turned around from its customary position of facing out into the street so that it was instead viewing inside Hancock's government office where the incriminating scene was filmed.[54] This had more than a whiff of the conspiratorial.

This impression was reinforced by subsequent events. Within a day of Hancock's resignation/sacking, Sajid Javid, right-wing neoliberal hardliner, former chancellor, and reputed supporter of the stillborn herd immunization strategy that the Cabinet briefly entertained as the first wave got started, was appointed as the new Health Minister. Javid wasted no time in declaring ("bullishly", as the ITN *News at Ten* put it)[55] that there was no prospect of anything but the full and complete termination of physical distancing on 19 July 2021. This was, as he put it, "irreversible". Nor would there be further lockdowns. This was because, since no date was risk-free, the Government would from now on be eschewing its allegedly "data, not dates" policy in favour of, as Javid put it, a "dates, not data" policy, so that thereafter the country would simply have to "learn to live with" the virus.[56] Now, this was complacency reinvigorated.

What of the immediate future? Irrespective of whether or not the post-19 July situation will lead to major increases in hospitalization in the UK, what is probable is that this will bring about a huge spike in transmission/infection rates, including and especially of the doubly mutated Delta variant that is viewed with concern worldwide. The UK is presently one of the world leaders in vaccination rates, well ahead of the EU and most of the rest of the developed world. This could mean that, just as restrictions on commerce and association within the UK are lifted, these will be radicalized on all things British across borders.

This is a scenario which is quite feasible as other countries seek to protect themselves from the import of new contagions from these shores, at least for the period of time that it will take for their vaccine programmes to achieve parity with the UK's, and perhaps beyond if many will still opt for physical distancing rules in some shape or degree. British exceptionalism would then be expressed as international isolation, as the country is red-flagged for COVID-19 hazard just as other national red flags are being lowered in countries where governments did not simply throw caution to the winds.

International isolation owing to British exceptionalism over COVID-19 containment policy would potentially place major obstacles in the way of the process of re-positioning UK corporate enterprise in the global marketplace. Such would not be good for business, to put it mildly, especially since the UK economy is more export-oriented than most of those in Europe, so that it has more vulnerabilities than they to the negative impacts of disruption of world trade. If so, the severe damage wrought on the UK economy by the pandemic and the shortcomings of the Government's response to it (which has been greater than that suffered by the other major advanced competitor economies) is likely to be ongoing and profound. Hard times beckon.

15 July 2021

Notes

1 Worldometer (2021). *COVID-19 Coronavirus Pandemic: United Kingdom*. Available at: www.worldometers.info/coronavirus/country/uk/. Accessed: 15/07/2021.

2   Worldometer (2021). *COVID-19 Coronavirus Pandemic: Reported Cases and Deaths by Country or Territory World*. Available at: www.worldometers.info/coronavirus/#countries. Accessed: 15/07/2021.

3   Scobie, S. (2020). *Measuring Mortality During COVID-19*. Nuffield Trust (online). (26 May). Available at: www.nuffieldtrust.org.uk/news-item/measuring-mortality-during-COVID-19-a-q-a?gclid=EAIaIQobChMIlNbIhd6z7AIV0N_tCh3T7gzqEAAYASAAEgKxiPD_BwE.

4   ONS (2020). *Coronavirus (COVID-19) in 10 Charts*. ONS (online). (24 September). Available at: www.ons.gov.uk/peoplepopulationandcommunity/healthandsocialcare/conditionsanddiseases/articles/coronavirusCOVID19in10charts/2020-09-24. Accessed: 28/04/2020.

5   Worldometer (2021). *COVID-19 Coronavirus Pandemic: Reported Cases and Deaths by Country or Territory: United Kingdom – Daily New Deaths in the United Kingdom*. Worldometer (online). Available at: www.worldometers.info/coronavirus/country/uk/. Accessed: 03/07/2021.

6   Raleigh, V. (2020). *Deaths From COVID-19 (Coronavirus): How They Are Counted and What They Show?* The Kings Fund (online). (19 August). Available at: www.kingsfund.org.uk/publications/deaths-COVID-19.

7   *ITV News* (2020). 'UK coronavirus death toll increases to 33,164 as further 428 deaths confirmed'. (14 May).

8   Dalton, J. (2020). 'UK coronavirus death toll increases to 31,587'. *Independent*. (10 May).

9   Lovett, S. (2020). 'Coronavirus: nearly 51,000 excess deaths in UK during COVID-19 pandemic'. *Independent*. (12 May).

10 Oliver, D. (2021). 'Mistruths and misunderstandings about COVID-19 death numbers'. *British Medical Journal* (online), 372 (8279). (10 February). Available at: www.bmj.com/content/372/bmj.n352.

11 Kitt, H. (2020). 'Contact tracers could deal with five people a week before scheme ended'. *Evening Standard*. (31 March); Tapper, J. (2020). ' "Recruit volunteer army to trace COVID-19 contacts now", urge top scientists'. *Guardian*. (4 April).

12 *Channel 4 News* (2020). 'Can we rely on COVID-19 death figures'? (13 April).

13 Oliver (2021).

14 Booth, R. (2020a). 'Care home fatalities to be included in daily coronavirus death tolls'. *Guardian*. (28 April).

15 Booth, R. (2020b). 'Half of coronavirus deaths happen in care homes, EU data suggests'. *Guardian*. (13 April).

16 Booth (2020a).

17 Holt, A. and Butcher, B. (2020). 'Coronavirus deaths: how big is the epidemic in care homes'? *BBC News*. (15 May).

18 The Health Foundation (2020). *Care Homes Have Seen the Biggest Increase in Deaths Since the Start of the Outbreak*. Available at: www.health.org.uk/news-and-comment/charts-and-infographics/deaths-from-any-cause-in-care-homes-have-increased. Accessed: 29/04/2020.

19 Booth, R. (2020c). 'Coronavirus: real care home death toll double official figure, study says'. *Guardian*. (13 May).

20 University of Stirling (2020). *Care Homes in England Had Greatest Increase in Excess Deaths at Height of the COVID-19 Pandemic*. University of Stirling, Management School. (30 August). Available at: www.stir.ac.uk/news/2020/august-2020-news/care-homes-in-england-had-greatest-increase-in-excess-deaths-at-height-of-the-COVID-19-pandemic/.

21 Worldometers (2020). *COVID-19 Coronavirus Pandemic: World*. Available at: www.worldometers.info/coronavirus/. Accessed: 15/10/2020.

22 Worldometers (15 October, 2020).

23 Worldometer (2021). *COVID-19 Coronavirus Pandemic: World*. Accessed: 15/07/2021.

24 Worldometer (2021). *COVID-19 Coronavirus Pandemic: World*. Accessed: 15/07/2021.

25 Worldometer (2021). *COVID-19 Coronavirus Pandemic: Reported Cases and Deaths by Country or Territory: United Kingdom*. Available at: www.worldometers.info/coronavirus/country/uk/. Accessed: 15/07/2021.

26 Worldometer (2021). *COVID-19 Coronavirus Pandemic: Reported Cases and Deaths by Country or Territory: United Kingdom – Daily New Deaths in the United Kingdom*. Accessed: 15/07/2021.

27 Worldometer (2021). *Reported Cases and Deaths by Country or Territory: United Kingdom*. Accessed: 03/07/2021.

28 Worldometer (2021). *Reported Cases and Deaths by Country or Territory: United Kingdom*. Accessed: 03/07/2021.

29 Worldometer (2021). *Reported Cases and Deaths by Country or Territory: United Kingdom*. Accessed: 03/07/2021.

30 Duncan, P., McIntyre, N. and Barr, C. (2021). 'UK's excess death toll since start of COVID pandemic passes 100,000'. *Guardian*. (2 February).

31 Scobie, A. (2021). *Measuring Mortality During COVID-19*. Nuffield Trust, Evidence for Better Health (online). (24 March). Available at: www.nuffieldtrust.org.uk/news-item/measuring-mortality-during-COVID-19-a-q-a.

32 Oliver. (2021).

33 See: Duncan, P. and Barr, C. (2021). 'UK official COVID death toll has always undercounted fatalities, analysis shows'. *Guardian*. (22 January).

34 This was actually presented in a government press release as an example of how the old counting methods could potentially be over-estimating pandemic casualties.

35 Duncan and Barr (2021); Oliver (2021).

36 Scobie (2021); Lovett, S. (2021). 'Not a single case of flu detected by public health England this year as COVID restrictions suppress virus'. *Independent*. (25 February); Pearce, C. (2021). 'No flu cases detected in England this year to date'. *Pulse*. (23 February).

37 Conway, E. (2021). 'How does the UK's death total really compare with other countries'. *Sky News*. (24 March). See also: Barr, C., McIntyre, N. and Duncan, P. (2021). 'UK COVID deaths pass 150,000 milestone, analysis shows'. *Guardian*. (27 March).

38 *ITV News* (2021). 'UK COVID cases rise by almost 50,000 in one day – highest increase since January 15'. (15 July).

39 Barr et al. (2021).

40 NHS (2021). *Long-Term Effects of Coronavirus (Long COVID)*. Coronavirus (COVID-19). Available at: www.nhs.uk/conditions/coronavirus-COVID-19/long-term-effects-of-coronavirus-long-COVID/. Accessed: 12/07/2021.

41 Which of these (third or fourth wave) is a matter of dispute based on whether one counts the dip in cases owing to the circuit-breaker lockdown of November 2020 as ending the second wave.

42 Worldometer (2021). *Coronavirus COVID-19 Pandemic: Countries: United Kingdom*. Available at: www.worldometers.info/coronavirus/country/uk/. Accessed: 15/07/2021; GOV.UK (2021). *Coronavirus (COVID-19) in the UK: Deaths Within 28 Days of Positive Test by Date of Death*. Available at: https://coronavirus.data.gov.uk/details/deaths. Accessed: 15/07/2021; GOV.UK (2021). *Coronavirus (COVID-19) in the UK: Cases in United Kingdom: Cases by Specimen Date*. Available at: https://coronavirus.data.gov.uk/details/cases. Accessed: 15/07/2021.

43 PHE (2021). *COVID-19 Vaccines Have Prevented 7.2 Million Infections and 27,000 Deaths*. Press Release. (28 June). Available at: www.gov.uk/government/news/COVID-19-vaccines-have-prevented-7-2-million-infections-and-27-000-deaths. These estimates were derived from analysis by PHE modellers and those of Cambridge University's MRC Biostatics Unit using their real-time pandemic surveillance model. Other pandemic modellers estimate smaller but still major gains.

44 De Maio, G. (2021). *Order From Chaos: EU Learns From Mistakes on Vaccines*. Brookings Institute (online). (20 May). Available at: www.brookings.edu/blog/order-from-chaos/2021/05/20/eu-learns-from-mistakes-on-vaccines/; *BBC News* (2021). 'COVID: what

is happening with the EU vaccine rollout'? (21 June); Oltermann, P., Giuffrida, F. and Wilsher, K. (2021). 'It's such a relief': how Europe's COVID vaccine rollout is catching up with UK'. *Guardian*. (19 June).

45 Our World in Data (2021). *Coronavirus (COVID-19) Vaccinations*. (12 July). Available at: https://ourworldindata.org/COVID-vaccinations.

46 Worldometers (2021). *COVID-19 Coronavirus Pandemic: Countries – United Kingdom*. Available at: www.worldometers.info/coronavirus/country/uk/. Accessed: 12/07/2021.

47 De Maio (2021); Oltermann et al. (2021).

48 *BBC News* (2020). 'COVID-19: PM announces four-week England lockdown.' (31 October).

49 Elgot, J. (2021). 'Losing "freedom day" is galling for Boris Johnson, but things could get worse'. *The Guardian*. (14 June).

50 Elgot (2021).

51 Campbell, L. and Sparrow, A. (2020). 'UK coronavirus: Johnson suffers biggest commons revolt since election as MPs back new COVID tiers by 291 to 78 – as it happened'. *Guardian*. (1 December); Fisher, L. (2021). 'Boris Johnson told his leadership will be "on the table" without exit strategy from restrictions'. *Telegraph*. (14 January); Hope, C. (2020). 'Headache for PM as dozens of conservative MPs set up COVID recovery group to fight lockdowns'. *Telegraph*. (10 November); Morris, S. (2021). 'COVID-19: Boris Johnson survives conservative rebellion as MPs back delay of lockdown easing until 19 July'. *Sky News*. (17 June); Press Association (2021). 'Tory MPs tell Johnson to commit to lifting COVID restrictions by end of April'. *Guardian*. (13 February); Rayner, G., Fisher, L. and Yorke, H. (2020). 'Tories in revolt over Boris Johnson's COVID tiers'. *Telegraph*. (30 November); Walker, P. (2020). 'Coronavirus: Johnson faces Tory revolt over stricter tier plan for England'. *Guardian*. (22 November).

52 Hughes, T. (2021). 'Hancock "sat on vaccine data" before freedom day delay'. *Evening Standard*. (20 June); Malnick, E. (2021). 'Matt Hancock kept Boris Johnson in dark over COVID vaccine success'. *Telegraph*. (19 June).

53 Harrison, E. (2021). 'Matt Hancock quits as health secretary after breaking social distance guidance'. *BBC News* (26 June); *Sky News* (2021). 'Matt Hancock resigns as health secretary after admitting breaking COVID rules'. (27 June).

54 Devlin, K. (2021). 'Security camera in Hancock's office which caught his affair was "outlier" and not general policy, government says'. *Independent*. (29 June).

55 *ITN* (2021). 'News at ten'. (28 June).

56 Allegretti, A. (2021). 'Sajid Javid: COVID restrictions in England must end on 19 July'. *Guardian*. (29 June); Cameron-Chileshe, J. and Parker, G. (2021). 'UK must "learn to live" with COVID, says new health secretary'. *Financial Times*. (28 June); Courea, E. and Swinford, S. (2021). 'Bullish Sajid Javid is confident that COVID restrictions will end on 19 July'. *Times*. (29 June); Jain, A. (2021). 'Javid "confident" of 19 July lockdown end, as NHS boss urges him to show "caution"'. *Independent*. (28 June).

1

THE ROAD TO LOCKDOWN

In the previous chapter, I set out the purely empirical dimensions of the British pandemic. This is the pandemic enumerated – a narrative of caseloads, hospitalizations, and deaths as statistics. The numbers alone make for sobering reading. They reveal a horrific record of failure of the Government to minimize damage to the life chances of its citizens. Now, acknowledgement of this state of affairs has not yet come to us courtesy of Boris Johnson's government. Nor is this likely to happen. To this day, despite all that has happened (which this book will document), and despite a mountain of evidence to the contrary, the Government brazenly insists that its handling of the crisis has been correct in essentials. Matt Hancock, Health Secretary since before the start of the pandemic up until mid-June 2021, was readily available in the run up to the first lockdown and thereafter to rule out as either premature or pointless every potential public protection measure (flight suspensions, travel bans, airport temperature screening, tighter physical distancing rules, mask-wearing, restrictions on mass gatherings, community lockdown, etc.) that were being brought in by other countries facing major COVID-19 outbreaks.[1]

The benefit of hindsight has since done little to alter his perspective. Responding to the comments of Professor John Edmunds – who lamented the tardiness of the first UK lockdown, seeing this as coming three weeks too late, and thus being responsible for thousands of unnecessary deaths – Hancock was simply dismissive: "We did the right thing at the right time".[2] In a refrain that was repeated *ad infinitum* throughout the course of the pandemic's first wave, ministers sought to legitimize this cocktail of governmental non-action and deferred action by insisting that this was based on the authority of "the science". This perpetuated the myth of a unitary science, as if scientists spoke with one voice (when clearly they did not), and as if decisions about which scientific guidance to listen to (and which not to) and how to respond to it were not political ones.

DOI: 10.4324/9781003275039-2

The PM, in his broadcast to the nation on 10 May 2020, which announced the start of the UK's scaling-down of the first lockdown, offered the most dogmatic and bullish affirmation of the party line, which has not since been modified or retracted – neither by him nor by his ministers or press officers. This was also remarkable for its temerity in asserting that, were it not for the effectiveness of the Government's actions (and the British public's co-operation with them), *hundreds of thousands* would have died in the first wave. This would have been the case, Johnson asserted, because of the seriousness of the threat posed by the disease. As he put it:

> Though the death toll is tragic and the suffering immense, and although we grieve for all those we have lost, it is a fact that by adopting those measures we prevented our country from being engulfed by what could have been a catastrophe in which the reasonable worse-case scenario was half a million deaths.[3]

At the time of Johnson's 10 May address, the "official" global death toll from COVID-19 stood at 292,000.[4] So, on Johnson's logic, the British public ought to have thanked its lucky stars that his government's response to COVID-19 was so effective that the UK had at that point avoided suffering *almost twice as many deaths as the rest of the world put together*. The staggering disingenuousness of this statement ought to be clear to anyone whose recollection extended only as far back as the start of March that same year (as the UK pandemic began to build) or who had taken the slightest interest in the global impact of the virus up to that point.

On the eve of the crisis

Back at the tail end of January and through to mid-March 2020, as the new coronavirus rapidly crossed borders and continents, *en route* to British shores, some of us (myself included) were experiencing a steadily rising feeling of horrified dismay at what appeared to be an almost complete lack of ministerial interest or concern over the potential crisis to come. I wrote several letters to the *Metro* towards the end of January, during February, and at the start of March, in which I expressed this concern and the reasons for it. Not a single one of these was considered worthy of publication. I did not take this personally, however, since not a single letter penned by anyone else (and there surely must have been plenty) was published in the *Metro* over this period, or not that I detected. Alas, the media was seemingly no more interested in the issue than was the Government. In the period from 20 January to 20 March, the dominant perspective of reporting the pandemic in the UK by the bulk of the corporate press was characterized by *complacency* and *acquiescence*. This was complacency in the sense of downplaying the threat posed to public health by the virus. This was acquiescence in the sense that government inaction was not challenged or scarcely questioned.[5]

There appeared to be no plan or strategy for the UK at all for managing the upcoming pandemic – not until one was unveiled with the belated publication (on 3 March 2020) of *Coronavirus: An Action Plan – A guide to what you can expect across the UK*.[6] This, as it transpired, was largely hefted from long-standing flu pandemic planning documents rather than representing anything new linking specifically to COVID-19. This document spanned a total of 27 pages, but it did not get around to laying out "planning principles" for dealing with a COVID-19 outbreak until p. 9, or actual plans to deal with the virus until p. 10. It manifested the glacial complacency that had characterized the Government's response up to that point:

> The UK is well prepared for disease outbreaks, having responded to a wide range of infectious disease outbreaks in the recent past, and having undertaken significant preparedness work for an influenza pandemic for well over one decade (e.g. our existing "flu" plans). Our plans have been regularly tested and updated locally and nationally to ensure they are fit for purpose. This experience provides the basis for an effective response to Covid-19, which can be tailored as more specific information emerges about the virus.[7]

Coronavirus: An Action Plan cautioned only that it was "*more likely than not* [my emphasis] that the UK will be significantly affected", despite the fact that known impacts elsewhere may be better described as major rather than merely significant, and ministers were aware that its own Scientific Advisory Group (SAGE) was of the view that the reports and studies from China were likely to be majorly downplaying its impacts on public health. The document made frequent references to the similarity of the impact of COVID-19 compared to seasonable flu viruses, even the common cold. Thus:

> Among those who become infected, some will exhibit no symptoms. Early data suggest that of those who develop an illness, the great majority will have a mild-to-moderate, but self-limiting illness – similar to seasonal flu.[8]

> . . . a minority of people who get COVID-19 will develop complications severe enough to require hospital care, most often pneumonia. In a small proportion of these, the illness may be severe enough to lead to death. So far the data we have suggest that the risk of severe disease and death increases amongst elderly people and in people with underlying health risk conditions (in the same way as for seasonal flu).[9]

> . . . The majority of people with COVID-19 have recovered without the need for any specific treatment, as is the case for the common cold or seasonal flu – and we expect that the vast majority of cases will best be managed at home, again as with seasonal colds and flu.[10]

All of this was, of course, speculative. It simply was not possible to offer sound judgements on the likely or probable depth and magnitude of public health harms, the proportions of people who would have no ill effects, or who would experience inconsequential or minor symptoms, and of those who would experience major and life-threatening illness. It was also one-sided: speculation on the side of optimism rather than on the side of pessimism. And so, for example, although a "small minority . . . *will* [my emphasis] develop complications" that would require hospitalization, for "a small proportion of these . . . the illness *may* [my emphasis] be severe enough" to cause death.

This was basically how ministers wanted it to play out – and so, it seemed, for that reason, this became for them the likely scenario. And so government forecasts were riddled with Panglossian assumptions, or the appearance of them. These were that only a tiny proportion of the population would likely experience significant symptoms (less than 1 percent of those infected). These were that as little as 0.1–0.2 percent would die from the illness (i.e. one or two in every 1,000 people). These were that "only" the elderly and infirm and those with underlying serious health conditions would be vulnerable to serious illness or dying from the illness.[11] These rose-tinted judgements, which were already being confounded by the Italian experience, were perhaps informed by the conclusions of a study by an Oxford University-based group of mathematical modellers that made headline news in March 2020 in a number of newspapers, which indeed predicted a mortality rate of 0.1 percent.[12]

Remarkably, despite its manifest complacency and lack of details, the Government's Action Plan was sufficient to dissolve anxieties within the right-leaning corporate press over the Government's approach that were finally, belatedly, manifesting by the start of March. Print media opinion-formers allowed themselves to be reassured that the Government's rejection of radical physical distancing measures such as were being implemented everywhere else was the "sober" and "sensible" response. Popular themes of press coverage regarding the Government's Covid strategy in the three weeks leading up to the U-turn that delivered the first lockdown became:

- *Decisive leadership* (Johnson's – for holding the line against those calling for lockdowns);
- *Over-reaction* (of foreign governments and politically motivated scaremongers at home who were calling for tougher physical distancing regulations);
- *Deference to expertise* (i.e. of the need of the public and politicians to accept the recommendations of the Government's scientific experts, just as the Government was supposedly doing – who were not supporting more radical physical distancing policies);
- *Herd immunity* (i.e. lending support to what appeared to be the Government's strategy of allowing the virus to spread unchecked in society at large whilst "shielding" the old and vulnerable from community outbreaks in order to build up natural immunity.[13]

Back in the real world, as the first wave tapered off before mid-May, there were 219,000 confirmed cases of COVID-19 infection in the UK alongside 31,855 confirmed deaths – a mortality rate of 14.5 percent approximately relative to these officially "known" cases.[14] Of course, the real number of cases would have been much higher than the count for recorded cases. This was owing to asymptomatic transmission (estimated as being anywhere between 20 and 60 percent of all cases) and, as noted earlier, because the Government had for a long period of time limited testing to hospitals and (to a lesser extent) care homes. This was also because, for reasons stated earlier, the attribution of COVID-19 fatalities in the community and care homes to other causes on death certificates must have led to a significant undercount.

Thus, estimating the real mortality rate relative to infection rate during the first wave with any degree of accuracy, given the lack of real data, is impossible. But loose estimates, within fairly elastic boundaries, are at least feasible. Data released by the ONS on 28 April 2020 indicated that the real mortality rate of the virus was 55 percent higher than the Department of Health and Social Care's (DHSC's) official count, estimating that 33,596 people had already died from it. On 24 April, four weeks after lockdown, Chris Whitty, the UK's Chief Medical Officer, estimated that at least 10 percent of Londoners (900,000 people) had already contracted the virus, but he considered that the infection rate was much lower outside the capital.[15]

Assuming, conservatively, a fairly high national infection rate of 8 percent by the time that the first surge of COVID-19 began to recede (on Whitty's estimates it was likely much lower), this would mean a mortality rate from COVID-19 in the UK of between 0.5 percent and 0.8 percent of those infected – which was *five-to-eight-times higher than the Government's initial "expectation"* of fatalities. This would be broadly consistent with the estimates of mortality rates drawn from studies in other countries and internationally. UC Berkeley researchers estimated, on the basis of first-wave data, a mortality rate of 0.85 percent for Italy and of 0.5 percent in New York State, for example. An Imperial College London study estimated that the global fatality rate from the disease up to mid-May 2020 stood at 0.66 percent, to offer a further example. The mortality rate from common flu, by contrast, is, according to data from the USA, around 0.1 percent.[16]

The March Action Plan

The "strategy" or "plan" for dealing with the COVID-19 outbreak in the UK that was set out in *Coronavirus: An Action Plan* was stated as follows:

> The fundamental objectives are to deploy phased actions to Contain, Delay, and Mitigate any outbreak, using Research to inform policy development. **Contain**: detect early cases, follow up close contacts, and prevent the disease taking hold in this country for as long as is reasonably possible. **Delay**: slow the spread in this country, if it does take hold, lowering the peak impact and pushing it away from the winter season. **Mitigate**: provide the best care possible for people who become ill, support hospitals to maintain essential services and ensure ongoing support for people ill in the community to minimise the overall impact of the disease on society, public services and on the economy.[17]

Pages 12–14 outlined what was currently being done under the "contain" stage. At the core of it, of course, was contact tracing – "case finding and isolation of early cases"[18] – with those found to have been infected (but without symptoms) or infected but with minor symptoms being required to stay home until the illness manifests and those symptoms pass. But what else? Here there were plenty of references to the unspecified work of "expert teams" (including that of Border Force, port operators and carriers), and to the equally unspecified "established . . . procedures" or "well-rehearsed plans" (all of course "tried and tested") of public health agencies and authorities, and also to the "cascading" of information between various teams and organizations and to all health professionals. There was also reference to an unspecified "public communications plan".[19] Needless to say, this was all rather hazy and impressionistic, the stuff of buzzwords, an exercise in impression management.

The Action Plan cited "new powers" under "public health legislation" in England that permits "medical professionals, public health professionals and the police . . . to detain and direct individuals in quarantined areas at risk or suspected of having the virus".[20] In Scotland and Wales, health boards or local authorities may draw upon equivalent powers if they wish. Yet citing existing powers under legislation to take certain actions was not of course itself any kind of action or plan of action. Powers to act are neither actions nor action plans.

Finally, a little more concretely, there was this:

> As part of the port health measures, direct flights arriving into the UK from countries within the UK's CMOs' case definition are required to provide a declaration (General Aircraft Declaration) to airport authorities stating that all their passengers are well, 60 minutes prior to landing. Similarly, The Maritime Health Declaration Form is required for all vessels arriving from any foreign port. For Scotland parallel measures are in place.[21]

Remarkably, this was the *whole* of the UK government's border-protection policy. People planning to travel back and forth overseas were simply asked to seek out the advice and guidance of the Foreign and Commonwealth Office (FCO).[22]

The outline of strategy and action plans for the "delay" stage was even more threadbare than for the "contain" stage. This contained just a few bullet points, the larger of which was simply a restatement of the definition and purpose of the stage:

> Delaying the spread of the disease requires all of us to follow the advice set out below. The benefits of doing so are that if the peak of the outbreak can be delayed until the warmer months, we can reduce significantly the risk of overlapping with seasonal flu and other challenges (societal or medical) that the colder months bring. The Delay phase also buys time for the testing of drugs and initial development of vaccines and/or improved therapies or tests to help reduce the impact of the disease.[23]

As for the rest: "Many of the actions that people can take themselves – especially washing hands more; and the catch it, bin it, kill it strategy for those with coughs and sneezes – also help in delaying the peak of the infection". This pretty much exhausted the content of the "plan", as far as guidance up to then was concerned. Looking ahead, if necessary, increased publicity on the need for good hygiene and of the need of people to stay home for the duration of their symptoms was promised. And there was mooted the possibility that "population distancing strategies" may need to be used in order "to slow the progress of the disease through the population" (e.g. "school closures, encouraging greater home working, reducing the number of large social gatherings").[24] Notably, no general community lockdown or even local lockdowns were being entertained here as even a *potential* scenario.

Nor was there clarity on the status of the stages of the Action Plan – contain, delay, and mitigate. Were these actually stages at all? Chris Whitty appeared to have trouble translating the Action Plan into something publicly intelligible, as he briefed MPs on 7 March. This was because he was trying to read it as setting out a sequence and was floundering with the task, because there were on his reading no stages as such. "We are now, basically, mainly in delay, but we are maintaining some elements of contain; we are mainly in the second stage at this point".[25] A problem with the Action Plan, therefore, was not simply that it was remarkably lacking in substance and coherence. This was as intentions were presented as plans, as plans were alluded to but not set out, and as objectives were counted as actions. Rather, part of the problem was that even the *semantics* of the Plan were misleading – even to those (like Whitty) who ought to know the difference between a goal and an action.

Up until and beyond the release of *Coronavirus: An Action Plan*, on 3 March 2020, it was clear that, in place of a strategy or plan for managing a UK outbreak of coronavirus, there was evidence only of an attitude of complacency, bordering on neglect, in effect "wait and see – and hope for the best", in ruling circles. As *Coronavirus: An Action Plan* states: "Based on experience with previous outbreaks, it may be that widespread exposure in the UK is inevitable; but slowing it down would still nonetheless be beneficial".[26] "Inevitable" is a strong word. That the Government considered widespread infection to be a likely *inevitability* was instructive, since that assumption may encourage the complacency of fatalism. Such fatalism most likely would have stemmed in part from Johnson's government's love affair with neoliberalism and corporate-capitalist "globalization", which meant it simply was blind to the possibility of a border-control defence policy. I will return to this issue later in greater detail.

Disregarded warnings

Whatever the reasons for it, the evidence for reckless complacency is plentiful. For a start, the Government's own scientific advisers, the SAGE group, did not meet to discuss the unfolding pandemic-in-the-making for the first time until 22 January 2020. This was hardly proactive. There was of course plenty of evidence of a potentially major crisis in the making several weeks before then. This is clear from the timeline by which events unfolded. This evidence was apparent not simply in known facts but also in potential facts that may reasonably be suspected – and which it is the job of SAGE and its advisory subgroups to be carefully monitoring.

As we have seen, the Chinese government reported the new disease to the WHO on 31 December 2019. This was a disease that was reportedly causing "severe, undiagnosed pneumonia" in people in Wuhan.[27] Such was a major cause for concern because pneumonia is life-threatening but usually treatable by antibiotics, yet these treatments and others for flu-type viruses were apparently ineffective. By 8 January 2020, China's Centres for Disease Control and Prevention (CDC) had confirmed this was a coronavirus, of the same family as Severe Acute Respiratory Syndrome (SARS), originating in bats.[28] Again, this was for scientists profoundly worrying, because human diseases originating in bats are plentiful and harmful. These include not only SARS, but also rabies, hepatitis C, Ebola, and Middle East Respiratory Syndrome (MERS), to name but a few.

> In April 2020, researchers reported six kinds of coronavirus previously unknown to science in bats in Myanmar. That adds to the 400-odd found already in China. In 2017, a survey of all known gene sequences of coronavirus found there were a hundred "clusters", essentially family groups, of the viruses. Ninety-one of those live in bats, making bats the world headquarters of coronavirus evolution.[29]

At that point, the Chinese authorities were reporting that there was no evidence that the new virus was capable of intra-species human transmission, just as it was claiming a low caseload in Hubei (of just 41). But all of this was viewed with considerable scepticism by international scientists, for a number of reasons. First, there were reports of community infections in the city and of arrests of people for discussing the disease on online platforms. This was alongside government censoring of the content of online group chats on which Wuhan medics discussed the virus as well as the reprimanding of healthcare staff for circulating "unfounded rumours" of intra-human transmission and a potential pandemic. Second, there was a lack of speedy public health information being released by Beijing on the subject of the illness's transmissibility. Finally, there was the CDC's delay in publishing the disease's genome sequence. This was done only after a Shanghai-based laboratory went public with its own sequencing without official permission and was promptly closed down by the regime for its troubles.[30]

Based on this sequencing, and on analysis of airline passenger statistics, Neil Ferguson's team of mathematical epidemiologists at Imperial College London estimated (in their report of 17 January 2020) that there were likely as many as 1,723 cases or so in Wuhan already. This appeared rather more than would be expected of a virus that was not capable of, as Ferguson put it, "self-sustaining human-to-human transmission".[31] By 20 January, it was apparent that the virus had escaped Hubei, with new cases not only popping up all over China, but also in Japan,

Thailand, and South Korea, so that human-to-human transmission was undeniable. On the same day, the Chinese government finally, belatedly, conceded that the new coronavirus was being spread by person-to-person contact. Within two days Wuhan was put into community quarantine and the whole of Wuhan was locked down a day after that.[32]

The rapidity of these radical measures ought to have spurred governments (and their scientific advisers) everywhere to sit up, take notice, and subject their public health pandemic protection policies to emergency review. These measures themselves were indicative of a mass outbreak. This was especially the case since the ideology of "globalization" has been virtually hegemonic among state-power actors for 30 years (as this has been borne by capitalist internationalization), so that the potential for a global pandemic ought to have had alarm bells ringing and warning lights flashing for governments across the world.

Neoliberal politicians who had long since ideologized globalization as a de-territorialized world market ought to have been highly sensitive to the danger of infectious diseases being carried across those open borders by the various great people-flows of traders, tourists, and migratory workers. Moreover, if that was not enough to trigger such a response, the fact that China's Hubei lockdown was already too late to isolate and choke off the virus in Wuhan certainly ought to have done so. Before curfew, between 11 and 23 January 2020, around 4.3 million people left the province, bound for all of China's great cities, to celebrate Lunar New Year.[33] Given China's pre-eminence as a major hub of ASEAN capitalism, this made cross-border transmission highly probable. So-called globalization was bound to do the rest. The UK – a major trading partner of China and a popular tourist destination for Chinese travellers – was amongst those countries especially vulnerable to catching this particular cold.

Despite the potential threat of COVID-19 to these shores, no specific recommendations for government actions emerged from SAGE's deliberations of 22 January 2020. Subsequently, PM Boris Johnson did not see fit to chair or attend several successive meetings of COBRA (the Government's emergency management group to which SAGE reports). He missed no fewer than five such meetings on the eve of the crisis. As the *Guardian* later reported:

> The five meetings Johnson missed came during a period in late January and February [2020] where he spent an entire parliamentary recess out of sight at his official country retreat of Chequers, prompting Labour to accuse him at the time of being a "part-time prime minister".[34]

In another COBRA meeting during this period, Johnson attended, but only briefly, and he left without contributing.[35]

Long prior to that, leaked confidential cabinet papers demonstrate that the Government received, in December 2019, clear and detailed advance warnings about the threat a viral pandemic posed to public health plus recommendations on how the UK should advance prepare for such an outbreak, whether of influenza or a novel coronavirus outbreak. This was the National Security Risk Assessment, a cabinet office briefing document spanning some 600 pages, which was commissioned by government and compiled by its own public health appointees.[36] Here the Government was warned:

> A novel pandemic virus could be both highly transmissible and highly virulent . . . Therefore, pandemics significantly more serious than the reasonable worst case . . . are possible.

A coronavirus pandemic comparable SARS or MERS – diseases far deadlier than COVID-19 (though much less efficient at transmission), with fatality rates of between 33 and 50 percent – was considered a reasonable case scenario.[37] Such an outbreak was considered likely to unfold in three waves or spikes. And, unless the major advance preparations were made, it was estimated that this could cause almost 66,000 deaths, cost the economy £2.35 trillion, and perpetrate major damage on health and care services for many years afterwards. Recommendations included "the need to stockpile PPE (personal protective equipment), organize advanced purchase agreements for other essential medical kit, establish procedures for disease surveillance and contact tracing, and draw up plans to manage a surge in excess deaths". That is, all of the things that were recommended were manifestly those that were not done.[38]

If that was not enough, Johnson ought to have been aware that three years earlier, Exercise Cygnus, a simulation exercise conducted in order to model the strain that would be placed on the NHS by a major novel flu pandemic, had concluded that the UK, lacking preparedness, would not be able to cope in the event of such a crisis. As was reported in the *Telegraph*:

> Ministers were informed three years ago that Britain would be quickly overwhelmed by a severe outbreak amid a shortage of critical care beds, morgue capacity and personal protective equipment (PPE). . . . Despite the failings exposed by Cygnus, the government never changed its strategic roadmap for a future pandemic, with the last update carried out in 2014.[39]

Even before the peak of an infection wave was reached, according to Cygnus's simulation modelling, "hospitals and mortuaries across the country were already being overwhelmed". This also exposed insufficient PPE for medical staff, whereas the NHS was set to collapse "due to a shortage of ventilators and critical care beds".[40] Four key policy recommendations (which remain confidential) based on Exercise Cygnus were brought by the New and Emerging Respiratory Virus Threats Advisory Group (NERVTAG – a subgroup of SAGE) to the attention of Theresa May's Conservative government. These were highly likely to include exactly the kind of advance preparations – stockpiling of PPE and testing equipment, the boosting of laboratory testing capacity, and so on – which were reiterated by way of warning in the Cabinet Office briefing document of December 2019, to no avail.[41]

Delayed lockdown

On 2 March 2020, the SPI-M group (one of the specialist groups of expert scientists that feed information and guidance up to SAGE) presented a COVID-19 risk-assessment to the latter that was sobering in the extreme. A sustained transmission of the virus in the UK was found to be "highly likely" already. The report highlighted that the virus was highly contagious, with each person who caught it being estimated to pass it on, on average, to three others. Unless "stringent" measures were put in place, it was concluded, up to 80 percent of the UK population (or 53 million people) were likely to catch the disease, with a likely death rate of between 0.5 percent and 1 percent (or 250,000 to 500,000 people). Of those hospitalized by the disease, it was estimated that 12 percent were likely to die, including 50 percent of those who were placed on mechanical ventilators.[42]

A week later, on 9 March, a government paper (informed by SAGE) stated that the best way of containing a UK outbreak would be physical distancing and other special measures to protect vulnerable groups. Therefore: "a combination of individual home isolation of symptomatic cases, household isolation and social distancing of the over 70s could have a positive effect". This positive outcome would be earned by "delaying the onset of the peak; reducing the number of cases during the peak; and reducing the total number of cases". Despite this, remarkably, the paper stopped short of actually proposing or recommending that physical distancing measures be implemented.[43] Yet the Government still did not act. Instead, Johnson made a point, in his press statement of 3 March, of publicising the fact that, when visiting a hospital "where I think there were a few coronavirus patients", he "shook hands with everybody". He advised the public: "We should all basically go about our normal daily lives. . . . The best thing you can do is wash your hands with soap and hot water while singing Happy Birthday twice".[44]

Only from mid-March 2020 did Johnson's government begin issuing the first physical distancing guidance – and this was merely advisory. There was during this long intervening period no public-protection information being broadcast by the Government across media outlets about how people might engage in precautionary self-care. There were no public announcements at airport terminals or rail stations or other congested public spaces advising people to hand-wash regularly, avoid close physical proximity with each other, and so on. There was no mass distribution of face masks to public-facing employees, as there was in some south-Asian countries.[45] This was the situation right up to mid-March, long after the first community cases were confirmed (on 29 January), and following on from the rapid climb in infections and mortalities after that. Consequently, people and organizations, lulled into sleepwalking, simply carried on as usual.

Despite Johnson then acknowledging that COVID-19 constituted "the worst public health crisis for a generation", public health guidance remained tepid and self-limiting in the extreme. The PM's address to the nation on 12 March 2020 stated: "I must level with the British public: many families are going to lose loved ones before their time". Yet the actual guidance offered to the public did not at all reflect the gravity of the situation implied by his words. People should, according to the Government's guidance, consider avoiding public gatherings where they could, stay at home if they experienced specific symptoms, and avoid unnecessary travel. Folks over 70 should avoid cruiser-line holidays, and schools should not send students on overseas trips. There would be no travel restrictions, however, either in the UK (i.e. within national borers) or beyond (i.e. across national borders) – and of course everyone has a good reason to travel.[46]

Simultaneously, as announced on 12 March, contact testing and tracing was abandoned (having barely been started), contrary to guidance from the World Health Organization (WHO) and the policy-practice of other countries. That was tantamount to disregard of the WHO's recommended strategy for containment of the virus, which placed the UK government out on a limb. This WHO guidance was clear since it was "based on decades of experience and widely accepted by public health leaders around the world". It may be summarized thus: test and isolate cases, trace and quarantine contacts, and accelerate public hygiene measures. Instead, as ministers made clear, testing would be limited to only those with symptoms in hospitals owing to the higher risk of contagion and of serious harm in those settings.[47] This marked the shift from the UK's supposed "containment" stage to its "delay" stage. The "delay" stage, which commenced on 12 March, was not intended, as already noted, to push back the virus, to reduce or curtail its spread, but to slow its rate of transmission. This was so that its peak was pushed into late spring or early summer, where it was surmised (without evidence) that the warmer climes would slow its transmission rate, and where hospitals would be less busy dealing with the ill-effects of seasonal flu, in order to reduce pressure on the NHS.

However, this guidance was inadequate. People who had symptoms ("a new persistent cough – one that continues over three or four hours" and/or "a temperature of 37.8C and above") were advised to stay home for just seven days. This seven-day period, the Government stated, was "based on people being infectious just as their symptoms start to show and for a week afterwards".[48] Yet the opinion of many scientists and health experts was that the incubation period could be at least two weeks, and that transmission may occur prior to symptoms displaying, whereas of course some of the infected would be asymptomatic. People without symptoms who had been in contact (or who thought they may have been in contact) with those who had contracted the disease were not, at this point, specifically advised to self-isolate. Physical distancing was a decision for individuals, not a matter of government policy. Public gatherings of more than 500 people were not banned. Major events, right up to 16 March 2020, were allowed to continue.[49]

As reported in *The Guardian*: "The week is remembered for the mega-events that went ahead: the Cheltenham Festival of horseracing, the Liverpool versus Atletico Madrid Champions League tie, the Stereophonics concert in Cardiff".[50] Right up until mid-March, the Government did not even see fit to ask organizers to cancel major public events that would pull together huge numbers of people – football fixtures, rugby internationals, festivals, and so forth – let alone advise them that they ought to consider it.[51]

> The government believes that banning large gatherings is one of the least effective measures a country can take, reducing the peak of the coronavirus by less than 5%. The virus is just as likely to spread within a smaller group such as those watching football in the pub as it would in a large crowd.[52]

Schools and colleges were to carry on as before.

> While school closures can be effective in the case of a flu pandemic, large-scale shutdowns are not thought to be an obvious next step in dealing with the virus in the UK. . . . Closures would have to be at least 13 weeks long to reduce the peak of Covid-19 by 10–15%.[53]

The high streets remained open for business. Universities not only continued with face-to-face classes but also ran their usual alumni and out-reach events (despite the misgivings of some staff), because they were following the Government's steer. This was the case for my university, the University of the West of England (UWE), for example. There was no national TV ad campaign or billboards to convey the distancing message, only pay-walled articles and a 5 pm press briefing throwing out confused and contradictory messages.[54]

The logic of much of this was peculiar. Banning large social gatherings was deemed ineffective "in reducing the peak" whereas banning smaller ones may not be – even though the virus was "just as likely" to spread in both. Doubtless, the thought informing this was that there are innumerable small groups where the virus may be transmitted but few larger ones and that contacts between people in the former would be more fleeting than in the latter. But, on the other hand, in a vast densely packed crowd, every single person may each come into close physical proximity with a large number of others, which would not always be the case in a typical local pub or club. Moreover, mass gatherings are not simply agglomerations of strangers, who mix intermittently, but include friends and peers who would cluster within these larger groups, thereby forming innumerable intimate subgroups that would accelerate transmission. Even if only one person in ten in a crowd of 10,000 at the start of the gathering had the virus, and each of them then infected only one other, who then each only infected one other (whereas, if in a more intimate setting, each person would, by comparison, infect two or three others) that is still 3,000 newly infected people heading home from one event to families, to local pubs and clubs, and to workplaces.

In any case, one would have thought that measures which, on the Government's own reckoning, would reduce the peak of transmission by almost 20 percent (hence saving many lives and significantly easing pressures on NHS staff and resources) ought to have been entertained rather than summarily dismissed. The fact that they were not, this throws into sharp relief the underlying purely economic cost-benefit considerations that were being applied to decision-making in the run-up to the first lockdown. It was not considered enough for a specific control measure (whether closing schools or shutting-down a big crowd event or limiting access to the high street) to merely *reduce* transmission. Rather, transmission must be reduced by x in order to be considered desirable, where x denotes the balance sheet of likely economic costs set against public health benefits. From the perspective of substantive value-rationality, by contrast, all measures that would generate some advantage in preventing deaths, easing pressure on health and care services, and reducing community transmissions, would be thrown into the mix.

The Government's tardiness in closing schools warrants particular scrutiny. Aside from the general reasons for delay set out above, further reasons were that children were considered a low transmission risk and that closing schools would empty hospitals of staff needed to cope with COVID-19 admissions as they were forced home to look after the stay-away children. Or, if the latter was to be avoided, this would be as health keyworkers delegated childcare duties to grandparents, which would render those who faced the greatest risks of illness from COVID-19 at greater risk of catching it. These rationales were endorsed by a *Telegraph* editorial of 17 March 2020.

> Some argue that should be done as a precaution but if you don't know what role children play in spreading the disease it could also make matters considerably worse. Also relevant is the fact that an estimated 30 per cent of the NHS and social care workforce in Britain have school-age children. Close the schools, and you may take them out of work too.[55]

Yet none of these "known unknowns" rendered sensible the Government's general resistance to school closures. Resistance based on the lack of knowledge of the infectiousness of children was manifestly reckless, not least because there were cases of children being infected, just as children were least capable of physical distancing, and because the rationales for not erring on the side of caution were threadbare. The fact that children were seen as potentially acting as silent spreaders of the virus (precisely because they were less vulnerable and therefore less likely to display symptoms) was exactly why school closures worldwide were being implemented. In fact, faced with the community breakout of COVID-19, fewer public health risks would be posed by school closures than by keeping them open, despite the fact this would create a demand for children to be supervised by grandparents as parents continued to work.[56] This was for reasons that ought to be obvious.

First, in the event of school closures, the risks (of infection of the elderly) would be confined to small self-isolating familial units benefiting from general distancing protections, whereas by contrast outbreaks of infection in schools could be readily transmitted to many families concurrently, leading to rapid community-level spikes. Second, there was the option of closing schools to all children except those of frontline health workers, running these with a skeleton staff, thereby solving the problem of pulling NHS staff away from the virus frontline into childcare. This too would have made physical distancing far more feasible within schools than if they were still packed to the rafters with the children of all parents.

Third, school closures as part of a general lockdown policy that included furloughing non-essential workers would in any case minimize the danger of grandparents being deployed as child care support. This was owing to the fact that the number of parents freed up by furloughing to do this work would ensure a large majority of children were catered for. Fourth, it would be a logical requirement of distancing rules that they strongly discourage working parents from delegating to grandparents childcare responsibilities. Instead, these would steer or instruct them to devolve these to other household or family members, or to switch to shift working so that in two-parent households there would be at least one parent on hand for care duties. Finally, most parents of school-age children would themselves voluntarily seek to absolve their own parents from childcare duties wherever possible in order to minimize their risk of catching the virus. Such is impelled by the family bond and this thing called love. Despite its obviousness, this apparently did not occur to ministers or the Government's scientific advisers, although they were supposedly basing their strategy on behavioural science.

Later on, bit by bit, physical guidance was tightened, in an *ad hoc*, piecemeal fashion, as the Government shifted from mere "delay" to draw in its supposed "mitigation" phase. "Mitigation" was really just another level of "delay", the escalation of delay tactics. Whereas "delay" meant people should self-isolate for seven days if they experienced symptoms consistent with COVID-19 infection, "mitigation" extended this to so-called "household isolation" – or isolation that extended to all persons resident with those who had the symptoms, and extending the period of isolation from 7 to 14 days. Under "mitigation", the emphasis of government guidance also shifted towards warning the elderly and vulnerable people to socially isolate themselves.[57]

SAGE guidance issued on 16 March 2020 recommending that the Government bring in "additional social distancing measures . . . as soon as possible" elicited no further response for several days. Patrick Vallance, the Government's Chief Scientific Officer, was then rebuked (or in his own words "told off") by officials and by Chief Medical Officer Chris Whitty for arguing for a nationwide lockdown.[58] On 18 March, ministers announced that schools would close, albeit two days later, on 20 March. Then, on 20 March, they instructed that entertainment, hospitality and indoor leisure venues must also be closed. Everything else, however, was to remain open for business. People were asked to avoid travelling from their home places to other locations unless for work or other essential purposes, to maintain two-metre distancing when outside, and so on.[59] Yet "essential" remained loosely defined, open to interpretation, and the guidance was morally prescriptive rather than normatively binding.

People, faced with this incrementalism and ambivalence, predictably continued to disregard physical distancing *en masse* – flocking to the beaches, parks, pubs, shops and clubs in large numbers. The press, social media and the Government declared its outrage at the "selfishness" of the hundreds of thousands of people who headed for the coast during the weekend of 21–22 March, for example.[60] The moralistic reporting style of *The Metro* was typical: "DISGRACE! The people flocking to public places in their thousands!"[61]

Media and politicians made folk devils of the non-compliant, individualizing responsibility for community spread, deflecting critique from government non-policy and communicative failures, having themselves for a long time tacitly encouraged this attitude of "it's only a flu, what's the fuss about?" in the public mind. After all, if the virus was a hugely serious matter, surely ministers would be ordering compulsory shutdowns, community quarantines, and police enforcements of curfews, just as it would be circulating public health warnings on primetime TV and offering systematic guidance to public-facing service providers on how to keep themselves and their clients safe – as had been happening for weeks on the continent? Since none of these things were happening, the public were given reasons for thinking the crisis was a bit of a storm in the teacup. Johnson's addresses to the nation over the weekend of 20–21 March, by means of which he was supposed to be offering clear guidance on physical distancing, did not ask the public to avoid heading for the beaches. On the contrary, he advised people to "enjoy themselves" in the "parks and open spaces".[62]

Finally, only on 23 March did the Government (with obvious reluctance) declare the start of the first compulsory lockdown. This started the following day.[63] Along with that, starting with Johnson's press conference statement to the nation on 12 March, the whole tenor of the Government's press conferences abruptly changed. These shifted away from emphasizing that the virus would cause serious ill-effects in a tiny proportion of the population, and instead emphasizing that many would die and no one was immune from serious harm.[64] But even this belated lockdown was piecemeal in its roll out, since at the start there was no order issued for shops to close; only for pubs, clubs, leisure centres, libraries, cinemas and restaurants to do so.

There were also seemingly plenty of exemptions, including home and hardware stores, market stalls, convenience stores, newsagents, and vehicle hire businesses. Fast-food takeout bars and restaurants and cafes (if running only takeaway services) were also allowed to continue, as they would do throughout the whole of the lockdown, sucking in bigger numbers of people owing to the closure of other consumption opportunities. And, for them, it was a voluntary matter whether or not they switched to delivery-only or permitted customers to order and collect on-site.[65]

But, with certain exceptions and exemptions (including and especially essential industries or services), workplaces were closed. The pubic was instructed they must self-isolate in their households and were not permitted to leave their homes except for essential reasons. On 26 March, the lockdown restrictions were further clarified. People were barred from leaving home and from travelling other than locally without "reasonable excuse" – which would be for other than essential reasons. These essential reasons included solitary exercise in the locality; people were permitted to leave their homes for once-daily exercise, not for recreational or leisure purposes. Public gatherings were prohibited (albeit with certain exemptions). All high street or retail businesses were closed for on-site services except those that were essential (though included among the "essential" were some whose qualification was questionable). Retail and hospitality businesses that could operate remotely were permitted to switch to wholly online delivery.

The lockdown restrictions were backed by new laws, sanctions and powers of enforcement. The police were permitted to apply Fixed Penalty Notices (FPNs) to suspected violators. These allowed alleged rule-breakers the option to submit to on-the-spot fines rather than face prosecution through the courts.[66] However, the penalties were pitifully low (£60 fines for non-compliance). This would dilute the force of normative constraint in favour of reliance on people's moral compass to bind them to the rules.

To a major degree, this was all bolting the stable door after the horses were gone – or, rather, it was ordering the horses to return to the fold after they had already done so on their own volition. This is because long before the official lockdown, business owners and employers were making their own decisions to suspend their operations or switch to homeworking wherever possible. The Government's lockdown, therefore, appeared reactive, tailing the public and public-facing business response, turning into policy what was already happening in practice on the ground. This was all too little, too late. An understanding of this as such is no kind of wisdom derived from hindsight (as ministers and certain government scientific advisers would later claim). This was clear from the start.

This was also the period in which began the Government's frantic efforts to repair the shortfalls in PPE and virus testing kits and up-scale test centre capacity to process results.[67] Hence from this point started the paraphernalia of target-mongering that unfolded thereafter,[68] along with the wholly predictable cases of delivery failures,[69] missed targets and manipulated data,[70] poor-quality or unusable kit,[71] and the like, which flowed from the need to make good in haste what was neglected at leisure. In the meantime, as this unfolded, frontline health and care workers risked their own lives and those of their loved ones unnecessarily, owing to bottlenecks and shortages in and of testing equipment and PPE,[72] and were ordered not to whistle-blow to the media about these problems.[73] These are the consequences of British exceptionalism that will be explored later in this book.

Yet, in spite of all of these problems that stemmed from ill-preparedness, tardiness of response, paucity of policy-planning and communicative ambivalence, the Government has simply refused to admit error and has insisted without a hint of humility or embarrassment that it has done as well as could be reasonably expected. The UK is "one of the most prepared countries in the world for pandemics", this is the script its press officers routinely parroted throughout the first wave. "We have followed a science-led action plan to contain, delay, research and mitigate the outbreak and acted swiftly to save lives and support our NHS, including prioritising access to testing and PPE for the frontline".[74] This was an almost complete disconnect with the facts and is belied by the UK's terrible performance in holding down infection rates and fatalities.

Herd immunity?

The road to lockdown in 2020 appears to be paved with government complacency of the highest order. If so, how can this be explained? Initially, the Government refused to put out in the public domain the notes or minutes of the meetings that ministers held with its emergency scientific advisory group (SAGE) before and since the crisis began.[75] Such would presumably have cast light on the nature of the scientific advice and the degree to which this did or did not inform government policy. This information, ministers insisted for a long while, would be released only after the pandemic is over.

Under pressure from lobbyists, however, including members of the SAGE group itself, the Government finally backtracked and released in the first week of May 2020 a number of SAGE documents covering proceedings of the advisory group since February of that year. Those expecting illumination on the key issues from this release were to be disappointed though. The release was radically selective or partial, just 28 documents out of a total of 120. Many of those documents that were released were heavily censored or redacted, with large passages of text scratched out. Included among the omissions were those documents that included discussions about border controls through flight suspensions to and from specific countries and about contact-tracing before ministers abandoned the policy.[76]

In the absence of transparency that would allow us to grasp how the Government seemingly sleep-walked into the crisis, conjecture must carry the burden. The critique that began to emerge on these shores in the spring of 2020 attributes this to a misbegotten (and quickly retracted) policy of allowing the virus to spread relatively unimpeded in the population, on the grounds that this would ultimately protect the community by building "herd immunity". That such a strategy of building herd immunity *may* be government policy was seemingly affirmed for the first time on 11 March 2020, when David Halpern, a behavioural psychologist connected to the Cabinet Office, offered the following press statement:

> There's going to be a point, assuming the epidemic flows and grows, as we think it probably will do, where you'll want to cocoon, you'll want to protect those at-risk groups so that they basically don't catch the disease, and by the time they come out of their cocooning, herd immunity's been achieved in the rest of the population.[77]

This was seemingly hinted at earlier by Chris Whitty, the Government's Chief Medical Officer. This was on 3 March, in the first of what were to become regular televised addresses hosted by Boris Johnson, alongside Patrick Vallance, the Government's Chief Scientific Adviser. Whitty stated that the Government was preparing for a worst-case scenario in which up to 80 percent of the UK population would be infected.[78] On Radio 4's *Today* programme, on the same day, Patrick Vallance elaborated:

> Our aim is to try and reduce the peak, broaden the peak, not suppress it completely. . . . Also, because the vast majority of people get a mild illness, to build up some kind of herd immunity, so more people are immune to this disease, and we reduce the transmission. At the same time, we protect those who are most vulnerable to it. Those are the key things we need to do.[79]

Later, on 5 March, the PM ventured the opinion, on the *This Morning* TV show, that "one of the theories" of how to manage the pandemic was

> that perhaps you could take it on the chin, take it all in one go, and allow the disease, as it were, to move through the population, without taking as many draconian measures. I think that we need to strike a balance.[80]

In an interview Vallance gave on the *Sky* news channel, on 13 March, when responding to a question, he surmised that "60 percent or so" of the UK population would need to catch the disease in order for herd immunity to be achieved.[81]

This (building up herd immunity) plan or strategy, if that is what it was, may then even be interpreted as the purpose or goal of the initial "contain" phase, and also the "delay" and "mitigation" stages to follow, as these were outlined in the Government's March 2020 strategy document. If so, I might add, this would also explain why there was no obvious stage prior to these that might be termed a *prevention* stage. That is, it would explain why there was no strategy of border-controls to prevent the virus getting a foothold in the national community (i.e. temperature screening at airports, the quarantining of those with symptoms, and flight suspensions and other travel restrictions) or of systematic community testing and tracing. This would also explain why the intention was to avoid mandatory physical distancing in favour of tepid guidance that people might consider doing so. The idea, on this reading, would be as follows. As community spread was allowed in a controlled way through the gradual ratcheting-up of distancing recommendations (hence allowing population immunity to build among the vast majority who would be relatively unharmed by exposure), the NHS would act to protect the tiny minority (especially the old and vulnerable) who experienced the serious ill-effects.

If that was the strategy, then what *appears* as complacency or even neglect was in fact *policy*, albeit an ethically indefensible one. On this reading, the Government's subsequently abrupt abandonment of this strategy, and its immediate denial thereafter that it ever was a strategy, would have been motivated by the dawning awareness of its political architects that the impact of COVID-19 on larger sectors of the population was going to be far more serious than predicted. This would, if the plan was put into effect, lead to hundreds of thousands of deaths and millions of hospitalizations, consequently overwhelming the NHS. Such would also risk a collapse of public support for the ruling party in adopting such a morally dubious high-risk strategy in the first place. After all, "herd immunity" as policy would mean turning the British population into laboratory test rats, in pursuit of a goal that most scientists considered would come at too high a cost in terms of loss of life, and which others considered unlikely to be achieved at all. Herd immunity, as virologists point out, is typically an objective to be pursued by mass vaccinations, not by simply allowing a new virus to let rip.

Thus, as the crisis unfolded in the spring of 2020, with rapidly escalating case-loads and deaths, criticisms of this supposed government policy, previously muted, burst forth. The dam of suspended critique finally burst. Rather late in the day, in the view of this author, the Government's whole approach to the pandemic (eschewal of testing and tracing and of ramping up test capacity, resistance to physical distancing controls, refusal to countenance controlled borders, ambivalent public health messaging) was vilified in the liberal-left press at home and drew upon itself shocked incredulity from overseas.[82] Yet, it is not clear to me that this strategy (building herd immunity) ever was the clear policy goal. Press releases around mid-March were certainly suggestive that it was, but without this ever being made absolutely clear-cut. Communicative ambivalence abounded.

Perhaps instructively, the Government's *Coronavirus: An Action Plan*, released in early March 2020, makes no mention of herd immunity as either goal or effect of government policy. Nor was there any other mention of the concept anytime else up to mid-March. Not only that, no minister ever stated that there was such a strategy. The affirmative statements about herd immunity all came from the Government's supposedly independent health and medical advisers. Moreover, the politicians themselves did not take long to begin stating their own denials. This started with Matt Hancock, the Secretary of State for Health. On 15 March, just a few days after Halpern's and Vallance's press statements apparently committing the Government to herd immunity, Hancock issued his rebuttal:

> We have a plan, based on the expertise of world-leading scientists. . . . Herd immunity is not a part of it. That is a scientific concept, not a goal or strategy.[83]

This may be considered as evidence of sorts that if indeed there was a coherent plan of government to manage the pandemic, this did not include a strategy of allowing mass spread of the disease in order to build natural population resistance.

But, of course, Hancock's statement was disingenuous. Herd immunity is a scientific concept, true. But a policy of permitting mass community infection in order to build it has nothing to do with science. Contrary arguments may draw attention to the fact that ministers took several days to retract those statements of the Government's own medical and scientific advisers that were seemingly affirmative of the strategy. It is odd that statements of supposed policy goals that were so obviously wrong from the perspective of government (as we are told they were)

were allowed to circulate unchallenged in the public domain for two to four days. However, that could simply be attributable to incompetence. This may be indicative of a government that was simply paralysed faced with a rapidly growing crisis.

Further evidence that would support the idea that the Government was set on a herd immunity strategy, however, would be that Hancock's public denial of the policy was released almost immediately after a vast number of scientists (more than 500 in total) went public in condemning it for posing astronomical public health risks and without necessarily achieving its objective. Their open letter dismissed herd immunity as untenable and called on the Government to introduce radical distancing measures in its place. It is possible, certainly credible, that this letter (widely reported in the media) spooked the Government into a U-turn.[84]

But perhaps not. If the open letter did generate a policy shift, it hardly did so promptly. Although there was initially Hancock's verbal disavowal of herd immunity, there was no corresponding tightening-up of physical distancing rules accompanying the rebuttal. Not even the publication on 16 March of an Imperial College paper by Professor Neil Ferguson predicting that the Government's "delay" and "mitigation" measures would not prevent the NHS being overwhelmed by millions of cases and leading to hundreds of thousands of deaths prompted an immediate policy shift. Distancing guidance remained merely advisory as well as loose and permissive. No other policies were declared. It is possible, therefore, that the Government was hitherto and still at this stage set on the path of herd immunity, in spite of its enormous predicted costs. If so, Hancock and company simply lied, because they found it prudent to claim otherwise faced with negative publicity. In short, it is definitely feasible that the Cabinet for a little while longer sought to slip herd immunity policy "under the radar", practising what they were not preaching.

Yet, again, however, and at the risk of repetition, it is also quite possible that none of these events (the timing of Hancock's retraction, the continued feet-dragging over physical distancing) evidence any such policy. Instead, this could be indicative of nothing other than a negligently unreflective and ill-prepared government which was either in denial of the crisis to come or frozen before it. What supports the latter interpretation is simply that it is preposterous that any government except perhaps those which are not hemmed-in by a need to be accountable to a mass electorate would embark on such a policy. And one would like to think that preposterous government must encounter limits. This is not only in the moral sense (after all, even neoliberal governments are peopled by human beings), but for reason of strategic self-interest. Herd immunity as policy would risk human catastrophe and thus (for its architects) political suicide. By contrast, a complacent government, with other things on its mind, with a view of national "best interest" that simply does not put public health at the head of the queue, inclined to a laissez-faire approach to health policy, may sleep-walk into what resembles a policy of herd immunity. This is by virtue of failing to wake-up to its full consequences, especially when lulled by the depersonalized technical language of science.

But a final piece of evidence in favour of the herd-immunity-as-government-policy thesis is that, if such a policy did exist, it was abandoned in a practical sense only on 23 March 2020. This was with the introduction of the full nationwide community lockdown. The timing of the lockdown may be instructive. This was owing to a political intervention by French president Emmanuel Macron. On Friday 20 March, Macron relayed to Johnson by way of a personal phone conversation that the French government would act with immediate effect to close its borders with the UK unless Johnson's government introduced stringent physical distancing measures that aligned with those on the continent.

This would at the very least have shut down all tourism travel from the UK to the continent, costing the economy billions. This, if indeed it included the shutting-off as well of freight trade, would have extinguished the UK's business with the EU altogether, rendering the economy untenable. This is because it was expected that the other EU countries would fall into line behind the French government's policy. This telephone conversation followed on from the declaration of France's PM Edouard Phillipe earlier in the week that British nationals would be denied access to France unless Johnson's government introduced a community lockdown. Reportedly, by the conclusion of Macron's and Johnson's aforesaid dialogue, Macron had withdrawn his border-closure threat. This, presumably, was because Johnson had reassured him sufficiently that imminent action would follow. Action, of course, did then imminently follow. Three days after the conversation Johnson finally ceased his feet-dragging over mandatory physical distancing and announced the start of the UK's national lockdown.[85]

The pressure exerted by the French government, therefore, may well have been the straw that finally broke the back of the PM's herd immunity policy. The fact that Johnson announced the lockdown right at the start of the week following Macron's weekend intervention is certainly suggestive of this possibility. Yet the evidence is a long way from being decisive. For, although this pressure may well have bullied Johnson into a lockdown he did not want and was inclined to resist, it does not demonstrate that his resistance to the lockdown was motivated by any intent to implement a herd immunity-building policy in the first place. Rather, Johnson's grudging acquiescence was as likely motivated simply by an instinctual, visceral preference to place economic considerations before public health ones.

That is why it was likely the threat of economic sanction that was probably decisive in breaking Johnson's stubborn refusal to lockdown the UK. When weighing-up the ledger of, on the one side, *certain* major economic damage that would arise from national lockdown, and on the other side, the rather more *uncertain* (i.e. more conjectural or theoretical and debatable) public health deficits that would arise from keeping the economy "open", it is feasible that ministers would be strongly inclined to settle the scales in favour of the latter. Such a settling of accounts would be attractive for a government and party of business and free enterprise, facing an uncertain post-Brexit future. That would especially be so given the wiggle-room that there was for varying interpretations of how much public health harm COVID-19 would actually cause, and given the penchant of politicians to evade conclusions that do not fit with their ideological presuppositions. However, Macron's intervention placed on the public health side of the ledger also economic considerations. If Macron's threat had materialized, the UK's economy would have been worse affected than by even a nationwide lockdown.

To summarize, although a misguided and inhumane policy of herd immunity may be the explanation for what *appears* as appalling complacency and neglect (or alternatively indecision) by government with regard to the task of public protection in the run-up to the first lockdown in the spring of 2020, it could be that the appearance was the reality. That is, it is conceivable that the reasons for the predicament faced by the UK at the start of its own pandemic was really either just mundane, complacent neglect by political leaders, or their incompetent dithering. For me, the jury is still out on this issue, though later evidence may settle it.[86] But, if the former, this would be sanctioned by the Government's laissez-faire attitude to social and public policy, and it would be underscored by the instinctual or "gut" default politics of neoliberal politicians that always priorities economic (i.e. capitalist) interests above all else.

Such would be the only explanation that could fit the facts *if* a misbegotten strategy of going for herd immunity through "controlled" community spread was not being entertained. If an attempt to build herd immunity through the gradual manipulation of physical distancing controls was *not* a plan of government, the brief flurry of talk about it flying around in the media in mid-March would have been no more than a pathetic attempt (no sooner advanced than withdrawn) to cover-up the fact that there was no real coherent plan at all to protect the public from COVID-19, not unless laissez-faire and "suck it and see" can be counted as a plan. If this was so, this raises the question of why there was this complacent "wait and see, or hope for the best" attitude. This could hardly be described as an approach, let alone a policy. How might this be explained? I will return to this question in the Conclusion of this book.

12 June 2020 (updated 22 December 2021)

Notes

1 Bull, M. (2020). 'Coronavirus: why UK borders will remain open despite ongoing coronavirus crisis'. *Daily Express*. (10 April); Truelove, S. (2020). 'London coronavirus: Hancock defends decision not to test for Covid-19 at airports as Heathrow and Gatwick remain open'. *My London*. (16 April); English, O. (2020). 'No checks please, we're British: indefensible UK border policy'. *ByLines Times*. (19 May); Sky News (2020). 'Government won't rule out banning large gatherings over coronavirus fears'. (1 March); Wood, V. (2020). 'Coronavirus: government should close schools and sort "half-hearted" response, Rory Stewart says'. *Independent*. (9 March).
2 Line, H. and Smith, D. (2020). ' "We took the right decisions at the right time". Hancock defends covid record against expert who says lockdown came too late'. *Wales Online*. (7 June). Available at: www.walesonline.co.uk/news/uk-news/we-took-right-decisions-right-18378258.
3 *BBC News* (2020). 'Johnson: full speech on coronavirus lockdown plan'. (10 May).
4 Worldometer (2020). *Covid-19 Coronavirus Pandemic: World: Death Toll – Total Deaths (Linear Scale)*. Available at: www.worldometers.info/coronavirus/coronavirus-death-toll/. Accessed: 10/05/2020.

5 See: Creaven, S. (2020). *Corporate Press Coverage of the UK Government Response to Covid-19: A Newspaper Content Analysis*. UWE Bristol. Department of Health and Social Sciences. (April 2020), pp. 1–72. (Unpublished).

6 Emergency and Health Protection Directorate (2020). *Coronavirus: Action Plan – A Guide to What You Can Expect Across the UK*. London: Department of Health and Social Care.

7 EHPD (2020), pp. 8–9.

8 EHPD (2020), p. 5.

9 EHPD (2020), p. 5.

10 EHPD (2020), p. 6.

11 Rahhal, N. and Blanchard, S. (2020). 'Coronavirus may be far deadlier than we think: the virus could kill up to 8-times more patients than official fatality estimates say – and 0.5% of infected people in New York city will die, new model predicts'. *Mail*. (27 April).

12 Lourenco, J., Gfarhari, M., Paton, R., Kraemer, M., Thompson, C., Simmonds, P., Klenerman, P. and Gupta, S. (2020). *Fundamental Principles of Epidemic Spread Highlight the Immediate Need for Large-Scale Serological Surveys to Assess the Stage of the SARS-CoV-2 Epidemic*. Oxford: University of Oxford.

13 Creaven (2020), pp. 12–32.

14 *ITV News* (2020). 'UK coronavirus death toll increases by 269 to reach 31,855'. (10 May).

15 Blanchard, S. (2020). 'How many people in London have really had coronavirus? Antibody surveillance studies suggest up to 2.6 million residents could have already caught it as professor Chris Whitty admits he thinks at least 10% of the capital has been infected'. *Mail*. (24 April).

16 Rettner, R. (2020). 'How does the new coronavirus compare with the flu'? *Live Science*. (14 May); Rahhal and Blanchard (2020).

17 EHPD (2020), p. 10.

18 EHPD (2020), p. 14.

19 EHPD (2020), p. 12.

20 EHPD (2020), p. 12.

21 EHPD (2020), p. 12.

22 EHPD (2020), p. 13.

23 EHPD (2020), p. 15.

24 EHPD (2020), p. 18.

25 Nuki, P. and Newell, S. (2020). 'Confusion over advice adds to public's anxiety; coronavirus "contain, delay, research and Mitigate" is awkward but UK response may yet be enough to contain outbreak'. *Daily Telegraph*. (7 March).

26 EHPD (2020), p. 18.

27 MacKenzie, D. (2020). *Covid-19: The Pandemic That Never Should Have Happened and Now to Stop the Next One*. London: Bridge Water Press, p. 6.

28 MacKenzie (2020), p. 8.

29 MacKenzie (2020), pp. 90–91.

30 MacKenzie (2020), pp. 5, 7, 8, 10, 17–18.

31 Ferguson cited in MacKenzie (2020), p. 9.

32 MacKenzie (2020), pp. 9, 10, 14.

33 MacKenzie (2020), pp. 13–14.

34 Walker, P. (2020). 'Boris Johnson missed five coronavirus cobra meetings, Michael Gove says'. *Guardian*. (19 April).

35 Conn, D., Lawrence, F., Lewis, P., Carrell, S., Pegg. D., Davies, H. and Evans, R. (2020). 'Revealed: the inside story of the UK's Covid-19 crisis'. *Guardian*. (29 April).

36 Hopkins, N. (2020). 'Leaked cabinet office briefing on UK pandemic threat – the key points'. *Guardian*. (24 April).

37 Pegg, D. (2020). 'What does the leaked report tell us about the UK's pandemic preparations'? *Guardian*. (24 April).

38 Hopkins, N. (2020). 'Revealed: UK ministers were warned last year of risks of coronavirus pandemic'. *Guardian*. (24 April).

39 Nuki, P. and Gardner, B. (2020). 'Exercise Cygnus warned the NHS could not cope with pandemic three years ago but "terrifying" results were kept secret'. *Telegraph*. (28 March).

40 Nuki and Gardner (2020).

41 Doward, J. (2020). 'Government under fire for failing to act on pandemic recommendations'. *Observer*. (19 April).

42 Conn et al. (2020).

43 HM Government (2020). 'OFFICIAL: potential impact of behavioural and social interventions on a Covid-19 epidemic in the UK'. *GOV.UK* (online). (9 March). Available at: https://assets.publishing.service.gov.uk/government/uploads/system/uploads/attachment_data/file/874290/05-potential-impact-of-behavioural-social-interventions-on-an-epidemic-of-covid-19-in-uk-1.pdf

44 Conn et al. (2020).

45 For example, in the Philippines.

46 Stewart, H., Proctor, K. and Siddique, H. (2020). 'Johnson: many more people will lose loved ones to coronavirus'. *Guardian* (online). (12 March).

47 Proctor, K. (2020). 'UK government's coronavirus advice – and why it gave it'. *Guardian*. (12 March).

48 Proctor (2020).

49 Stewart et al. (2020); Proctor (2020); Conn et al. (2020).

50 Conn et al. (2020).

51 Stewart et al. (2020); Proctor (2020); Conn et al. (2020).

52 Proctor (2020).

53 Proctor (2020).

54 Temperton, J. (2020). 'Across the UK, this past weekend was a coronavirus horror show'. *Wired*. (23 March).

55 Nuki, P. (2020). 'There are things we know – but there are also known unknowns'. *Daily Telegraph*. (17 March).

56 Here it is worth noting the fundamental contradiction in the government's rationalisation of its non-closure school policy. Proposition A: Schools should not close because very small numbers of children become ill from coronavirus. And this could mean they are low risk to catch it and/or to transmit it. Proposition B: Schools should stay open because, if they did not, grandparents would be the ones to supervise the children so that parents could continue to work. This would hence expose grandparents to unnecessary danger of catching from their grandchildren the virus, which is bad because the elderly are in high risk of serious illness or death if they contracted coronavirus. On the one hand, then, schools should stay open, because the kids are not risky. But, on the other hand, the schools should not close, because the kids are risky.

57 Conn et al. (2020).

58 Kermani, S. (2020). 'Chief scientist "told off" for lockdown plea'. *BBC News*. (14 September).

59 Conn et al. (2020).

60 Sparrow, A., Campbell, L. and Rawlinson, K. (2020). 'UK coronavirus: Boris Johnson announces strict lockdown across country'. *Guardian*. (23 March).

61 Harper, P. (2020). 'Disgrace! The people flocking to public places in their thousands'! *Metro*. (22 March).

62 Sparrow et al. (2020); Temperton (2020).

63 *BBC News* (2020). 'Coronavirus: strict new curbs on life in UK announced by PM'. (24 March).

64 Proctor (2020).

65 *BBC News* (24 March, 2020); Proctor (2020).

66 Brown, J. and Kirk-Wade, E. (2021). *Coronavirus: A History of English Lockdown Laws*. Briefing Paper No. 9068. (22 December). London: House of Commons Library, p. 6.

67 Schraer, R. (2020). 'Coronavirus: what tests are being done in the UK'? *BBC News*. (14 May).

68 *BBC News* (2020). 'Coronavirus: are these seven targets being hit'? (15 May).

69 Mason, R., Rawlinson, K., Proctor, K. and Sabbagh, D. (2020). 'Government confirms 400,000 Turkish gowns are useless for NHS'. *Guardian*. (7 May).

70 Mason, R. and Campbell, D. (2020). 'Pressure on Johnson as UK's daily coronavirus testing target missed again'. *Guardian*. (7 May).

71 Dean, E. (2020). 'COVID-19: nurses say they are not getting adequate PPE'. *Nursing Standard* (online). (10 April). Available at: https://rcni.com/nursing-standard/newsroom/analysis/covid-19-nurses-say-they-are-not-getting-adequate-ppe-159881.

72 Booth, R. (2020). 'Residential homes "desperate" for PPE, as two care workers die'. *Guardian*. (6 April).

73 Campbell, D. (2020). 'NHS staff "gagged" over coronavirus shortages'. *Guardian*. (31 March).

74 Doward (19 April, 2020).

75 Adam, D. (2020). 'UK's coronavirus science advice won't be published until pandemic ends'. *New Scientist* (online). (17 April). Available at: www.newscientist.com/article/2241082-uks-coronavirus-science-advice-wont-be-published-until-pandemic-ends/.

76 *ITV News* (2020). 'Sage publishes evidence behind advice on lockdown following calls for more transparency'. (5 May); Wilcock, D. (2020). 'The secret SAGE files the government doesn't want you to see: advice on wearing masks, stopping flights from specific countries and the impact of school closures among documents still not revealed – with mysterious passages missing from others'. *Mail*. (5 May); Lewis, P. (2020). 'UK scientists condemn "Stalinist" attempt to censor Covid-19 advice'. *Guardian*. (8 May).

77 Boseley, S. (2020). 'Herd immunity: will the UK's coronavirus strategy work'? *Guardian*. (13 March).

78 Conn et al. (2020).

79 O'Grady, C. (2020). 'The U.K. backed off on herd immunity. To beat COVID-19, we'll ultimately need it'. *National Geographic*. (21 March).

80 Shaw, M. (2020). ' "Herd immunity and let the old people dies" – Boris Johnson's callous policy and the idea of genocide'. *Discover Society* (online). (23 March). Available at: https://archive.discoversociety.org/2020/03/23/herd-immunity-and-let-the-old-people-die-boris-johnsons-callous-policy-and-the-idea-of-genocide/.

81 Conn et al. (2020); Yong, E. (2020). 'The U.K.'s coronavirus "herd immunity" debacle'. *Atlantic*. (16 March).

82 Boseley, S. (2020). ' "Absolutely wrong": how UK's coronavirus test strategy unravelled'. *Guardian*. (1 April); Conn et al. (2020); Guerrera, A. (2020). 'Italians are looking on aghast at the UK's coronavirus response'. *Guardian*. (10 May); Helm, T., Graham-Harrison, E. and McKie, R. (2020). 'How did Britain get its coronavirus response so wrong'? *Guardian*. (19 April); Perraudin, F. (2020). 'UK government's coronavirus response beset by mixed messages and U-turns'. *Guardian*. (14 April); Ryan, F. (2020). 'Don't just blame the public over social distancing. Look to the government'. *Guardian*. (24 March); Shabi, R. (2020). 'The Myth of Great Britain must finally end when our government has failed us so badly over coronavirus'. *Independent*. (14 April).

83 Cited in Conn et al. (2020).

84 Conn et al. (2020).

85 Allen, P. and Dresch, P. (2020). 'Coronavirus: UK lockdown began after France "threatened to shut border with Britain"'. *Mirror*. (21 March); *Euractive* (2020). 'Macron threatens UK entry ban in lieu of more stringent measures'. (22 March). Available at: www.euractiv.com/section/uk-europe/news/macron-threatened-uk-entry-ban-without-more-stringent-measures/; Islam, F. (2020). 'PM had to soothe concerns over UK virus strategy'. *BBC News*. (22 March); Milmo, C. (2020). 'Coronavirus: Emmanuel Macron threatened Boris Johnson with closure of French border without more stringent UK

Measures'. *I-News*. (22 March); Sheridan, D. (2020). 'Emmanuel Macron "Threatened to close border with UK unless it stiffened coronavirus measures"'. *Telegraph*. (22 March).

86 Shipman, T. and Wheeler, C. (2020). 'Coronavirus: ten days that shook Britain – and changed the nation for ever'. *Times*. (22 March). The reporters claim insider information to the effect that Dominic Cummings had towards the end of February acknowledged that the UK was committed to a herd immunity strategy for dealing with the virus, even at the price of pensioner lives. As Cummings reportedly said, "herd immunity, protect the economy and if that means that some pensioners die, too bad". The reporters also cite another senior Tory who is similarly quoted as saying simply: "Herd immunity and let the old people die". If these reports are trustworthy, the conclusion that herd immunity policy was a firm undertaking of government is probably true. In that case, ministers who made that decision ought to be facing criminal proceedings.

2
NHS SHORTAGES AND THE VENTILATOR CHALLENGE

In the first quarter of 2020, spanning the period from January right through to March, that is, as the new coronavirus began to internationalize, the British government made no large-scale procurement of PPE for frontline workers in the NHS or in social care.[1] This was even though ministers could draw on the experience of other affected countries to inform its own best practice. If the PM's former Chief Adviser Dominic Cummings is to be believed, not only were advance preparations for the pandemic not made, but the Health Secretary Matt Hancock misled the Cabinet and PM that these were well developed and were comprehensive – "including pandemic levels regularly prepared and refreshed, CMOs and epidemiologists, . . . stress testing", etc. These assurances were "basically completely hollow", as Cummings later put it.[2]

Now, if Hancock had uttered such assurances, these would indeed have been empty, because undoubtedly the "plans" were totally inadequate, as events were to show. But to attribute responsibility for the inadequacy of the "plans" solely to Hancock is implausible, since managing a pandemic can hardly be laid exclusively at the door of the DHSC. The DHSC's proposals to manage the pandemic ought to have undergone the wider and deeper scrutiny of ministers and government officials. If that had happened, this would have exposed their hollowness. It was also clear that the chronic lack of pandemic advance planning preceded Johnson's leadership of the Government.

Not only did the Government make no such advance preparations for the pandemic, but it also reduced its capacity to deal with one. This was by selling 279,000 items of PPE to the Chinese,[3] and of millions of others to EU countries, including Germany, Italy, and Spain.[4] No impending public health crisis was going to interfere with the sacred duty of a neoliberal state to conduct trade for commercial advantage (or to prevent UK companies from doing so) when opportunity presents.

DOI: 10.4324/9781003275039-3

Companies which were exporting or who were set to export PPE that was in short supply in the UK asked ministers if they should proceed with the exports, or agree new export sales, in effect offering the Government the opportunity to step in as an alternative buyer. But these companies were given the green light to carry on, since apparently business contracts must be honoured, and new ones signed up for, even if at the cost of public health.[5]

The ventilator challenge

Simultaneously, on the brink of the UK crisis, and as it began to gather steam, it became clear that the NHS was saddled historically with a chronic insufficiency of ventilators. Mechanical ventilators are high-tech life-saving equipment, typically found in Intensive Care Units (ICUs), which function as artificial lungs for people experiencing acute respiratory distress. The shortage was both in actual numbers and compared with the healthcare systems of other OECD countries. This was also a story of a basic long-standing insufficiency and relative paucity of emergency care beds in ICUs in which such equipment would commonly be found.[6] The experience of the Wuhan outbreak appeared to show that COVID-19 caused acute breathing difficulties, leading to respiratory failure, so that ventilators *en masse* were necessary to evade huge numbers of fatalities. For that reason, the Chinese government had mass-produced them, and other countries began to procure (and where possible manufacture them) in large volumes, leading to bulging order books for companies that specialized in these medical technologies.[7]

Yet going into the crisis there was "no pre-existing plan in place for how to increase the number of ventilators available to the NHS". This was even though, as the DHSC put it, the "NHS is not run . . . with spare capacity".[8] On the brink of the UK pandemic, the Government had not even collected data from NHS providers on the number of ventilators that were in use in its hospitals, let alone sought out emergency procurements. On the contrary, a request for information on ventilator numbers was not circulated until late in February 2020. "As a result, the DHSC did not start its programme to secure additional ventilators until 3 March, despite the WHO announcing a 'public health emergency of international concern' on 30 January".[9]

By mid-March 2020 it was apparent that the number of ventilators in NHS hospitals was pitifully small, with estimates varying from 5,000 to 7,400.[10] This number included "some that would not normally be used to treat patients in a hospital bed such as ventilators from ambulances".[11] This was projected by mathematical modellers to be enough to meet but a fraction of the possible or potential demand of the first wave, estimated initially on 12 February (based on modelling data from the Chinese experience) as requiring 59,000 units.[12] There then followed a bewildering series of seemingly *ad hoc* recalculations of likely need, some of which may have been motivated as much by the failures of procurement than the real situation on the ground.

Projected demand was adjusted up to 90,000 by the start of March, "before reducing to 17,500 on 24 March, and again (in what seemed a remarkable spurt of optimism) to just 6,200 by 8 April".[13] (The Government had declared that 30,000 ventilators would be needed on 26 March.)[14] On 5 April this was again re-adjusted to 18,000 (which was to be achieved by mid-April).[15] This mid-April target was missed. "On 15 April, after the peak of COVID-19 hospitalizations, the Department [of Health and Social Care] set targets of 18,000 ventilators by 30 April and 30,000 by 30 June to prepare for a potential second wave".[16] These targets too were missed. By the end of July, only 24,000 ventilators had been acquired,[17] whereas by mid-August this was only 26,000.[18]

Thus, over a month after the WHO declared the new coronavirus a global health emergency, the Government began its desperate last-ditch scramble to repair the shortfall in intensive-care equipment, on prohibitively tight timescales, faced with global shortages stemming from high international demand on suppliers, and having entered the procurement market far too late.[19] The Government's apparent strategy, as reported by *The Guardian*, was threefold: "buy proven devices from the few small firms that made them, import some from overseas and, most importantly, look to . . . [a] ventilator challenge to deliver thousands more machines".[20] Not included as part of the strategy, owing in all likelihood to the pervasive influence of gung-ho anti-EU Brexit-mongering in government circles, was participation in a EU-wide procurement scheme for intensive care equipment. This scheme included procurement of tried-and-tested models of mechanical ventilators and was delivering supplies across the continent.

When this story reached the press, provoking a minor media storm, the Government's initial response was to claim that non-participation was deliberate, a matter of choice, because the country was no longer in the EU and preferred to "make its own efforts".[21] That was likely the truth of it. But, if so, telling the truth was bad PR, given the Government's procurement struggles and other evident failures of preparation, including the failure to stockpile PPE. Therefore, the official story was changed, so that the failure to join the scheme was attributed to mischance – the accidental missing of the deadline (supposedly owing to not having received an invitation email from the EU) to register for it. Whatever the truth, the error (whether miscommunication or dogma-driven recklessness) ensured that the UK "missed out on benefiting from the collective buying power of the EU . . . [and] its clout to source large numbers of ventilators and protective equipment".[22]

In any case, faced with growing competition for ventilators on the world market, the Government "usually had to pay up front, and in some cases more than typical market rates, accepting the risk that products may be unsuitable" – as indeed some were. Established NHS suppliers "were paid an average of £20,000 for each of the . . . new intensive care unit mechanical ventilators, while [those] . . . bought from new suppliers [were for] . . . £30,100 apiece".[23] The FCO tasked British embassies to urgently seek out suppliers abroad. Requests for donations or sales (it is not clear which) were made of foreign governments – and were received, in dribs and drabs, courtesy of China, the USA, Taiwan, and Germany.[24] The DHSC even requested that veterinary surgeries loan the NHS their animal ventilators.[25]

This too motivated the Government's so-called "Ventilator Challenge", launched officially on 16 March 2020.[26] This was an SOS-style appeal to UK manufacturers to deliver from scratch thousands of serviceable ventilators within just two weeks. This was desperate stuff because the manufacturers mostly had no knowledge or experience of making these specialized products – the R&D for which may take several years.[27] The Government even rushed out (on 20 March) its own specification for a "minimally clinically acceptable" ventilator, which soon turned out not to be minimally acceptable. This was based on an outmoded 1960s machine, which non-specialist companies were advised they may use to manufacture units to speed up the process.[28] The goals set for the ventilator challenge were completely unrealistic, not simply because the timescale was utopia, but also because of the Government's worship of competitive laissez-faire markets. This meant that companies were allowed an option of competing among themselves to innovate wholly new designs rather than being steered to co-operate with each other drawing on existing designs and the expertise of specialists.

Millions of pounds were destined to be wasted on blind alleys along a road of failed and abandoned designs, simply because it was unfeasible for non-specialist companies to turn themselves almost overnight into specialist ones, particularly those set on "going it alone" in competition with others. As an anonymous industry insider put it:

> It's easy to say you can just design a ventilator, but the safety isn't just in the design, it's about how you make them, the quality management, servicing them. It's not an innovation programme, it was there to meet a clinical need. And that need was always most likely to be met by scaling up manufacture of existing devices.[29]

Or, as Craig Thompson, Head of Products at medical equipment manufacturers Penlon (of the UK Ventilator Challenge Consortium), put it: "The idea that an engineering company can quickly manufacture medical devices, and comply with the rules, is unrealistic because of the heavy burden of standards and regulations that need to be complied with". Much more feasible, Thompson opined, would be to focus on "existing medical device companies increasing supply of ventilators",[30] whereas non-specialist companies wanting to produce machines, according to Dick Elsey (Chairperson of the Challenge UK Consortium), would have a better chance of success by liaising with specialist ones, drawing on their knowledge and product designs.[31]

Predictably, given the reactive tardiness of the Government's approach to procurement and its basic lack of coherence, the strategy delivered slim pickings on the timescales considered necessary to avoid a health disaster.[32] By the start of May 2020, scarcely more than 800 ventilators had been procured from overseas.[33]

Alison Pittard, Dean of the Faculty of Intensive Care Medicine, declared a month before that the Government's own proposed ventilator specification unfit for purpose, on the grounds that there was little value in a machine that could stabilize a patient for just a few hours.[34] The Government placed big orders for new machines with non-specialist companies (e.g. Dyson – vacuum cleaner manufacturer) that had not demonstrated they had usable prototypes let alone submitted these for clinical approval.[35] None of these had by May "reached the final stages of testing and the majority – including those made by Sagentia and Dyson – have proved surplus to requirements".[36]

In the end, hardly any of the non-specialist companies that undertook to produce their own prototypes came up with a usable machine, and none did so on a usable timescale.[37] By contrast, the Ventilator Challenge UK Consortium did, by focusing efforts on established designs and drawing on the expertise of specialist manufacturers. These companies received ministerial approval to produce machines for the NHS but would not be ready to start manufacturing them before the first COVID-19 wave had passed its peak.[38] By early April 2020, the NHS had 9,000 ventilators – but not one was by virtue of the ventilator challenge.[39] By 18 May, there were still only 11,900 ventilators in UK hospitals. As of 4 May, only 344 of these were "provided by new suppliers responding to . . . the ventilator challenge", whereas 118 were produced by specialist UK firms, the others from overseas.[40] By 20 May, the Ventilator Challenge had coughed up a total of 2,000 machines for the NHS.[41]

Workers on the frontline: PPE shortages in the NHS and social care

The ventilator crisis was symptomatic of the wider crisis of basic shortages of essential medical kit in the NHS. Of biggest concern for NHS frontliners, of course, was the paucity of PPE. The result was that COVID-19-facing hospital and care workers grappling with rapidly escalating caseloads throughout the first wave were doing so without the necessary safeguards of their own (or of their families') health and safety which they had a right to expect from their employers. Not only that, as they were doing so, they were also being served gagging orders by their bosses, under pain of disciplinary sanction, to deter them from bringing these issues to the attention of the media.[42]

Labour MP, Nadia Whittome, who was helping as a volunteer carer at the Lark Hill retirement home, was sacked by the Extra Care Charitable Trust for doing just that.[43] The predictable ill-effects of this for them included massive levels of stress, anxiety, emotional or psychological distress, as well as high risk of COVID-19 infection, together with large numbers of deaths of these frontline workers from the virus. By mid-July 2020 at least 540 health and care workers had died from COVID-19, 268 of them care staff, with 60 percent of them identified as of minority BAME ethnicities, and with overseas workers from South Asia particularly over-represented.[44] The number of equivalent fatalities worldwide at the time was estimated at 3,000. This placed the UK in second place internationally for COVID-19 deaths of care and health frontliners.[45]

An article published in *The Atlantic* journal on 24 March 2020 by an emergency physician on the US pandemic frontline relayed a host of issues that were emblematic in the UK context,[46] as revealed by a host of reports emanating from whistle-blowers, initially in hospitals, latterly in care homes. These included: absence of staff training for coping with pandemic situations; chronic shortages of basic self-protective kit (surgical gloves, masks, visors, goggles, gowns, and so on); and the strains of witnessing colleagues becoming sick and occasionally dying, and of patients dying unnecessarily owing to shortages of critical-care beds or ventilation units. Throughout the first wave, shortages of PPE were acute.

According to the Doctors' Association UK (DAUK), in the latter part of April 2020, at the peak of the first wave of the pandemic, three-quarters of doctors said that "they cannot access a mask when they need one, and nearly half of clinicians attending to the highest-risk cases say they cannot access the correct gowns".[47] Moreover, nurses in the NHS during the first wave reported being compelled to mock-up their own PPE, reutilize single-use kit, and seek out their own supplies. This was as stock never arrived, or being insufficient was quickly exhausted.[48] As Samantha Batt-Rawden, President of the DAUK, reported:

> Many doctors have told us they have also had to buy their own respirator masks from hardware stores, while others have reached out to schools and laboratories for protective glasses. Some have approached 3D printing companies to have batches of visors made.[49]

Yet scarcity of PPE was strenuously denied by Hancock's DHSC in favour of attributing blame to distribution problems or to frontline workers using up "too much" kit.[50] This was the Government's media spin on the crisis that would in due course be exposed as lies. Later on, of course, Dominic Cummings, Johnson's former Chief Adviser, offered testimony to the Parliamentary Select Committee that revealed Hancock's efforts to blame these PPE shortages (which he had previously said did not exist) on the Treasury and on the boss of NHS England for blocking orders. These allegations, Cummings testified, were also shown to be false. On Cummings' account, No. 10 was also frustrated with Hancock's procurement efforts.[51]

If anything, the crisis of under-protected staff (and hence of under-protected clients), across the duration of the first wave of the virus, was even more acute in the social care sector than it was in the NHS.[52] In contrast to frontline healthcare workers, upon whom ministers have copiously lavished their gratitude, they have been among the relatively forgotten heroes of the pandemic. This is because they are in the wrong tier of a two-tier care system in terms of status and reward – and a tier that has been even more radically run-down than the NHS under austerity. Care home and domiciliary care staff are poorly paid (at minimum wage). They work long hours (often 12-hour shifts – especially during the first wave of the pandemic, since many became ill, so that others had to deputize). A quarter of them are on zero-hours contracts, and 55 percent of them are without entitlements to statutory sick pay, so that (as essential workers without furlough protections) they have been under pressure during the pandemic to go to work even if they themselves are unwell.[53]

Matt Hancock, discoursing on "selfish" workers, who for some reason thought it was "acceptable to soldier on and go into work if you have flu symptoms", thereby infecting colleagues with the virus, might have paused to reflect on the causes of this "selfishness" that he found so perplexing. This may quite plausibly be, as Owen Jones suggests, because UK workers "stricken with coronavirus have the lowest mandatory sick pay of the OECD industrialised nations as a proportion of average earnings".[54] Indeed, mandatory sick pay rates in the UK are less than ten percent of the value of average wages, whereas across the OECD as an aggregate these make up 70 percent.[55] Consequently, even where workers have entitlements to statutory sick pay, which many (two million according to the Trade Union Congress (TUC) – including a third of zero-hours contracted workers) do not,[56] this is not enough to pay the bills. The threat this particular exemplar of British exceptionalism poses to public health faced with pandemic outbreaks (the source of which of course resides in neoliberal austerity politics) is so obvious it hardly needs spelling out.

Social care staff are also recruited disproportionately from BAME groups and from overseas – especially from South Asia but also from certain EU countries – just as are many NHS staff.[57] Alarmingly, under the Government's new post-Brexit immigration rules, care workers from the EU would not even be eligible to work in this country, since their incomes fall below the salary baseline (£23,040) that would qualify them for entry as "skilled professionals". Care workers typically earn less than £20,000 a year. Nor, indeed, would a majority of EU-recruited workers in the NHS – including porters, cooks, canteen staff, cleaners, even nurses – be eligible to work in the UK under these Brexit immigration rules.[58] Yet, these workers, just as much as NHS medical staff, were (and are) on the pandemic frontline, risking their lives in the service of the virus's victims, just as they have faced terrible anxieties over the uncertain status of their UK residency. I will address these issues in more detail in the next chapter.

For the better part of six weeks, at the start of the British pandemic, in the spring of 2020, as the virus spread rapidly through UK care homes, virtually without media attention or ministerial acknowledgement, care residents (the latter of whom were of course the most vulnerable of community members) became ill and died in unaccounted numbers. This eventually prompted accusations that ministers were "airbrushing" older victims out of the pandemic.[59] When quizzed about this, on 23 April, in the House of Commons, Dominic Raab, Secretary for Foreign and Commonwealth Affairs, admitted that the Government did not know how many care residents had lost their lives to COVID-19. This was because the only deaths that were being counted were in hospitals.[60] It was not until 29 April, after concerted lobbying by care providers and others, that the statistics for deaths and infections in hospices and in care homes were totted up for inclusion in the Government's daily bulletins.

COVID-19-linked deaths of care home residents it then transpired were being recorded on death certificates as being caused by pneumonia or even dementia. This was for two main reasons. Firstly, lack of testing to confirm the actual causes. Secondly, political and economic incentives to minimize the scale of the crisis: of private-sector care home owners to keep their facilities "open for business"; and of government to ease pressure on the NHS by fast-tracking admissions from care homes back into residential care, indeed shifting NHS patients into care homes, in order to make room for COVID-19 admissions into hospitals struggling to accommodate escalating caseloads.[61] Confronted with the NHS crisis, it was basically *this* decision of officials in Hancock's DHSC – that is, to discharge NHS patients into social care settings without COVID-19 exit screening and without adequate quarantine safeguards in place for them – that exported the virus from hospitals into residential homes.[62] From the start of the pandemic in Britain up until 15 April 2020, the DHSC's published guidance for NHS hospitals was that "negative tests are not required prior to transfers or admissions into the care home".[63]

Johnson's former Chief Adviser, Dominic Cummings, rightly claimed that "one of the worst failings in Feb/March, less discussed than lockdown, was the almost total absence of a serious plan for shielding social care".[64] As data provided by NHS England showed, more than 25,000 people were discharged from hospitals to care homes in the (largely pre-testing) period from 17 March to 16 April 2020. This was in spite of dire warnings by health professionals that the care sector was ill-prepared and ill-equipped to cope with a major outbreak of the virus.[65] This unleashed the disease to prey on those who were known to be at greatest risk of being killed by it, just as it left a workforce that was among the poorest paid and in possession of the fewest entitlements in the UK to cope with the fallout. Tens of thousands of the most vulnerable members of society – the very old, the already sick, those with major infirmities or disabilities, those with mental health ailments such as dementia that made it impossible for them to respect physical distancing – were to forfeit their lives owing to this negligence.

According to ONS data, the pandemic's first UK wave (March to September 2020) was responsible for 20,664 deaths in care homes whereas the second wave (September 2020 to April 2021) was responsible for a further 21,677 deaths. That was around 23 percent of all pandemic deaths during the first wave and almost 26 percent of all during the second wave.[66] However, the real death rate in the first wave was likely much higher than in the second wave owing to radical under-counting.

> Caution is advised comparing between the two waves since the higher proportion of deaths involving COVID-19 in wave two could be attributed to undiagnosed COVID-19 cases in the first wave. By contrast, there were more total deaths of care home residents above the five-year average in wave one (27,079 excess deaths) than in wave two (1,335 excess deaths).[67]

The excess death rate in care homes during the first wave was owing to political decision-making that was in effect (whether owing to incompetence, or callous disregard for the lives of those superfluous to the economy and profit-making, or both) potentially genocidal.[68] If Cummings is to be believed, this was indeed a mixture of both. According to his testimony, Johnson had opined (in the autumn of 2020) that COVID-19 was a disease that was "only killing 80-year olds".[69] This was why he was set against a second lockdown as the second wave began to build. But why would elderly lives be the "only" in Johnson's calculus? Why would they be deemed as of lesser important than younger lives? Presumably, because care home residents are not the biggest participants in the consumer culture, and nor do they add value to the productive economy.

But Cummings has claimed that Health Minister Matt Hancock categorically assured the PM that elderly hospital patients "would be tested before they went back to homes; we only subsequently found out that that hadn't happened".[70] Hancock's failure to deliver on that undertaking reputedly earned him a summons to No. 10 to explain the debacle amid accusations of negligence. This was denied by Hancock and by Hancock's allies and senior aides at the DHSC. Nor did Johnson support Cummings' version of events. According to Hancock, he had committed to testing those dispatched from hospitals into social care settings only when testing capacity was increased, since lack of testing capacity ensured that the NHS front-line had to be prioritized.[71] In doing so, Hancock tacitly conceded Cummings' main point of critique, despite explicitly disavowing it. This was that it was indeed true that he had given NHS managers the green light to shift tens of thousands of untested former patients from hospitals jam-packed with COVID-19 unwell into care homes where staff lacked the healthcare expertise and protective equipment to protect their charges from the inevitable outbreaks.

This was a rather peculiar method of "placing a shield" around the residential care sector, as Hancock claimed to have done, when giving his evidence to the parliamentary select committee. This definition of "shielding" was certainly given short shrift by Nadra Ahmed, executive chairperson of the National Care Association:

> There was no shield. . . . He put social care on the altar to be slaughtered while we worked on the mantra that the NHS must be protected. I absolutely understand why we needed the NHS to be running in the way that it was because we didn't know what was coming round the corner. I think what we didn't know was the consequence of ignoring social care.[72]

However, even if Hancock led Johnson to believe that elderly people would be tested for the virus before being released into residential care, and even if (as Cummings also claimed) Johnson regarded Hancock as "totally f****** hopeless" (owing to his failure to build up testing capacity or procure PPE),[73] neither his general lack of competence nor his disastrous failure to shield the elderly and infirm was deemed sufficient to remove him from his post. This too is fairly compelling evidence that a lesser value was being placed on the currency of elderly lives compared to younger lives. Saving these lives was deemed a much lesser priority than saving those of others – as was protecting the lives and wellbeing of those trusted to care for these lives.

History should remember social care staff as those who fought to shield the most vulnerable from the virus with meagre resources at their disposal. For the most part, during the first wave, they were without medical training and clear guidance on how to self-protect or protect those in their care.[74] They were, across the first wave, twice as likely to die from the virus as NHS workers, according to ONS statistics.[75] They were also, in the thick of the first wave, right at the back of the queue for testing and the distribution of PPE, owing to the prioritization of the NHS under conditions of acute shortages. This would account for their higher vulnerability to being killed by the virus compared to healthcare workers. "We have thermometers – that's about it", as a residential care worker put it. Or as another put it:

> How do we contain it in a home? We have people with dementia and we can't keep them in their rooms. All we have for PPE is the generic paper mask, gloves and plastic aprons. We are risking our lives. It makes us feel like we are cannon fodder.[76]

As a domiciliary care worker reported: "For a week, we only had four masks. We had 300 masks delivered from the pandemic stockpile about three weeks ago. If we wore PPE as we should, that wouldn't even last us a day. We carry out 344 calls a day". Or, as another explained: "We now have to wear the same very sub-standard mask all day instead of changing it for every domiciliary visit". In some cases, during the first wave, care home managers and staff resorted to mocking up their own homemade protective kit, whereas some home managers tried to go it alone in ordering their own supplies, bypassing the usual procurement process. "I've been begging, stealing and borrowing, buying, making masks and stuff for my staff, because we're not given it".

Other workers reported feeling frightened to hug and kiss their children before or after a work shift because of the lack of PPE or test kits. Others reported being required by managers to work even though they had underlying health conditions that would expose them to high COVID-19 risk and of being asked to bring in their children to work if they were unable to find childcare. Even after the first wave had receded, for much of the summer (of 2020), residential and domiciliary care workers still found that they could not get hold of the COVID-19 test kits they needed due to the continuing shortages. They also found they had to travel to and from test centres that were often many miles away, exposing themselves to the risks and expense of public transport to get there and back. Most care workers simply cannot afford a private car.[77]

The question posed by the author of the *Atlantic* piece – "what happens if we don't show up?"[78] – was doubtless testament to the astronomical mental fatigue that frontline health and care workers were experiencing faced with these first-wave pressures without the resources to cope with them. This was venting the feelings of those pushed to the brink of endurance by the crisis, so that simply walking away was a highly attractive option, whether for their own sake or for the protection of their own families. But this question was also a pertinent one for another reason.

This is simply that health and care staff are not obliged by their professional codes of public service to play roulette with their own health or lives (or that of their loved ones) owing to under-resourcing and the resultant lack of the most elementary of self-protective equipment.

Now, it is one thing for frontliners to risk their own lives and health (and those of loved ones) in the service of care for unknown others. But it is quite another to be doing that (as frontline health and care workers were doing as the first wave of the virus ran amok) *unconditionally*, which is exactly the choice that the lack of appropriate safeguards forced on them if they were to carry on. Yet that is what they did, in the teeth and claw of the first wave. Even though frontline medics reported being subjected to bullying and moral shaming by their line managers,[79] to pressurize them to carry on regardless despite the deficiencies of PPE, this behaviour was for them much more a source of moral repugnance than it was a motivating factor.

As journalist Sam Earle rightly pointed out, Boris Johnson began eulogizing NHS staff as "the beating heart of this country" just as the death toll began to mount and the health system was stretched and strained to the limit. But, at the same time, he also abstained from acknowledging the failures of government that placed these staff under intolerable pressures and needlessly exposed them to risk. NHS staff, Earle opined, deserved better than to be used as a kind of "human shield" for politicians to use to deflect public attention from their own policy failures – "a lockdown that arrived too late; and a chronic lack of NHS equipment, staff and preparation predating the pandemic".[80] For frontline medical staff to then be accused of "not being adult" for raising these safety issues and voicing concern over having to make difficult rationing decisions over who to treat and who not to, who would live and who would die, was to add insult to neglect. This, remarkably, was UK's Deputy Chief Medical Officer Jenny Harries' response to the whistleblowers, whose press briefing of 18 April was also notorious for her reassertion of the Government line that the UK was an "international exemplar in preparedness" for the pandemic.[81]

The fact that the NHS avoided collapse, and more-or-less coped with the crisis, as the first wave of the pandemic built towards its early-April to mid-April 2020 peak, was especially remarkable, given the circumstances. These circumstances were those stemming from the health service being radically underfunded for years under the impact of an especially brutal round of public sector cutbacks dating back to the election of the Lib-Con coalition government in 2010. Indeed, even before then, the NHS had gone through funding ups and downs for more than 30 years, which had left it relatively under-resourced and resorting to "stop-gap" measures to plug all manner of shortages, including by drawing on a pool of hourly- and poorly-paid "Gig" workers.[82] This meant that on the eve of the COVID-19 crisis the healthcare system in the UK was in a dire state of neglect and disrepair that was unparalleled in the postwar period, just at a time when it needed to be at its most robust to cope with the biggest national emergency since World War II.

That the NHS managed, by the skin of its teeth, to weather the first wave of the pandemic (and in doing so save tens of thousands of lives), despite its own state of disrepair, was testament to the resilience, fortitude, and dedication to the cause of public health of its frontline professionals and of its ancillary and support workers (many of them out-sourced, on bare minimum wage, without entitlements, and on zero-hours contracts) who toiled in the backroom to keep the show on the road.[83] This was a triumph of collective subjective will over adverse institutional objectivity, and like all such triumphs, it was won against the odds. Indeed, it would not have been won at all without the intervention of a large dose of good fortune. The good fortune in question was simply that far fewer mechanical ventilators were necessary than the public health experts (and therefore ministers of state) imagined in their wildest hopes would be needed:

> Luckily for Covid-19 patients – not to mention the ministers overseeing the ventilator challenge – external factors came to the rescue. Only about half of Covid-19 patients admitted to intensive care with breathing difficulties were being put on mechanical ventilators.[84]

This was because COVID-19 does not always attack the lungs, but has diverse avenues of attack on multiple organs, whereas alternative less invasive and radical methods of supporting patients with breathing difficulties were unexpectedly found to be effective in treating many with acute symptoms. These included, for example, simpler CPAP devices, of which there were several thousand that could be used. But, if this had not been the case, or if even only a *small fraction* of the expected number of ventilators had been needed, the NHS would have been overwhelmed, and what Boris Johnson considered his "reasonable case scenario" of at least 100,000-plus deaths from the first wave would have come to pass.

Nonetheless, even putting aside the ventilator issue, thousands of people were to die unnecessarily from COVID-19 in the first wave. This was owing to the Government's general mishandling of the pandemic, of which the ventilator panic was emblematic. Hancock repeatedly denied that anyone died unnecessarily during the first wave due to a lack of PPE or other shortages of life-saving equipment. This has been the Government's official position ever since, despite the UK's outlier status in terms of pandemic fatalities and the testimony of frontline whistle-blowers. Dominic Cummings, No. 10's former Chief Adviser, has since revealed that Hancock's denials were known to be false in ministerial circles.

> He [Hancock] knew that was a lie because he'd been briefed by the chief scientific adviser and chief medical officer about the first peak. We were told explicitly that people didn't get the treatment they deserve. Many people were left to die in horrific circumstances.[85]

Cummings also testified before the parliamentary select committee (in May 2021) that Hancock had offered assurances to the PM and himself in a cabinet office meeting in the midst of the first wave in mid-April 2020 that "everything is fine with

PPE, we've got it all covered".[86] This was one example, said Cummings, of Hancock's blatant lies to deny his own incompetence over the course of the pandemic.

However, it was hard not to read Cummings' exposes as motivated by his attempt to distance himself from responsibility for the shortages debacle. For, if Hancock did offer these assurances, it was remarkable that they were accepted. They were, after all, already radically at odds with the facts. The PPE crisis was, of course, already manifest before mid-April 2020, or as Cummings put it, "we were actually completely short, hospitals all over the country were running out".[87] The PM's recognition of Hancock's "incompetence" (on Cummings' account), and Hancock's supposed exposure as a liar in government circles for misleading the PM over the adequacy of PPE provisions (on that same account), remarkably did not cost him his job. This is surely instructive, in that it evidences the collective failure of government to manage the supply issue. Or, at the very least, it evidences Johnson's (and Cummings') negligent complicity with the Health Secretary's errors. Back in the world of verifiable facts, the official ministerial line throughout the pandemic was that PPE supplies were perfectly sufficient.

Assuredly too, the public health of a population was placed in jeopardy by a form of political governance (neoliberalism) that had for decades systematically undermined the public sector systems (of social welfare and healthcare) that would defend it. The politics of austerity and of neoliberalism did not simply deliver a terrible public health outcome that would otherwise have been avoided, but these also threatened a public health catastrophe many times bigger than that which transpired – and which only the beyond-the-call-of-duty exertions of hundreds of thousands of NHS workers plus blind luck averted. The extent of the crisis of social care and healthcare on the eve of the pandemic and the special role of neoliberal politics in generating these crises will be addressed in the next chapter. This will verify in a quite empirical way just how exposed the population of the UK was to a magnitude of public health disaster many times greater than the one that transpired owing to chronic vulnerabilities generated in these frontline services of an increasingly threadbare welfare state.

21 June 2020 (updated 28 July 2021)

Notes

1   *BBC News* (2020). 'Coronavirus: UK failed to stockpile crucial PPE'. (28 April); Foster, P. and Neville, S. (2020). 'How poor planning left the UK without enough PPE'. *Financial Times*. (1 May); Gardner, B. and Nuki, P. (2020).'Exercise Cygnus warned the NHS could not cope with pandemic three years ago but "terrifying" results were kept secret'. *Telegraph*. (28 March); Booth, W. (2020). 'Boris Johnson and his ministers accused of bungling coronavirus response, unleashing disaster'. *Washington Post*. (20 April); Hopkins, N. (2020). 'UK ministers were warned last year of risks of coronavirus pandemic'. *Guardian*. (24 April); Hopkins, N. (2020). 'Leaked Cabinet Office briefing on UK pandemic threat – the key points'. *Guardian*. (24 April); Doward, J. (2020). 'Government under fire for failing to act on pandemic recommendations'. *Observer*. (19 April).

2 Booth, R. (2021). 'Dominic Cummings' key accusations against Matt Hancock'. *Guardian*. (27 May).

3 Devlin, K. (2020). 'Coronavirus: delivery of 84 tonnes of vital protective kit for NHS staff delayed'. *Independent*. (19 April).

4 Gardner, B. (2020). 'Millions of pieces of PPE being shipped from Britain to Europe despite NHS shortages'. *Telegraph*. (24 April).

5 By contrast, the Taiwanese government imposed, as did many others, an immediate ban on manufacturers exporting vital medical equipment that could be mobilized to combat the virus at home. See: Maizland, S. and Felter, C. (2020). 'Comparing six health-care systems in a pandemic'. *Council on Foreign Relations* (online). (15 April). Available at: www.cfr.org/backgrounder/comparing-six-health-care-systems-pandemic

6 Murphy, S. and Wunsch, H. (2012). 'Clinical review: international comparisons in critical care – lessons learned'. *Critical Care*, 16, pp. 2–7; Prin, M. and Wunsch, H. (2012). 'International comparisons of intensive care: informing outcomes and improving standards'. *Current Opinion in Critical Care*, 18 (6), pp. 700–6. Murphy and Wunsch found that the UK was at the bottom of the OECD "league table" for ICUs where comparisons were possible.

7 Miller, J. (2020). 'Exclusive: UK faces "massive shortage" of ventilators – Swiss manufacturer'. *Reuters*. (18 March).

8 House of Commons Public Accounts Committee (2020). *Covid-19: Supply of Ventilators*. Twenty-Seventh report of Session of 2019–21. (25 November). London: House of Commons, Committee of Public Accounts, p. 9.

9 HCCPA (2020), p. 5.

10 Davies, R. (2020). 'The inside story of the UK's NHS coronavirus ventilator challenge'. *Guardian*. (4 May); Balogun, B. (2020). *Coronavirus: Ventilator Availability in the UK*. Briefing Paper No. CPB 8904. (3 June). London: House of Commons Library, p. 8.

11 HCCPA (2020), p. 10.

12 HCCPA (2020), p. 3.

13 HCCPA (2020), p. 5.

14 Balogun (2020), p. 8; Jack, S. (2020). 'Coronavirus: Government orders 10,000 ventilators from Dyson'. *BBC News*. (26 March).

15 Balogun (2020); BBC One (2020). *The Andrew Marr Show*. 'Matt Hancock: outdoor exercise could be banned if people flout rules'. Interview: Matt Hancock. (5 April).

16 HCCPA (2020), p. 5.

17 National Audit Office (2020). *Investigation Into How Government Increased the Number of Ventilators Available to the NHS in Response to COVID-19*. NAO (online). (25 September), p. 8. Available at: www.nao.org.uk/report/increasing-ventilator-capacity-in-response-to-covid-19/.

18 HCCPA (2020), p. 3.

19 Sabbagh, D. and Davies, S. (2020). 'UK scrambles for foreign-made ventilators ahead of coronavirus peak'. *Guardian*. (8 April).

20 Davies (2020).

21 Davies (2020).

22 Mason, R. and O'Carroll, L. (2020). 'No 10 claims it missed deadline for EU ventilator scheme'. *Guardian*. (26 March).

23 Roberts, M. (2020). 'Coronavirus: NHS well stocked for ventilators this winter'. *BBC News*. (30 September).

24 Balogun (2020), p. 8.

25 *BBC News* (2020). 'Coronavirus: NHS asks vets to donate animal ventilators'. (25 March).

26 GOV.UK (2020). *Call for Business to Help Make Ventilators*. (16 March). Available at: www.gov.uk/government/news/production-and-supply-of-ventilators-and-ventilator-components.

27 Andreas Wieland, Chief Executive of Hamilton Medical in Switzerland, the world's largest ventilator maker, was dismissive of the scheme. "I wish them the best of luck . . . [But] . . . I do not believe anything will come of it. These devices are very complex. It takes us four to five years . . ." to develop a new product (Miller, 2020).

28 Balogun (2020), p. 10.
29 Quoted in Davies (2020).
30 Quoted in Balogun (2020), p. 16.
31 Davies (2020).
32 Davies (2020).
33 Davies (2020).
34 Balogun (2020), p. 10; Foster, P. and Pooler, M. (2020). 'Ventilator standards set out for UK makers "of no use" to Covid patients'. *Financial Times*. (15 April).
35 Davies (2020); Sabbagh and Davies (2020)
36 Davies (2020).
37 Balogun (2020), p. 13.
38 Balogun (2020), pp. 10–11.
39 Davies (2020).
40 Balogun (2020), p. 8.
41 Balogun (2020), p. 12.
42 Amnesty International (2020). *Exposed, Silenced, Attacked: Failures to Protect Health and Essential Workers During the Pandemic.* (13 July). Available at: www.amnesty.org/en/documents/pol40/2572/2020/en/; Campbell, D. (2020). 'NHS staff "gagged" over coronavirus shortages'. *Guardian*. (31 March); Dyer, C. (2020). 'Covid-19: doctors are warned not to go public about PPE shortages'. *British Medical Journal* (online). (21 April). Available at: www.bmj.com/content/369/bmj.m1592; Earle, S. (2020). 'Boris Johnson: the hollow priest of the NHS'. *Al-Jazeera*. (21 April); Haynes, C. and Clayton, J. (2020). 'Coronavirus: doctors "told not to discuss PPE shortages"'. *BBC News*. (15 May); Lintern, S. (2020). 'Coronavirus: surgeons told not to discuss lack of PPE'. *Independent*. (10 August).
43 Bartlett, N. (2020). 'Labour MP Nadia Whittome sacked as carer for speaking out about PPE shortages'. *Mirror*. (6 May).
44 A reason for this asymmetry of human tragedy is likely owing to the fact that the BAME workers are over-concentrated in the lower-status role-positions in the health and care sectors whose occupants have not been prioritized for PPE (where this is in short supply and tightly rationed) yet who are exposed to significant levels of exposure to coronavirus infection. This may also be linked to duration of exposure risk. Lower-paid health and care staff (porters, cleaners, laundry workers, caterers, nurses, care assistants, etc.) are those more likely than those better placed (doctors, consultants, care managers, etc.) to work extended shifts and longer working weeks.
45 Amnesty International (2020).
46 Kirsch, T. (2020). 'What happens if health-care workers stop showing up'? *Atlantic*. (24 March).
47 Earle (2020).
48 *Al-Jazeera* (2020). 'UK: coronavirus deaths near 10,000; PM Johnson makes progress'. (11 April); Campbell, D. (2020). 'Doctors lacking PPE "bullied" into treating Covid-19 patients'. *Guardian*. (7 April); Campbell, D. (2020). 'UK hospital tackles PPE shortage by making 5,000 visors a day'. *Guardian*. (17 May); Carrell, S. (2020). 'Care home operators ask army and GPs to tackle coronavirus deaths'. *Guardian*. (7 April); Chakelian, A., Grylss, G. and Calcia, N. (2020). 'How the UK's care homes were abandoned to coronavirus'. *New Statesman*. (24 April); Gardner, B. (2020). 'Three nurses forced to wear bin bags because of PPE shortage test positive for coronavirus'. *Telegraph*. (8 April); Marsh, S. (2020). 'NHS staff making masks from snorkels amid PPE shortages'. *Guardian*. (1 April); *Guardian* (2020). 'Nearly half of England's doctors forced to find their own PPE, data shows'. (3 May); Savage, M. (2020). 'UK care homes scramble to buy their own PPE as national deliveries fail'. *Guardian*. (6 April).
49 Marsh (2020).
50 Perraudin, F. (2020). 'UK government's coronavirus response beset by mixed messages and U-turns'. *Guardian*. (14 April).
51 Lacobucci, G. (2021). 'Covid-19: PM's former chief aide accuses health secretary of lying over PPE and access to treatment'. *British Medical Journal* (online), 373 (1369). (26 May). Available at: www.bmj.com/content/373/bmj.n1369.

52 Booth, R. (2020a). UK care home staff "at breaking point" as coronavirus cases rise'. *Guardian*. (31 March); Booth, R. (2020b). 'Residential homes "desperate" for PPE, as two care workers die'. *Guardian*. (6 April); Savage (2020).

53 Chakelian et al. (2020).

54 Jones, O. (2020). 'Really, Matt Hancock, do you not know why people work when they're ill'? *Guardian*. (26 November). Jones interviewed a number of Covid keyworkers about their plight. As "Hannah", care assistant in a nursing home, explained: "If I catch it and have to isolate, I won't even be able to make rent, never mind all of the other bills that I would be expected to pay". Similarly, as "Sarah", care assistant in a private care home, instructed her: "We have had a number of staff test positive for Covid . . . We also have staff carrying on working who are high risk, as they can't afford not to. I feel like we're forgotten about."

55 OECD (2020). *Paid Sick Leave to Protect Income, Health and Jobs Through the COVID-19 Crisis*. (2 June). Available at: https://read.oecd-ilibrary.org/view/?ref=134_134797-9iq8w1fnju&title=Paid-sick-leave-to-protect-income-health-and-jobs-through-the-COVID-19-crisis.

56 Klair, A. (2020). *Sick Pay for All – Why the Benefits System Isn't the Answer*. TUC (online). (9 March). Available at: www.tuc.org.uk/blogs/sick-pay-all-why-benefits-system-isnt-answer.

57 Chakelian et al. (2020).

58 Gostoli, Y. (2020). 'As Brexit nears, EU workers fortify UK's coronavirus front lines'. *Al-Jazeera* (online). (20 April).

59 Swerling, G. (2020). 'Fears half of coronavirus deaths may be in care homes as officials accused of "airbrushing out" older people'. *Telegraph*. (13 April).

60 McIntyre, N. and Duncan, P. (2020). 'Care homes and coronavirus: why we don't know the true UK death toll'. *Guardian*. (14 April).

61 Chakelian et al. (2020).

62 Reality Check Team (2021). 'What happened to care homes early in the pandemic'? *BBC News*. (28 May). As reported by the BBC's R.C.T. On 19 March 2020, NHS England instructed that "unless required to be in hospital, patients must not remain in an NHS bed". What this meant for the care sector was clarified on 2 April: "Negative [Covid-19] tests are not required prior to transfers/admissions into the care home". It was even permissible for elderly patients who had tested positive for coronavirus to be discharged into care homes, on condition that care staff were protected by PPE and there were quarantine protocols in place. But, of course, few staff were protected, owing to the chronic shortages of PPE during the first wave, and care home managers and staff were unknowledgeable of how to protect their charges and each other.

63 Booth, R. (2022). 'Covid care home discharge policy was unlawful, says court'. *Guardian*. (27 April).

64 Stewart, H. (2021). 'Dominic Cummings says PM had no plan to protect vulnerable people from Covid'. *Guardian*. (25 May).

65 Lintern, S. (2021). 'More than 25,000 patients discharged to care homes in crucial 30 days before routine testing'. *Independent*. (2 June).

66 ONS (2021). *Deaths Involving COVID-19 in the Care Sector, England and Wales: Deaths Registered Between Week Ending 20 March 2020 and Week Ending 2 April 2021*. GOV.UK (online). (11 May). Available at: www.ons.gov.uk/peoplepopulationandcommunity/birthsdeath-sandmarriages/deaths/articles/deathsinvolvingcovid19inthecaresectorenglandandwales/deathsregisteredbetweenweekending20march2020andweekending2april2021.

67 ONS (11 May, 2021).

68 Chakelian et al. (2020); Savage, M. and Tapper, J. (2020). 'Patients were sent back to care homes without Covid test despite bosses' plea'. *Guardian*. (29 May).

69 Woodcock, A. (2021). 'Pressure mounts on Matt Hancock with claim he was summoned to see PM over care home tests'. *Guardian*. (30 May).

70 Booth (2021).

71 Woodcock (2021).
72 Woodcock (2021).
73 Pickard, J. and Cameron-Chileshe, J. (2021). 'Cummings reveals Johnson messages calling Hancock's efforts "hopeless"'. *Financial Times*. (16 June).
74 Booth (2021).
75 Holt, A. and Butcher, B. (2020). 'Coronavirus deaths: how big is the epidemic in care homes'? *BBC News*. (15 May).
76 Booth (2020a, 2020b).
77 Chakelian et al. (2020).
78 Kirsch (2020).
79 Campbell (2020).
80 Earle (2020).
81 Tapsfield, J. and Wright, J. (2020). 'Furious doctors threaten to stop treating patients as ministers admit 84 tonnes of crucial coronavirus PPE has failed to arrive from Turkey with supplies running out – but medical officer Jenny Harries complains critics are not being "adult" about problems'. *Mail*. (19 April).
82 King's Fund (2020). *NHS Funding: Our Position*. (22 October). Available at: www.kingsfund.org.uk/projects/positions/nhs-funding. See also: King's Fund (2020). *NHS Workforce: Our Position*. (26 October). Available at: www.kingsfund.org.uk/projects/positions/nhs-workforce.
83 Indeed, a significant proportion of NHS nursing staff were also casualized workers provided by employment agencies. The paradox this presents is that those workers who were protecting the public from COVID-19 were simultaneously pressurized by their precarious position in a two-tier NHS to report for work even if they were experiencing Covid symptoms, thereby simultaneously protecting and endangering lives. Jones (2020) cites the case of his interviewee "Christopher":

> If I don't go to work I don't get paid, so in normal times I need to be pretty unwell not to go in . . . Also, when we call in sick we are often . . . made to feel very guilty about it, so again, unless you're very unwell the pressure is on you to come in anyway.

84 Davies (2020).
85 Lacobucci (2021).
86 Booth (2021).
87 Booth (2021).

3

NEOLIBERALISM AND THE CRISIS OF WELFARE

In the previous chapter, I addressed the chronic shortages of PPE and other health-care resources in the NHS and in social care at the start of the pandemic and throughout its first wave. As we have seen, these problems threatened to undermine the cause of public safety in the teeth and claw of the crisis. NHS workers were forced to cope with mass hospitalizations without sufficient critical care beds or mechanical ventilators or self-protective gear to manage the huge demands that were placed on the healthcare system and on themselves. NHS and social care frontliners were forced to accept unacceptably and unnecessarily high personal health and safety risks when dealing with the sick due to the paucity of PPE.

At one level, these sorts of issues have arisen from the complacency or disregard of the present government and its predecessor, as these have continued a politics of austerity that have long outlasted the rationales that were originally given for them. But, at a more fundamental level, these have arisen from a deeply entrenched crisis of the welfare state in Britain. The origins of this crisis predate the Great Financial Crisis of 2007/2009 and the policy responses to it of successive governments by several decades. Rather, this is as much a story of the long-standing neoliberal reshaping of state and government in the UK over the past 40 years. A fundamental aspect of this reshaping has been a thoroughgoing retrenchment of public and social services, including those of health and social care. The purpose of this chapter is to explore this contemporary crisis of public welfare in its political and historical contexts. This serves to help make sense of the magnitude of the pressures placed on the public health and care systems by the pandemic.

Neoliberalism in Britain

Neoliberalism as ideology is thoroughly permeated by neo-classical economics and classical liberal social theory. According to these, only private ownership of the

DOI: 10.4324/9781003275039-4

means of production and the operation of unrestricted markets in goods and services and labour power can deliver economic efficiency and material prosperity. This is because these not only release individuals to pursue their rational self-interest as buyers and sellers (thereby allowing economic freedom to flourish), but also foster in them self-reliance, by compelling them to take responsibility for their own welfare. In the absence of the incentives generated by private ownership and market rewards, and protected from the pressures these impose by generous welfare states that are intended to abolish social injustice, individuals would be deflected from the work ethic, from economic enterprise, and from self-reliance Moreover, private ownership and the market mechanism, according to economic liberalism, also safeguards individual liberty, by acting as a bulwark against the encroachments of state power on civil society and on the rational pursuit of self-advantage. To wit, these also have the virtue of imposing cost-efficiency on the functions of public administration.[1]

Neoliberalism as political governance may be identified with a specific set of policies that were intended to deliver on the prescriptions of neoliberalism as ideology. Pioneered by right-wing governments in the UK and the USA in the 1980s, neoliberalism was internationalized in the 1990s and 2000s, just as corporate free-trade capitalism became globally consolidated with the crisis and subsequent demise of communism or state socialism.[2] Neoliberalism as state policy sought to reinvigorate national economic competitiveness by placing itself unambiguously and enthusiastically in the service of mega capital and corporate enterprise. This has committed ruling parties to a form of class warfare from above whereby the political process is converted into a mechanism to squeeze welfare systems, emasculate the trade unions, promote labour market flexibility, liberalize finance and trade, empower multinational companies (MNCs), privatize public goods and services, reduce taxation on business and wealth, and "modernize" (i.e. financialize and commodify) society and the state.[3] Ultimately, the secret of capitalist renewal, from the neoliberal perspective, is to bring about an anti-egalitarian redistribution of allocative resources. This is away from labour or from income from wages and the "social wage" (i.e. welfare benefits) towards capital.

The neoliberal assault on public services as an ideologically driven political project in Britain began in earnest under the Conservative New Right governments of the 1980s. Thatcherism as a political project was intent on dismantling so-called Butskellism (the loose post-war consensus of mixed-economy of state and market, of a corporatist welfare state offering universal entitlements and services, of legally empowered unionized labour, of regulated employment and other markets, and of progressive and high rates of taxation in order to fund expansive public services. This was on the grounds that this was stifling capitalist enterprise and locking Britain into a spiral of relative economic decline *vis-à-vis* competitor states.[4] Thatcherism as a political programme thus energetically pursued a portfolio of policies intended to restore the fortunes of British capitalism. Most notably, these included:

(*a*) deregulation of the labor and financial markets . . .; (*b*) privatization and marketization of the main utilities . . . and state enterprises . . .; (*c*) promotion of home ownership (including the widespread sale of public housing stock under the "right to buy" scheme); (*d*) curtailing of workers' and trade union rights (e.g., bans on the "closed shop"; obligatory membership ballots before any industrial action; restrictions on the right to picket, including a ban on secondary picketing; and removal of trade union immunity from damages); (*e*) promotion of free-market ideology in all areas of public life (including health-care and the civil service); (*f*) significant cuts to the social wage via welfare state retrenchment (e.g., a 7% reduction in state expenditure on social assistance between 1979–1989; removal of 16- to 18-year-olds from entitlement; reductions in state pensions; abolition of inflation-link for welfare benefits); (*g*) acceptance of mass unemployment as a price worth paying for the above policies; and (*h*) large tax cuts for the business sector and the most affluent.[5]

A fundamental strand of this project was the neoliberalization of social and public policy that has continued to this day. "Public spending is at the heart of Britain's . . . economic difficulties", announced the Thatcher government's first White Paper on its election into government in 1979.[6] The declared objective of the New Right on winning office was to "roll-back" the state.[7]

This was not the state "in general" (since spending on the criminal justice system, on the penal system, and on the military tended to increase) under the watch of Conservative governments from 1979 to 1997. Rather, this was of the "economic state" (publicly-owned utilities and enterprises – such as the railways, steel, coal, water and sewerage, gas, electricity, telecommunications, postal services, airports, and so on – all of which were sold off to big corporations at bargain-basement prices)[8] and of the social-welfare and (initially) educative functions of the state.[9] Nor was this roll-back of the state in the sense of a project of outright abolition of public systems of healthcare and welfare and education, in favour of market-based alternatives, or of their privatization (though some form of outright privatization was envisaged, though abandoned because impractical, for education and the NHS).[10] Instead, except for social housing (some of which was sold off to former tenants but mostly to housing associations)[11] and residential care (which devolved to privately owned care homes),[12] outright privatization and marketization was superseded by quasi-marketization whereby service provider units (e.g. hospital trusts, academies, school boards) were forced into competition with each other for tightly rationed public funds.[13]

New Labour in office was even more ideologically doctrinaire in extolling the virtues and extending the practices of neoliberal capitalist "globalization" than its New Right predecessors had been. This was

> evidenced in its welcome to inward investment, its active promotion of the international interests of British-based (but not always British-owned) financial, commercial, and industrial capital, and its support for the Washington Consensus on the benefits of free trade in services on a world scale.[14]

Even though New Right governments pioneered neoliberal agendas in economic, social, and welfare policy, these were continued in essentials by New Labour and by successor governments. New Labour was about *consolidating* and *routinizing* neoliberalism.[15] Privatizations were not reversed, whereas quasi-marketizations of public services were not only preserved but extended.[16] "This facilitated a plethora of private organisations entering the market to sub-contract to government, particularly in health, social care and housing",[17] but also in education.[18] Naturally, marketization and financialization of the public sector have been accompanied by the penetration everywhere of managerialism and the paraphernalia of performance surveillance mechanisms for exercising disciplinary control over staff and organizations and clients.[19]

To these private–public partnerships (PPIs) Blair's governments added Private Finance Initiative schemes (PFIs), which intensified the marketization and financialization of public goods and social services. These were intended to attract private capital into the public sector by inviting companies to run social services as commercial enterprises or by allowing them to fund public projects in return for income from rent or interest. This in effect turned public goods into private assets that were merely loaned to the state at astronomical cost to the taxpayer.[20] New Labour also stuck rigidly to the outgoing Tory government's radically stringent public spending and taxation thresholds for its first two years in office.[21] Thereafter, spending was increased in real terms, but this was targeted especially on health and education, whereas social care and social security continued to suffer.[22] This was as the commitment to a minimalist social charter continued so as to protect flexible labour markets.[23] The policy strategy of New Labour, as was ceded by Blair, was to raid budgets in certain areas of public spending in order to release funds for priority areas, rather than generate new investments.[24] Consequently, targeted austerity became a permanent feature of policy. Spending as a proportion of GDP did eventually increase beyond the level of the preceding New Right governments,[25] but this was undoubtedly exaggerated by the inclusion in public accounting of private financing from the bourgeoning PPI market.

A fundamental goal of the neoliberal project for New Right and New Labour governments alike was a thoroughgoing and permanent retrenchment of spending on the social welfare aspect of the public sector. This was so that total spending on welfare would not increase as a proportion of GDP, and ideally could also be reduced somewhat. This supported a commitment of state policy to holding down the general income-tax thresholds, especially on middle- and higher-earners, so that any greater investments in the public sector would have to be funded by inflationary government borrowing.[26] A further important goal of this neoliberal project was to embed "entrepreneurship" throughout the state sector. This was for reasons not simply of supposed "efficiency gains" (in reality reduced wage costs won from cheapening outsourced labour-power) but also for the ethical or normative virtue of "innovation".[27] This was based on the dogma that the only innovation possible must be that motivated by market competition and by money incentives and disincentives rather than by norms of public duty and community service.[28]

Naturally, this ensured that social policy could no longer be aimed at reducing inequalities of outcome, narrowing structural class divisions, by redistributing resources through the tax and welfare systems from haves to have-nots.[29] Rather, this must (in the jargon of Blair and the Third Way) be about promoting "equality of opportunity".[30] Or this must (in the jargon of Thatcher and the New Right) be about facilitating individual freedom as both self-interest and self-reliance.[31] This was equality of opportunity or personal freedom for an undifferentiated society of individuals, which would somehow be accomplished for the marginalized or socially excluded simply by weaning or coercing them off benefits and into jobs-training schemes, voluntary work, or paid work.[32]

If neoliberalism in the UK was initially, under the Tories, primarily about easing the immediate fiscal crisis of the state (as borrowing expanded in the absence of sufficient taxation income to support public services),[33] it rapidly evolved into a project to reconfigure society and state as both enabler and extension of the market – as *consumer society* and *business state*. Crucial to the success of this project was permanently scaling down the level of taxation of wealth and of corporations, since this was seen to be a barrier to international capitalist competitiveness, slowing growth and deterring inward investment, undermining the dynamism of the market.[34] Crucial to this project as well was ensuring that whatever "liberty" or "opportunity" is afforded to the less well-off and economically marginalized this does not upset the capitalist applecart by encouraging in them "unreasonable" aspirations for consumer success or economic security.

New Labour thus neither repealed nor substantially ameliorated Tory anti-labour laws that placed restrictions on industrial action to enhance or defend wages or working conditions. This was likely owing to fear that this would restore the confidence of unionized labour in collective projects of self-advancement and be a beacon call for the poor to join unions.[35] Instead, opportunity for many in the UK has been hemmed in by a national minimum wage that has for most of its existence since it was introduced by Blair's first Labour government in 1998 been pegged at less than half of the median income and which has functioned to depress incomes and reproduce and legitimize in-work poverty.[36] Consumer society needs *flawed* consumers as much as it needs *actual* consumers.[37] For the relentless cheapening of commodity goods and services that renders mass consumer markets viable is won in large measure at the expense of the incomes and occupational entitlements of the working poor – those who are to be found in the McJobs, or in the G-economy, at the wrong (deregulated) end of the labour market.

Neoliberalism and hyper-austerity

Reigning-in the welfare state has been integral to the neoliberal project in Britain since the rise to government of Thatcher and the New Right from the tail end of the 1970s. The project has been continued by governments of the right and of the centre and centre-left, with greater or lesser enthusiasm. In recent times, however, the assault on public welfare, or on the social aspects of the state, has been invested with renewed intensity and ferocity, under the rationale of austerity politics. Austerity politics are a continuation and acceleration of the broader project of curbing state expenditures. The immediate motivation behind this was to reduce a vast overhang of public debt generated by New Labour's bailouts of major British banks facing collapse owing to the Great Crash. However, what was doubtless seen initially as economic imperatives have been replaced by those which are more straightforwardly political, though the architects are incentivized not to acknowledge this publicly.

The cost of the rescue to the exchequer has been estimated at £456.33 billion, or the equivalent of 33 percent of the UK's GDP.[38] However, this is likely to be an over-estimate. The UK government earmarked £500 billion (US $718 billion to the bailouts), 41.6 percent of GDP, but spent "only" the equivalent of 26.8 percent of GDP, spread over multiple financial years.[39] This was because a large part of the bailout resource took the form of guarantees rather than actual monies or were for capitalization schemes that were never used. Moreover, not all of the actual spending was lost, since the Government could, up to a point, levy charges on the guarantees and recoup interest on loans, though the complexities and lack of transparency over the rescues rendered the task of calculating how much was repaid (and lost) and how much was still to be repaid speculative.[40]

A striking feature of the UK bailouts was that these exerted a heavier financial toll on the public purse than those of other countries. This was partly due to the greater degree of liberalization of finance capital in the UK compared to other high-income countries, especially those in the EU. UK banks, being more deregulated and internationalized than those on the continent, suffered greater exposure to the ill effects of the global financial crisis than was typical across the channel. The UK banking sector suffered, as a consequence, losses that were higher than those in every EU state. This was 6.3 percent of GDP compared to 3.1 percent in Spain, 2.4 percent in Germany, and 1.4 percent in France.[41]

But there was another reason why the bailouts wreaked a heavier toll on the UK's state finances compared to those of comparable others. This was simply because the British state, being far more absorbed by neoliberalism than the leading EU states, embraced a rescue strategy that was simply more unbalanced than theirs. This was inasmuch as this placed the burden of costs on the state rather than on private–public partnerships, so that these could not be devolved or spread as happened on the continent. The idea was to absolve private commerce completely from the task of paying towards the cost of the bailouts, so that the taxpayer would pick up the whole tab. Nonetheless, the net cost to the British taxpayer of the bank rescues in terms of written-off debts has been estimated as being equivalent to 1 percent of GDP. In the EU, only Ireland and Portugal incurred bigger losses. By contrast, several countries – France, Denmark, Greece, Sweden, Spain, and Belgium – not only recouped the costs of the bailouts but had turned these into government profits from interest repayments by 2011.[42]

In any case, the Great Crash and subsequent long recession was the outcome of untrammelled free-market capitalist internationalization (so-called globalization) and the neoliberal policies that drove it. The immediate drivers of the crisis were the deregulation of global finance markets and internationalization of banking (though accomplished to varying degrees by national banks in the major trading zones). But the underlying dynamic was a long-standing structural crisis of over-capacity and hence of reduced profitability in the real economy worldwide owing to the intensification of global capitalist competition in an over-saturated world market. The latter, by squeezing opportunities for profitable investment in material production and services, fed into over-capitalization in the finance sector. This led to the proliferation of irresponsible loans and commercial speculation (in housing, real estate, stock markets, popular consumerism) by banks seeking to put vast sums of idle capital to profitable use.[43] This plunged the world economy into a long period of recession and sluggish growth from which it had barely started to recover before the COVID-19 crisis struck.[44] This was the initial motivation behind what may be described as the shift towards *hyper*-austerity under the Tory-dominated Coalition government of 2010–2015, or at least part of the initial motivation.

However, this hyper-austerity has been extended well beyond its use-by date. It has been continued in the UK under successive governments long after less radical austerity cutbacks were eased in the USA and across the EU. Indeed, hyper-austerity has been continued after the deficit ramped-up by the bank rescues was finally brought under a measure of control, owing to revenues rolling-in to the state purse from the selling-back to the banks of shares that they had relinquished in the buyouts.[45] Hyper-austerity in the UK, in short, simply never went away – not under the Coalition government, nor under the Conservative governments that followed.

The reason for this is that austerity dovetails exactly with the radical anti-statism (or radical anti-*welfare*-statism) of the Tory brand of right-wing neoliberalism. Rather than being driven by economic necessity, the politics of deficit-driven hyper-austerity were a police move in ideology to legitimize policy preferences of government that could not in "normal times" be entertained let alone enacted in policy. And so hyper-austerity has continued for the better part of a decade irrespective of its impact on the public finances or on the economy. Initially, for the better part of three years, austerity cutbacks were accompanied with rising budget deficits, owing to the post-crash recession and sharply rising public claims on social security benefits. Latterly, however, hyper-austerity succeeded in reducing the budget deficit, at appalling cost to public services, yet was continued long after the deficit was reduced to a level below the post-war average.[46] The economic after-effects of the COVID-19 crisis (along with any other crisis that just happens to come along) will also be weaponized by radical neoliberals to legitimize a further indefinite perpetuation of the public sector squeeze.[47]

The political discourse on "killing the budget deficit" on a fast-track represented this as a moral duty of government on behalf of the citizenry and for the benefit of generations to come. This was on the grounds that balancing the books was indispensable to national economic performance. Yet budget deficit (which results from a government's immediate excess of expenditures beyond revenues on its current account) is potentially much less impactful on a country's economic fortunes than is government debt (which is a story of a state's total shortfall of revenues *vis-à-vis* expenditures over the long *duree*). This is because the latter would not only be larger than the former in purely fiscal terms and as a proportion of GDP but would also be much more intractable or incorrigible.

But significant if not major public debt is the typical situation of state finances.[48] In the UK, the bank bailouts almost doubled government debt, from 34 percent to 70 percent of GDP between 2009 and 2011. Thereafter, up until 2018, public debt continued to grow, peaking at 84 percent of GDP in 2017.[49] This was due to the impact of recession in driving up the social security budget, falling revenues from tax receipts, and of austerity itself in putting a break on demand-led recovery and hence contributing to several years of slow growth.[50] Yet, at the start of the 1950s, UK government debt was almost 200 percent of GDP, whereas by the start of the 1960s, this was still at around 105 percent of GDP. This was owing largely to the massive costs of the Second World War and of interest repayments on American loans for postwar reconstruction under the terms of the Marshall Plan.

It was not until the mid-1960s that the UK national debt as a proportion of GDP was reduced to a level below that generated by the financial meltdown of 2007/2009 and its aftermath. But none of this deterred British governments from building an expansionary welfare state almost from scratch or prevented the UK economy from growing at a faster rate than at any time during the 1980s, 1990s, and 2000s.[51] This shows that economic growth and prosperity can coincide with much higher levels of public debt than that caused by the recent bank bailouts. This lends support to the notion that the spectre of government debt and budget deficit was deployed as an ideological weapon by "hard" (right-wing) neoliberalism to legitimize radicalization of their 40-year project to roll back the welfare state.

Neoliberalism and crisis of healthcare

What are the consequences of neoliberalization on public services? Even prior to the current austerity era, UK governments have spent less on healthcare as a proportion of national income (or GDP growth) than is typical among the leading developed countries. Between 1975 and 1987, the UK devoted on average 5.5 percent of national income to healthcare. This is compared to 7.1 percent in France, 7.2 percent in Germany, 7 percent in the USA, and 8.6 percent in Sweden. Of the OECD countries, only Greece, Portugal, and Japan spent less over that period.[52] Between 1990 and 2000, the UK devoted approximately 6.8 percent of national income to healthcare. This is compared to 9.2 percent in France, 10.2 percent in Germany, 13 percent in the USA, and 8.4 percent in Sweden. This, too, was below the EU average of 8.1 percent and OECD average of 7.8 percent.[53] Between 2000 and 2018, the UK devoted an average of 9.2 percent of national income to healthcare spending. This is compared to 10.8 percent in France, 10.7 percent in Germany, 15.5 percent in the USA, and 10.5 percent in Sweden. This placed the UK (the world's fifth largest economy) in 13th place for health spenders among the OECD group. This was below the European average of 9.5 percent. This was also below the average for high-income countries of 11.2 percent.[54]

Over time, this relative under-investment in the NHS has likely led to a cumulative decline in the efficacy of the service by international standards and increased pressures on frontline delivery. This is in the context of increased demands on healthcare by an ageing population and rising prices for drugs and new medical technologies. The corporate ownership of drugs production and commodification of medicine in a deregulated market dominated by giant pharmaceutical MNCs is a fundamental but unacknowledged aspect of the crisis of healthcare. For this has meant that the prices of a wide range of healthcare commodities have grown much faster than general inflation,[55] just as corporate profits in the pharmaceutical industries are typically much bigger than in other large public companies with mark-ups estimated as being 6.1 percent higher.[56] Traditionally, the NHS's centralized purchasing system of drugs and other treatments has offered a measure of protection from cost inflation generated by corporate price-fixing,[57] whereas elsewhere, most notably in the USA, where healthcare is wholly privatized and commodified, the price of drugs increases relentlessly year on year, so that millions of the poorest Americans cannot afford health-sustaining treatments.[58] But, owing to the creeping marketization of healthcare in the UK, under successive neoliberal governments, these protections are ever in danger of being chipped away.

Investment in the NHS has increased on average by 3.7 percent annually since 1948.[59] Between 1955 and 1979, under the Conservative and Labour governments, the average yearly spending increase was around 4.3 percent. Under the New Right governments of the 1980s and 1990s, the average annual spending increase on the NHS was cut back to 3.3 percent,[60] and to just 3.1 percent during the Thatcher years,[61] so that resourcing of healthcare in the UK fell further behind OECD standards. Health spending under New Labour was then increased to a level much beyond the post-war average (overall, almost 6 percent per year adjusted for inflation from 1997 to 2010,[62] and 8.6 percent from 2001/2002 through to 2004/2005).[63] "This was particularly pronounced during the period of 2000–09", which saw a serious attempt to drag resourcing of the service closer to OECD standards and repair 18 years of relative Tory neglect, "reflecting the commitment of the Blair government to match UK NHS spending to the European average".[64]

However, the level of investments was not quite sufficient to match this goal, given the large gap that had been opened by almost two decades of funding shortfall. Under New Labour, therefore, per capita health spending remained below that of comparators. Thereafter, under the post-financial crash Coalition government of 2010–2015, the calamitous present era of radicalized, accelerated cutbacks began. This delivered five consecutive years of spending increases on the NHS of just 0.9 percent,[65] whereas owing to the increase in the size of the elderly population and population growth generally at least three times that level was necessary to maintain the system at its existing level of efficacy. The situation post-2015 has scarcely improved, with average spending increases between 2010/2011 and 2018/2019 of just 1.4 percent, and of just 1.6 percent between 2011/2012 and 2018/2019 owing to a 2 percent rise on the 2018/2019 round.[66]

A recent study published in the *British Medical Journal* of the performance of the UK healthcare system in comparison with those of other high-income countries (USA, Canada, Australia, France, Germany, Sweden, Denmark, the Netherlands, and Switzerland) revealed the extent of its relative funding disadvantages *vis-à-vis* the others:

> The UK spent the least per capita on healthcare in 2017 compared with all other countries studied (UK $3825 (£2972; €3392); mean $5700), and spending was growing at slightly lower levels (0.02% of gross domestic product in the previous four years, compared with a mean of 0.07%). . . . The OECD reports per capita spending for the UK to be $3943, which also reflects components of social care that are included in expenditures for other countries. Expressed as a proportion of gross domestic product (GDP), the picture was similar, with the UK spending approximately 8.7% of GDP compared with the study average of 11.5% of GDP in 2017. . . . From 2009 onwards, the growth in UK healthcare expenditure slowed to its lowest levels whereas health expenditure growth in the comparator countries was notably higher, averaging a rate of 0.08% of GDP per year over the period 2011–14 compared with an average annual decrease of 0.03% of GDP in the UK, and a rate of 0.07% of GDP over the period 2014–17 in comparator countries compared with a rate of 0.02% of GDP in the UK.[67]

Yet the Conservative government's five-year investment plan for the NHS released in the fall of 2017 was set on an even more stringent course than eventually transpired and one that would have tightened the financial ligature of the Coalition years. This committed £128.4 billion to the service over the course of five years – a paltry 0.7 percent average annual increase. But, as the King's Trust, Nuffield Foundation and Health Foundation pointed out, based on projections from the Office for Budget Responsibility (OBR):

> NHS spending would need to rise from £123.8 billion to at least £153 billion between 2017/18 and 2022/23 (a 4.3 per cent average annual increase) to keep pace with demographic pressures and other increasing cost pressures. . . . This falls a long way short of what is needed.[68]

Indeed. As it happened, these plans were softened. Healthcare austerity was eased fractionally. In the summer of 2018, Theresa May's Conservative government announced plans to increase spending on healthcare by £20.6 billion for the period from 2018/2019 to 2023/2024.[69] These were reiterated by Boris Johnson in January 2020 along with some additional *ad hoc* funds. This amounted to an annual spending increase of 3.3 percent over the five years. But, according to the Health Foundation's projections, this was enough only to prevent a further deterioration of the NHS rather than begin the job of repairing it.[70] Or, as the King's Fund put it, this was "less than the long-term average of 3.7 percent" and insufficient "to restore provider finances, improve performance against waiting time targets and kickstart the process of reform".[71]

Not only that, but excluded altogether from the new spends, in the manner of robbing Peter for the benefit of Paul, were areas of health (i.e. public health and health education) outside the remit of NHS England, so that the budget of the Department of Health as a whole was projected to rise by just £4.5 billion (or 0.9 percent) over the five years. Indeed, the budgets for public health and health education were to be cut by 20 percent to release funds for the NHS. Thus, by 2019, the budget for public health services was "£850 million lower than in 2015/16", whereas "by 2021 the budget will have been cut by 25% from its 2015/16 level in real-terms".[72] Spending on healthcare as a proportion of GDP consequently *fell* between 2010 and 2018, from 7.6 percent in Labour's last year in office to 6.8 percent.[73] This was historically unprecedented.

The spending crisis of healthcare has in recent years given rise to glaring resource shortfalls in frontline service delivery. Firstly, the NHS provider sector (NHS trusts and NHS foundations) has become increasingly mired in debt. This is due to a perfect storm of insufficient revenues to meet escalating demands for services and crippling interest charges on repayments under PFI and other government loan schemes that were intended to draw private capital into financing and running hospitals. In 2012/2013, NHS provider trusts were just about keeping their heads above water, with a surplus of around £577 million. However, by the 2015/2016 financial year, the sector had run up "a combined deficit of almost £2.45 billion",[74] and by 2019/2020 this had mushroomed to £13.4 billion.[75]

Naturally, this was blamed, as neoliberal free-market dogma insists it must, on inefficient public sector service delivery rather than on funding constraints and the vampire-like sucking of exorbitant sums of public money into the shareholder coffers of private companies.[76] Thus, indebted trusts and foundations were expected to demand improved productivity of frontline workers and services to recover their losses and service their debts. The Government's Five Year Forward Review of 2014 supposedly committed £30 billion to the NHS to plug the funding gap up until 2020/21, yet just £8 billion of this was to be new money, whereas the other £22 billion was to be made up from cost-efficiency savings.[77] This was even though the NHS had been labouring under various allegedly efficiency-boosting methods imported from the business sector for more than a decade. These included "reductions in reimbursement rates, staff freezes, and cuts to administrative and prescribing costs", all of which ensured that since 2009 "productivity in the NHS has risen faster than in other sectors of the British economy".[78]

Secondly, there has arisen in the NHS a basic insufficiency of specialized diagnostic equipment such as MIR and CT scanners as well as of general beds and acute-care and emergency-care beds. As reported by *BBC News*: "A comparison by the OECD . . . in 2014 – the last set of comparable figures – showed there were just 9.5 scanners per million head of the population, far below figures for Spain, Germany, France and Italy".[79] Although bed reductions are a general trend of contemporary healthcare systems over the past 30 years, their wastage in the NHS has been especially pronounced. Of the 21 OECD countries, only Denmark, Sweden, and Canada have fewer hospital beds per capita than the UK.[80] As reported by the King's Fund, this undoubtedly is a key barometer of the funding crisis.[81]

The British Medical Association (BMA) has estimated that the magnitude of the general shortage of beds is forcing four out of five NHS hospitals to use emergency surgical beds for routine patients. This is not simply for peak winter periods but all year round as well. This has contributed to increasing rates of postponement for surgical operations, routine and critical, and longer waiting times for operations, owing to the paucity of recuperation beds. The BMA further estimates that between 3,000 and 5,000 extra general care NHS beds are needed to end the misallocation of emergency surgery beds and to prevent trusts from having to find the money to fund so-called "escalation" beds to cope with winter surges in demand.[82]

The number of emergency-care beds in ICUs per 100,000 of the population in the NHS is far below the OECD and EU averages for healthcare systems. On the eve of the pandemic, there were 6.6 of them per 100,000 people in the UK system compared to 7.3 in Japan, 9.7 in Spain, 10.6 in South Korea, 11.6 in France, 12.5 in Italy, 29.2 in Germany, and 34.7 in the USA.[83] The same is true of acute-care beds more generally. The number of these across the WHO European region was 433 per 100,000 in 2014/2015, whereas the number of these across the EU was 461 per 100,000. This is compared to 228 per 100,000 in the UK. The number per 100,000 in Germany was 621, in Belgium 565, in France 428, in Switzerland 375, in Italy 273, in Denmark 248, in Spain 239, and in the Nordic countries 277.[84] The comparative paucity of acute-care beds in UK healthcare means that there is less leeway to cope with spikes in demand in critical periods (such as those generated by the present pandemic) so that acute or emergency care services are placed in danger of being overwhelmed.[85]

Thirdly, basic shortfalls in healthcare delivery have been revealed in recent years by missed targets on waiting times for hospital treatments following GP referrals and by declining A&E performance faced with escalating demands. As reported by *BBC News*, for 2018/2019,

> in cancer care patients are meant to start treatment within 62 days of an urgent GP referral. But that . . . is being missed, while waiting lists for routine treatments are rising. In England it has topped 4.4 million – the highest on record. Some 15% have waited more than the target time of 18 weeks.[86]

The crisis of emergency care is, with the benefit of hindsight, the most worrying aspect of the whole picture. This was to be exposed by the pandemic which pushed the NHS to the brink of meltdown. Here the escalating demands on the service, as reported by the King's Fund, have been relentless. A&E performance has been measured since the early 2000s against the "four hours" standard. "This refers to the pledge in the NHS Constitution that at least 95 per cent of patients attending

A&E should be admitted to hospital, transferred to another provider, or discharged within four hours".[87] But, again, as reported by the King's Fund:

> A&E waiting times have worsened substantially over the past decade, as the NHS has experienced a sustained period of financial austerity and staffing pressures. The NHS has not met the four-hour standard at national level in any year since 2013/14, and the standard has been missed in every month since July 2015.[88]

Up until December 2012, the four-hour standard was met, month by month, albeit on a declining curve. Thereafter, between December 2012 and July 2015, the pattern was that the standard was met, albeit fractionally, in the spring and summer months, but not so in the autumn and winter, where the shortfall was much bigger and progressively deepened. Since July 2015, the pattern has been not only failure to meet the performance target every month but steadily worsening performance, comparator month by month, season by season, year after year. In July 2015, 95.2 percent of patients attending A&E departments were processed within four hours, whereas in November 2015 this was 91.4 percent. By July 2019, 86.5 percent of patients attending A&E departments were processed within four hours, whereas in November that year it was 81.4 percent. The situation in Category 1 A&E departments (which are the major frontline ones providing 24-hour service with resuscitation facilities and which cater for a large majority of admissions) is the most precipitous, with only 73 percent of attendees being processed within four hours by February 2019.[89]

The pressures on A&E departments caught between the rock of underfunding and the hard place of rising demand has led to the annual carnivalesque spectacle of the NHS winter crisis. This is where largely predictable rises in the number of hospital admissions owing to spikes in the rate of seasonable infectious illnesses (and the negative impact of these on vulnerable populations) push A&E units to breaking point and beyond. Hence, the spectre of tens of thousands of patients stuck in the back of ambulances or in hospital corridors on trolleys awaiting beds, and of tens of thousands leaving A&E departments without having received treatment, which has become a big media event especially since the winter of 2013/2014, with each successive winter manifesting a bigger crisis than the preceding one.[90]

In the winter crisis of 2017/2018, for example, reportedly "a record 163,298 patients waited more than half an hour to be handed over to A&E departments".[91] This was accompanied by 10,375 unexplained "excess" deaths (i.e. beyond the seasonable average of the previous five years), which were not attributable to population ageing or unusually high numbers of mortalities from flu or influenza, and so were likely resulting from delays in receiving A&E treatment or owing to patients leaving the units without being seen because they were distressed or disenchanted by the delays.[92] How many of the COVID-19 ill who felt sufficiently ill to avail themselves of accident and emergency services may have been deterred by the stresses and strains of the long queues to stay put and get seen by a medical professional?

Finally, there is a growing shortfall of frontline healthcare professionals in the NHS, indeed of staff at all levels and of all job types. This is comparatively, that is, *vis-à-vis* international comparators, but also in real terms, with recruitment targets going unmet. Relative to OECD and EU averages, as well as to high-income countries, the UK has "among the lowest numbers of doctors and nurses per capita, despite having average levels of utilisation (number of hospital admissions)".[93] According to a study conducted by the King's Fund in 2018, and reported as headline news in the *Guardian*, the UK was found to have the third-lowest number of doctors and the sixth-lowest number of nurses in the OECD group of 21 countries, these being just 2.8 and 7.9 per 1,000 of the population, respectively.[94]

Recruitment deficits and staff shortages exist right across the board in UK healthcare – of GPs, of radiologists, of health visitors, of consultant physicians, of hospital nurses, and of midwives.[95] In recent years, either numbers have fallen, or increases have been too small to fill the necessary posts. The number of GPS fell by 1.6 percent in the year up to September 2018, leaving 15.3 percent of posts unfilled. The number of midwives increased by less than 1 percent (leaving 48 percent of midwife heads reporting that their teams were under-staffed) and the number of nurses and health visitors increased by less than half a percent between July 2017 and July 2018. Simultaneously, the "number of nurses and health visitors working in community health services has continued its long-term decline", falling by 1.2 percent over the same period.[96] There are presently 84,000 unfilled FTE vacancies (or one in ten positions), including 38,000 for nurses,[97] and 2,330 for hospital doctors.[98] For nurses, and for other job types, this is an improvement from the previous year (owing perhaps to a basic above-inflation pay rise), where the shortfall was 100,000 overall and of 41,000 nurses.[99] Nonetheless, this is of course nowhere near sufficient to ease pressures on chronically over-stretched staff. Staff shortages ramp up workload demands on keyworkers, lead to burnout and high rates of staff turnover, and impact negatively on performance.

The problem of under-recruitment for nurses (which is where recruitment shortfalls are most acute) is partly explainable by the lack of sufficient financial support for trainees, with cuts to nursing bursaries, and with grants replaced by means-tested maintenance loans that are pegged beneath bare subsistence levels. It has been estimated that this is reducing applications for places on university nursing courses by as much as a third.[100] This has also generated high rates of attrition, so that a quarter of trainee nurses abandon their studies.[101] But the poor recruitment situation generally is also explainable by relatively low salaries, including for nurses, as well as for non-medical staff, this impacting adversely on the attractiveness of careers in public sector healthcare.

Under the recent regime of cutbacks, pay in the NHS was capped or frozen from 2010/2011 to 2017/2018. This resulted in the real-term value of a nurse's starting salary decreasing by almost 10 percent over that period.[102] Though recently pay for nurses has been thawed, with an agreed pay rise of 6.5 percent spread over three years (from 2018/2019 to 2021/2022),[103] this has not repaired nor will come close to repairing the losses of the previous years. As for hospital doctors, these have recently been awarded a 2.8 percent pay rise under the latest DDBR. But, with inflation projected to rise to 1.2 percent in 2021, this constituted a paper-thin gain in real terms and again does very little to compensate medics for their much greater real income losses over a decade. The BMA estimates these as amounting to 8.8 percent in purely cash terms and more than 20 percent in real terms adjusting for inflation.[104]

Relatively low pay impacts not simply on recruitment but also on the retention of staff. One in nine staff left the NHS in 2017/2018 for reasons that included poor remuneration. Other reasons that certainly cannot be separated from the issue of the impact of under-funding included overwork, feeling undervalued, and encountering obstacles to delivering quality care.[105] A relatively recent online survey of 3,380 UNISON members working for the NHS found that 64 percent were working overtime whereas 58 percent were experiencing unwelcome increased workload volumes. Almost three-quarters of respondents felt that there was insufficient staffing in their workplace or on their ward or work team, with almost two-thirds having concerns about patient safety for this reason. The survey also showed that 70 percent of respondents

> are not paid when they work over their shift, two thirds rarely leave work on time and half (49%) are not able to take breaks because of their workload. More than three quarters (77%) said they are not at all satisfied with their pay and seven in ten don't feel valued by their employers despite the extra effort and goodwill NHS workers bring to the service. A staggering four in five (83%) NHS workers said they have to work more for less money and more than seven in ten (71%) said they had a poor work life balance.[106]

These results would certainly help explain the problems that the NHS is having in retaining staff – including and especially of nurses. And the exodus of nurses from the NHS is especially acute. A recent major study has shown that almost three-quarters quit the NHS within a year of qualifying, whereas 50 percent report that they are considering either leaving their trust or the NHS altogether. A further 34 percent report that they are unhappy with the job and 41 percent say that they do not feel valued by their employer. Just over 50 percent opine that "funding cuts have had a negative impact on their place of work, while 39 per cent admit that they have been personally impacted by pay caps". Three-quarters surveyed cited that "staff stress and burnout is a problem across their organisation", whereas 54 percent "admit that working long hours or being overworked is one of the biggest issues impacting their day-to-day job".[107] Yet it is not only nurses who have been feeling the pinch. According to the BMA's pay review of July 2021, "declines in doctors pay has had a damaging impact on . . . [their] morale. . . . This has contributed to a workforce crisis in the NHS and has had a detrimental effect on its ability to recruit and retain doctors".[108]

These were the public health workers upon which the gargantuan task of protecting millions of people from a highly infectious and for the old and vulnerable potentially deadly disease was to depend. Yet the state of morale of these workers could hardly have been at a lower ebb when the pandemic struck. This raised obvious potential for deficiencies and failings of care under the intense pressures wrought by the escalating caseloads. The fact that these workers somehow coped, more or less, with the demands placed on the healthcare system by the pandemic, despite the devaluing of their role and the almost intolerable stresses placed on their work by decades of under-resourcing (and indeed that the system itself did not unravel owing to the unprecedented strains that were placed on it *under these circumstances*) may be described as remarkable by way of understatement. Labouring under conditions wrought by neoliberal austerity, the feat appears almost miraculous.

The crisis in social care and social security

The crisis of healthcare is simply one aspect of the wider crisis of the welfare state. The impacts of neoliberal retrenchment and austerity have been experienced even more acutely in social care and social security. Although the public sector has overall endured financial retrenchment and austerity cutbacks over this period, these particular sectors of the welfare state have been especially targeted by successive governments. The main reason for this is clear enough. These are social services that have least efficacy for servicing the goal of capitalist performativity. Rather, the costs that these sectors levy on the public purse are, from the perspectives of a neoliberal polity, mere subtractions from corporate profits, and (owing to this) also constraints on economic growth. In contrast, funding of education and health as social services, from a capitalist point of view, are often recognized as "productive" costs, which may enhance capitalist performativity.[109] The reason for this is that if workforces are to be mobilized for success in international economic competition, the human resources that compose them must be rendered usable or exploitable, indeed ever more so.

Capitalism requires workers who are employable in that they are equipped with the requisite social and technical skills and attitudes towards work and authority that will render them productive and acquiescent. Employers also require workers who are motivated and enabled for flexibility, that is, who appreciate the need to continually upgrade and have the aptitude for adaptability that upgrading requires, so as to ensure their continued employability.[110] Indeed, countries which invest more in higher-skilled workforces may confer on themselves economic advantages over those which invest less.[111] Thus, in a capitalist world economy characterized by greater mobility of finance capital and ever-accelerating technological change, continual upskilling and reskilling of the workforce, or safeguarding the reproduction of "ready and able" graduates, has for state policymakers everywhere become regarded as indispensable to national competitiveness and to personal opportunity.[112] As Tomlinson notes: "In an effort to keep the . . . economy competitive, education and training are elevated to key positions; 'raising standards', 'learning to compete' and getting education 'right' [have become] major policy objectives".[113]

Capitalism also requires workers who are maintained in sufficient health to be capable of coping, day-by-day and week-by-week, with the physical and mental demands of intensive (high tempo) and extensive (prolonged) labour. This is just as capitalist internationalization requires that locally (i.e. nationally) based human resources are more-or-less comparable with regard to fitness for work where there are shared competitor markets.[114] This is necessary if labour-power is to be exportable and if a national economy is to attract investments from overseas in the employment of local labour power. Striving to secure competitive economic advantage over other national capitals on the world stage was doubtless a major incentive driving New Labour governments from 2001 to 2008 to ramp up investment in education and healthcare, just as hitherto under Conservative rule the NHS was at least relatively or partially shielded from the worst excesses of the broader austerity project.[115]

By contrast, social care and social security cater in the main for surplus populations – retired workers and unemployed workers. These are surplus in the sense that they are either marginal or superfluous to economic production and capital accumulation. Consider, firstly, the case of the unemployed. A reserve army of labour (i.e. the unemployed) is certainly functional for capitalism, inasmuch as this provides a surplus labour capacity that may be drawn upon in the event of rapid periods of economic growth, and also exerts a downward drag on overall wage rates (by rendering employed workers replaceable).[116] But reproducing the constituents of this reserve army at an income level equivalent even to the lowest paid of workers certainly is *not* functional to capitalism, since that would undermine work incentives. This necessitates that the unemployed must be given enough only to live, not to be included in the cultural life of a consumer society, to which access must be earned by submitting to the cash nexus. This is even though the labour power of the reserve army may often be superfluous, which is why it is not employed.[117]

Such is legitimized by ideologies of denigration of the workless as workshy malingerers. These contend that the unemployed or under-employed are demotivated to enter the labour market, not because jobs are unavailable or unattractive, but because welfare benefits are overly generous, making of them willing captives of the welfare state, "welfare dependents".[118] Such political discourses have become the common currency of successive governments in the UK over the past 40 years that are committed to welfare-to-work or workfare policies which make benefits entitlements contingent on the recipient accepting any kind of paid work available.[119] These are intended to force the "unemployed – including lone parents, the disabled, and those who had taken early retirement on benefits – into the labour market at entry-level, low-wage jobs in order to expand the labour pool and reduce wage-inflationary pressures".[120]

Consider, now, the case of the retired – the elderly and infirm, those no longer capable of working as productively as employers would like. The situation here is not dissimilar to the case of the unemployed, because there is no economic advantage to capitalism in maintaining people much above subsistence who can no longer function as exploitable human resources. In the UK, pensioners, like the unemployed, are disproportionately among those getting by on less than 60 percent of average income. There are 12 million people aged 65 years plus in the UK – 18 percent of the population. Of these, two million – or 16 percent of the total – are living on less than 60 percent of average income (i.e. in relative poverty), whereas a million of these are living in severe poverty, that is, on an income of less than half the average.[121] But the elderly make up 25 percent of the UK's eight million poorest adults.[122] Moreover, adults in workless households have a much higher rate of poverty than those who are not, so that approximately 46 percent of poor adults are in workless households, even though these make up only 8 percent of working-age households.[123] "In 2018/19, 51% of working-age adults in workless families were in poverty, compared with 15% of those in working families".[124]

The reason why these groups are over-represented amongst the poor is that large numbers of pensioners (i.e. those who did not earn enough during their working lives to make savings or invest in private or occupational pension schemes) and most of the unemployed or under-employed derive the bulk of their income from social security benefits that capitalism-sustaining polities have little incentive to align to average income levels. Indeed, they have rather stronger motives (i.e. easing the tax burden on profits and salaries) for pegging these at subsistence levels. This is why, over several decades, the economic situation of the unemployed in this country has steadily worsened, owing to the relentless downgrading of social security benefits.

The austerity-driven five-year benefits freeze (from May 2015 until April 2020),[125] which followed on from three years of 50 percent below price inflation benefit increases,[126] was simply the latest episode, albeit an accelerated one, in the long-run direction of travel of British welfare policy since the 1970s.[127] Long before the current round of austerity,

> the real value of basic out-of-work support in 2019–20 . . . [was] – at £73 a week (£3,800 a year) – lower than it was in 1991–92, despite GDP per capita having grown by more than 50 per cent since then. Even more starkly, child benefit for a second child or beyond . . . [was] worth less in 2019–20 than when it was (fully) introduced in 1979. . . . Relative to earnings, unemployment support has fallen to a record low of 14 per cent, down from 27 per cent at the emergence of the Beveridge system.[128]

In fact, since the 1980s, the value of unemployment benefit in the UK has been reduced by half in comparison with average household spending.[129] This occurred as Conservative governments committed to overall public spending reductions dissolved the link "between the value of social security benefits . . . and measures of other incomes or earnings", which subsequent (including New Labour) governments failed to restore. Such was accompanied by ever more stringent means-testing disqualifications of welfare claimants – as "dozens of rule changes . . . reduced entitlements to social insurance benefits for the unemployed". As a consequence, instead of "cash benefits rising with national prosperity at times of economic growth, they are . . . generally increased each year in line with price inflation", so that the value of income support benefits has been dwindling in relation to average earnings from employment ever since.[130]

The situation faced by large numbers of the elderly has not been more perspicacious. Pensioner poverty skyrocketed in the UK in the 1980s and early 1990s, under those New Right governments that were pioneering neoliberal policies, so that 45 percent of the elderly were then living below the official poverty line of less than 60 percent of median income.[131] This was owing to the devaluation of the state pension and drastic cutbacks in subsidies to the social housing sector. Pensioner poverty has been on the increase again in the UK in recent years, having been cut back significantly, though by no means curtailed, under 13 years of New Labour rule in the late 1990s and 2000s. This is the result of the deregulation of the private rental market (which has led to spiralling housing costs as landlords cash in) and the acceleration of the process of declining value of welfare benefits under austerity measures since the Great Crash.

> Around 20 percent of pensioners are now forced to privately rent their homes, and this proportion is increasing thanks to the lack of affordable housing. Sky-high rents mean that the poverty rate for these households is more than 35 percent, nearly double the level for pensioners in general. The freeze on housing benefit has exacerbated the problem.[132]

The proportion of the elderly living in severe poverty, that is, on incomes of less than 40 percent of the median, increased from 0.9 percent to 5 percent, so that this is now five times higher than it was in 1986.[133] This is according to Professor Bernhard Ebbinghaus's research based on data from the Luxembourg Income Survey presented at the August 2019 European Sociological Association conference in Manchester. As Ebbinghaus reported:

> British basic pensions are particularly low, 16% of average earnings, and require a long contribution period. Income-tested or means-tested targeted benefits are needed to supplement basic pensions and to lift them out of severe poverty – every sixth British pensioner receives such additional benefits.[134]

Even though the link between state pensions and average earnings was restored in 2007 (in the context of a rafter of austerity-driven cutbacks to welfare services), after this was scrapped in the 1980s,[135] the massive devaluation of the state pension (as this was tied to prices that rose much slower than incomes) that happened in the intervening period has not since been repaired. The state pension in the UK is currently set at £9,109 per annum.[136] The current median income is £31,461 per annum for full-time workers.[137] Average annual expenditure for a single-person pensioner household is £13,265.[138] This is a meagre amount (£1,020 per month approximately, or £255 per week), since many pensioners are by necessity well acclimatized to austere living. Yet the basic state pension leaves them short of this modest sum to the tune of £4,156 a year. As Ebbinghaus rightly says: "The United Kingdom is a good example of . . . historically [having] failed to combat old-age poverty". The "Beveridge-lite" system in the UK offers "ungenerous basic pensions with means-tested supplements, and this reproduces relatively high severe poverty rates among the elderly".[139]

The problem is likely to become exacerbated or further radicalized by the nature of the private sector pension provisions that successive neoliberal governments have encouraged people to take out to support them in retirement in this context of devaluation of statutory state pension entitlements. Pension companies in the UK invest a higher proportion of their funds in stocks and shares rather than in government bonds. The practice is not of course in the least bit discouraged or limited by governments in the UK for the usual and obvious political and ideological reasons of a doctrinaire nature. This places workers' pension entitlements at the mercy of the vagaries of the financial markets, and this has been during a period where these markets are increasingly unstable, with major downturns, most recently the credit crunch in the context of the Great Financial Crisis, which has eroded the value of investments made by the pension providers on behalf of their clients.

As Darren Philp, Policy Director at the National Association of Pension Funds, describes the matter: "UK funds are broadly in line with the global average but that is disappointing nonetheless". This was attributed by Philp to the "exceptionally weak worldwide economic environment".[140] Consequently, employees in the UK with private workplace insurance saw the size of their pensions decline by an average of 0.1 percent per year between 2001 and 2010. Yet, despite the weakness of finance capital generally, the pension pots of employees in most other countries saw increases over the same period, including in relatively poor countries such as Poland and Chile. Only two other countries saw a fall in the value of private occupational pensions over the same period – the USA and Spain.[141] This was because most providers invested much more in government bonds. By contrast, as Philp cautions, the "UK will struggle to pay for its retirement and the weak returns of recent years make it even more important that we improve these pensions".[142]

There is thus no mystery in the fact that unemployed and retired former wage workers under capitalism generally constitute the poorest and are often very poor. Nor is this surprising that this is especially the case in those countries, such as the UK, that under neoliberal governance are most committed to allowing markets free reign, just as they strive to reign in social-welfare state and public services and subject these to "efficiency gains". This is because surplus populations, being largely "unproductive" from a capitalist point of view, do not warrant the investment of resources. Nor, therefore, do the agencies or sectors of the welfare state that cater for them. For that reason, a particularly attractive focus or target for retrenching public spending has for neoliberal governments such as the UK's been the social security budget: pensions and other income-support benefits. So too is the social care sector since this caters largely for retired workers without sufficient savings (or revenues derived from private occupational pensions) to maintain an independent life in the community. Social care in the UK is thus ever the poor relation in a two-tier healthcare system, subordinate to the NHS in terms of social prestige and funding priority. This naturally translates into a lack of investment in the social care workforce.

This is why workers in the social care sector are amongst the lowest paid and least secure of those in the UK workforce. The other aspect of the neoliberal revolution, as I observed earlier, has been the cultivation of a low-wage economy, especially in the burgeoning services sector. Consequently, just as the phenomenon of out-of-work and post-work poverty has grown in Britain, so too has the phenomenon of working poverty. The number of Britain's working poor has increased rapidly in recent decades.[143] Workers in social care (residential and domiciliary) are, as I discussed in the previous chapter, very much a part of that sector. They are recruited disproportionately from BAME groups (24 percent of social care workers are BAME) and from overseas (18 percent of social care workers are from overseas, with 11 percent from outside the EU, especially from South Asia).[144] Median pay for care work (based on hourly rates) is barely above the statutory wage, with many care workers earning less than the minimum rate.[145] Around 35 percent of all social care workers (335,000) are on zero-hours contracts, with this rising to 58 percent of those working in domiciliary care.[146]

According to a survey carried out by the GMB in 2019, "of the 795,000 carers working in the private sector, more than half (55 per cent) are not entitled to a single day of sick pay a year".[147] Many care workers tend to work "flexible" (i.e. unpredictable) hours, alternating between excess and insufficient hours, based on the needs of care managers. Poor pay, low benefits, and unstable hours translate into a high annual staff turnover rate of 37.6 percent for care workers and 42.3 percent for domiciliary care workers. This also generates high rates of sickness-related absenteeism (6.5 million days lost in 2018, for example) and recruitment shortfalls (with 110,000 posts going unfilled in 2018, for example). These negative trends have radicalized in recent years. The rate of staff turnover has increased by 7.6 percent between 2012/2013 and 2017/2018, whereas the proportion of unfilled vacancies rose by 2.2 percent over the same period.[148]

Again, these were the workers who were to be thrust on to the pandemic frontline. For they were the ones who would shield that part of the public for whom COVID-19 was a deadly disease and who had been left as sitting ducks for infection by the Government's policy of discharging untested hospital patients into social care. If anything, the fact that these workers kept the care homes running under the prohibitively difficult circumstances of the virus's first wave, as this ripped through residential care facilities in the spring of 2020, was perhaps an ever greater accomplishment than that of the NHS frontliners who held together the healthcare system. These workers, as noted earlier, commanded much less status than those on the NHS frontline, and they were generally much worse paid. The risks they took with their own health and the health of family members under conditions where they were at the back of the PPE queue dwarfed the financial and symbolic rewards of keeping the care show on the road. Their achievement was, again, by way of understatement, remarkable. But the potential for these workers to respond to the horrific pressures of the pandemic by walking away in huge numbers was a real one. This was a risk made by neoliberal austerity and by capitalist disdain for those who cater for the "surplus" populations.

13 February 2021

Notes

1 Friedman, M. (1962). *Capitalism and Freedom*. Chicago: Chicago University Press; Hayek, F.A. (1949). *Individualism and Economic Order*. London: Routledge and Kegan Paul; Hayek, F.A. (1944). *The Road to Serfdom*. London: Routledge and Kegan Paul; Hayek, F.A. (1960). *The Constitution of Liberty*. London: Routledge and Kegan Paul; Seldon, A. (1967). *Taxation and Welfare*. London: Institute of Economic Affairs; Seldon, A. (1981). *Wither the Welfare State*. London: Institute of Economic Affairs.

2 Callinicos, A. (1991). *The Revenge of History: Marxism and the East European Revolutions*. Cambridge: Polity Press, ch. 2.

3 Duménil, G. and Lévy, D. (2004). *Capital Resurgent: Roots of the Neoliberal Revolution*. Cambridge, MA: Harvard University Press; Glyn, A. (2006). *Capitalism Unleashed: Finance, Globalization and Welfare*. Oxford: Oxford University Press; Harman, C. (2008). 'Theorising neoliberalism'. *International Socialism*, 117 (Winter), pp. 87–121; Harvey, D. (2005). *A Brief History of Neoliberalism*. Oxford: Oxford University Press; Klein, N. (2007). *The Shock Doctrine: The Rise of Disaster Capitalism*. London: Allen Lane; Miller, D. and Dinan, W. (2008). *A Century of Spin: How Public Relations Became the Cutting Edge of Corporate Power*. London: Pluto Press; Saad-Filho, A. and Johnston, D. (Eds). (2004). *Neoliberalism: A Critical Reader*. London: Pluto Press.

4 George, V. and Wilding, P. (1983). *Ideology and Social Welfare*, 2nd edition. London: Routledge and Kegan Paul, pp. 26–43.

5 Scott-Samuel, A., Bambra, C., Collins, C., Hunter, D.J., McCartney, G. and Smith, K. (2014). 'The impact of Thatcherism on health and well-being in Britain'. *International Journal of Health Services*, 44 (1), pp. 53–71 (p. 53).

6 HM Treasury (1979). *The Government's Expenditure Plans 1980–81*. Command (White) Paper, no. 7746. London: HMSO, p. 1.

7 Hills, J. (1998). *Thatcherism, New Labour and the Welfare State*. Case Paper No. 13. London: LSE, Centre for Analysis of Social Exclusion, p. 1.

8 For "efficiency" and "accountability" gains that were illusory. See Centre for Public Impact (2016). *Privatising the UK's Nationalised Industries in the 1980s*. Available at: www.centreforpublicimpact.org/case-study/privatisation-uk-companies-1970s/; Hart, P.E. (1996). 'Accounting for the economic growth of firms in UK manufacturing since 1973'. *Cambridge Journal of Economics*, 20 (2), pp. 225–42; Hall, D. (2014). *Public and Private Sector Efficiency*. PSIRU. Available at: www.psiru.org/sites/default/files/2014-07-EWGHT-efficiency.pdf; Letza, S.R., Smallman, C. and Sun, X. (2004). 'Reframing privatisation: deconstructing the myth of efficiency'. *Policy Sciences*, 37 (2), pp. 159–83; Seymour, S. (2012). 'A short history of privatisation in the UK, 1979–2012'. *Guardian*. (29 March).

9 The goal of the New Right in office to reduce public spending overall as a proportion of total GDP was accomplished. This was reduced from 49.6 percent in 1975/1976 to 39.6 percent in 1996/1997, placing the UK in 22nd place among the 28 OECD countries for public spending. See Chote, R., Crawford, C., Emmerson, C. and Tetlow, G. (2010). *Public Spending Under New Labour*. Institute for Financial Studies, Nuffield Foundation, p. 2. Available at: www.ifs.org.uk/bns/bn92.pdf).

10 Dearlove, D. and Saunders, P. (2000). *Introduction to British Politics: Analysing a Capitalist Democracy*, 2nd edition. Cambridge: Polity Press, pp. 585–86.

11 Renton, D. (2012). 'Housing – as it is, and as it might be'. *International Socialism*, 134 (Spring), pp. 127–31.

12 Hills (1998), p. 8.
13 Dearlove and Saunders (2000), pp. 586–88; Hills (1998), pp. 8–9.
14 Jessop, B. (2002). *From Thatcherism to New Labour: Neoliberalism, Workfarism, and Labour Market Regulation*. Lancaster University, Department of Sociology, p. 7. Available at: www.lancaster.ac.uk/fass/resources/sociology-online-papers/papers/jessop-from-thatcherism-to-new-labour.pdf.
15 Jessop (2002), p. 8.
16 Jessop (2002), p. 6; Buchanan, J., Froud, J., Johal, S., Leaver, A. and Williams, K. (2009). *Undisclosed and Unsustainable: The Problems of the UK National Business Model*. CRESC Working Paper, 75, pp. 1–21.
17 Alberton, K. and Stepney, P. (2020). '1979 and all that: a 40-year reassessment of Margaret Thatcher's legacy on her own terms'. *Cambridge Journal of Economics*, 44, pp. 319–42. For a forensic exploration of the systematic damage marketization has inflicted on the NHS, see: Pollock, A.M. (2005). *NHS plc: The Privatisation of Our Health Care*. London: Verso.
18 Ball, S.J. (2012). *Global Education Inc.: New Policy Networks and the Neoliberal Imaginary*. London: Routledge; Grant, N. (2002). 'Bottom of the class: labour's crude currency of success in education is the market'. *Socialist Review*, 266 (September), pp. 22–23; Hill, D. (1999). *New Labour and Education: Policy, Ideology and the Third Way*. London: Tufnell Press; Hatcher, R. (1999). 'Profiting from schools: business and education action zones'. *Education and Social Justice*, 1 (1), pp. 9–16; Rikowski, G. (2001). 'New labour and the business take-over of education'. *Socialist Future*, 9 (4), pp. 14–17.
19 Dorey, P. (2015). 'The legacy of thatcherism: public sector reform'. *Observatoire De La Société*, 17, pp. 33–60; Mazzucato, M. (2013). *The Entrepreneurial State: Debunking Public vs. Private Sector Myths*. London: Anthem Press.
20 Campbell, D. (2019). 'NHS hospital trusts to pay out further £55bn under PFI scheme'. *Guardian*. (12 September); El-Gingihy, Y. (2018). 'The great PFI heist: the real story of how Britain's economy has been left high and dry by a doomed economic philosophy'. *Independent*. (16 February); Evans, L. (2010). 'The Data Blog Guide to PFI'. *Guardian*. (19 November); Monbiot, G. (2007). 'This great free-market experiment is more like a corporate welfare scheme'. *Guardian*. (4 September); Triggle, N. (2010). 'Fears over £65 billion "NHS mortgage"'. *BBC News*. (13 August).
21 Jessop (2002), p. 6.
22 Spending on the NHS and education increased by an average of 5.7 percent and 3.9 percent per annum from 1997 until 2009 under New Labour compared to 3.2 percent and 1.5 percent under the Conservatives from 1979 until 1997. Spending on social security under New Labour declined from 13.1 percent of total public spending in 1996/1997 to 11.1 percent in 2007/2008. Chote et al. (2010).
23 Jessop (2002), p. 2.
24 Panitch, L. and Leys, C. (1997). *The End of Parliamentary Socialism: From New Left to New Labour*. London: Verso, pp. 251–52.
25 Public spending as a proportion of GDP stood at 41.1 percent when New Labour was first elected to office in 1997 (Hills, 1998, p. 24). It then fell to just 36.3 percent in 1999/2000 owing to radicalization of austerity policies, the lowest level it had been since 1958. After that, however, it increased to 47.9 percent of GDP by 2009/2010. Chote et al. (2010).
26 Hills (1998), pp. 21–24.
27 Somers, A. (2013). *The Emergence of Social Enterprise Policy in New Labour's Second Term*. Goldsmiths College, University of London. Available at: https://research.gold.ac.uk/id/eprint/8051/1/POL_thesis_Somers_2013.pdf
28 As Blair put it: "Competition is the sharpest spur to improve productivity and the best guarantee of reward for talent and innovation. A dynamic economy needs flexible, open markets . . . The Government must promote competition, stimulating enterprise, flexibility and innovation by opening markets" (Department of Trade and Industry (1998).

Our Competitive Edge: Building the Knowledge-Driven Economy (White Paper). London: DTI, p. 5, 8).

29 Under the New Right, the proportion of cash benefits going to the poorest fifth of households declined from "42 to 30 per cent of all benefit spending between 1979 and 1994/95" (Hills, 1998, p. 12).

30 Lister, R. (1998). 'From equality to social inclusion: new labour and the welfare state'. *Critical Social Policy*, 18 (55), pp. 215–25.

31 Bosanquet, N. (1983). *After the New Right*. London: Heinemann.

32 This meant that social policy must change to ensure that welfare would be, in Blair's words, "a hand-up not a hand-out . . . We have a responsibility to provide young people with life chances. They have a responsibility to take them". See: White, M. (1999). 'PM's 20-year target to end poverty'. *Guardian*. (19 March). Liberal-left rhetoric aside, this was an identical approach to tackling social exclusion to that pioneered by the New Right. See: Dolowitz. D.P. (1997). 'Reflections on the UK workfare system'. *Review of Policy Issues*, 3 (1), pp. 3–15. This was "hard workfare". New Labour's welfare-to-work policies, like those of the Conservatives, were not only tougher than those then running on the continent, but they were even tougher than those that were running in the USA (Jessop, (2002), p. 11, 12).

33 O'Connor, J. (1973). *The Fiscal Crisis of the State*. New York: St Martin's Press.

34 Aldred, J. (2019). ' "Socialism for the rich": the evils of bad economics'. *Guardian*. (6 June); Chapman, B. (2019). 'Corporation tax cut to cost UK public finances £6.2bn per year, HMRC finds.' *Independent*. (29 January); Clark, T. and Dilnot, A. (2002). *Long Term Trends in British Taxation and Spending*. Briefing note no. 25. Institute for Fiscal Studies. Available at: https://election2017.ifs.org.uk/bns/bn25.pdf.

35 Brown, W. (2011). 'Industrial relations in Britain under new labour 1997–2018: a post mortem'. *Journal of Industrial Relations*, 53 (3), pp. 402–13.

36 Statista (2020). *Average Hourly Earnings in the United Kingdom (UK) From 1995 to 2019, by Trade Union Membership Status*. Available at: www.statista.com/statistics/287260/hourly-earnings-united-kingdom-uk-by-union-membership-status/); Statista (2020). *Median Hourly Earnings for Full-Time Employees in the United Kingdom From 1997 to 2020*. Statista (online). Available at: www.statista.com/statistics/280687/full-time-hourly-wage-uk/.

37 Bauman, Z. (1997). *Postmodernity and Its Discontents*. Cambridge: Polity Press. (Ch.3: strangers of the consumer era); Bauman, Z. (2005). *Work, Consumerism and the New Poor*. Maidenhead: Open University Press; Marotta, V. (2000). 'The Stranger and Social Theory'. *Thesis Eleven*, 62 (August), pp. 121–34.

38 National Audit Office (2011). *The Financial Stability Interventions*. HM Treasury: The Comptroller and Auditor General's Report on Accounts to the House of Commons. Available at: www.nao.org.uk/wp-content/uploads/2011/07/HMT_account_2010_2011.pdf

39 Grossman, E. and Woll, C. (2013). 'Saving the banks: the political economy of bailouts'. *Comparative Political Studies*, 47 (4), pp. 574–600.

40 Curtis, P. (2011). 'Reality check: how much did the banking crisis cost taxpayers'? *Guardian*.

41 Grossman and Woll (2013).

42 Grossman and Woll (2013).

43 Brenner, R. (2006). *The Economics of Global Turbulence*. London: Verso.

44 The Great Crash chalked approximately $2 trillion off global GDP, or four percent of world output, between March 2008 and March 2009. See: Merle, R. (2018). 'A guide to the financial crisis – 10 years later'. *Washington Post*. (10 September).

45 UK Public Spending (2020a). *UK National Debt as Pct GDP*. Available at: www.ukpublicspending.co.uk/spending_chart_1950_2020UKp_17c1li011lcn_G0t_UK_National_Debt_As_Pct_GDP. UK government debt finally fell, by 3.59 percent, as a proportion of GDP, between 2017 and 2020.

46 The average size of the UK budget deficit since World War 2 has been roughly 2.8 percent of GDP. See Office of Budgetary Responsibility (2020). *Fiscal Sustainability Report*. (July). Available at: https://obr.uk/coronavirus-analysis/. By 2017, however, the budget deficit was reduced to 0.85 percent of GDP, and by the end of 2019, it was replaced with a budget surplus of £1.9 billion. See: UK Public Spending (2020b). *Recent UK Current Budget Deficits*. Available at: www.ukpublicspending.co.uk/uk_national_deficit_analysis

47 Francis-Devine, B. and Ferguson, D. (2020). *Public Sector Pay: Research Briefing*. UK Parliament: House of Commons Library. (2 December). Available at: https://commonslibrary.parliament.uk/research-briefings/cbp-8037/.

48 FRED (2020). *Central Government Debt, Total (% of GDP)*. Economic Research: Federal Reserve Bank of St Louis. Available at: https://fred.stlouisfed.org/tags/series?t=debt%3Bgdp%3Bworld+bank.

49 UKPS (2020a).

50 Clarke, D. (2020). *GDP Growth in the UK 1949–2019*. Statista (online). (November 12 2020). Available at: www.statista.com/statistics/281734/gdp-growth-in-the-united-kingdom-uk/.

51 Clarke (2020a). GDP annual growth in the 1950s averaged 3.18 percent whereas in the 1960s it averaged 3.44 percent. Thereafter, it has slowed considerably. In the 1980s annual average GDP growth was 2.66 percent. In the 1990s it was 2.33 percent. In the decade from 2000 to 2009 it was just 1.77 percent. From 2010 through to 2019 it was just 1.83 percent.

52 Scheiber, G.J. and Poullier, J-P. (1989). 'Overview of international comparisons of health care expenditures'. *Medicare and Medicaid Research Review*, (Supplement), pp. 1–7.

53 Huber, M. and Orosz, E. (2003). 'Health expenditure trends in OECD countries, 1990–2001'. *Health Care Financial Review*, 25 (1), pp. 1–22.

54 OECD (2020). *Health Expenditure and Financing*. (21 December). Available at: https://stats.oecd.org/Index.aspx?DataSetCode=SHA; World Bank (2020). *Current Health Expenditure (% of GDP)*. Available at: https://data.worldbank.org/indicator/SH.XPD.CHEX.GD.ZS.

55 Elvidge, S. (2016). 'UK government to tackle high drug prices'. *Pharmaceutical Journal* (online). (20 September). Available at: www.pharmaceutical-journal.com/news-and-analysis/news/uk-government-to-tackle-high-drug-prices/20201736.article; Ewbank, L., Omojomolo, D., Kane, S. and McKenna, H. (2018). *The Rising Costs of Medicines to the NHS*. The King's Fund (online). Available at: www.kingsfund.org.uk/sites/default/files/2018-04/Rising-cost-of-medicines.pdf?platform=hootsuite; Wickware, C. (2020). 'Generic drug price increases of up to 1,700% have cost the NHS £76m in 2 years'. *The Pharmaceutical Journal* (online). (27 November). Available at: www.pharmaceutical-journal.com/news-and-analysis/news/generic-drug-price-increases-of-up-to-1700-have-cost-the-nhs-76m/20208510.article?firstPass=false.

56 Anderson, R. (2014). 'Pharmaceutical industry gets high on fat profits'. *BBC News*. (6 November); Ledley, F., McKoy, S., Vaughan, G. and Cleary, E. (2020). 'Profitability of large pharmaceutical companies compared with other large public companies'. *Journal of the American Medical Association*, 323 (9), pp. 834–35; Mikulic, M. (2020). *Global Pharmaceutical Industry – Statistics and Facts*. Statista (online). (5 November). Available at: www.statista.com/topics/1764/global-pharmaceutical-industry/

57 Wickware (2020).

58 Meller, A. and Ahmed, H. (2019). *How Big Pharma Reaps Profits While Hurting Everyday Americans*. Center for American Progress (online). (30 August). Available at: www.americanprogress.org/issues/democracy/reports/2019/08/30/473911/big-pharma-reaps-profits-hurting-everyday-americans/; Minemyer, P. (2020). 'Here's how much faster drugs prices are rising compared to other healthcare services'. *Fierce Healthcare* (online). (17 September). Available at: www.fiercehealthcare.com/payer/here-s-how-much-faster-drug-prices-are-rising-compared-to-other-healthcare-services; Peter G. Petterson Foundation (2018). *How Will the Rising Cost of Prescription Drugs Affect Medicare?* Available at: www.kingsfund.org.uk/sites/default/files/2018-04/

Rising-cost-of-medicines.pdf?platform=hootsuite; Pew Charitable Trusts (2018). 'A look at drug spending in the United States: estimates and projections from various stakeholders'. *Factsheet* (online). Available at: www.pewtrusts.org/en/research-and-analysis/factsheets/2018/02/a-look-at-drug-spending-in-the-us; Rice, W., Clemente and Kitson, K. (2018). *Bad Medicine: How GOP Tax Cuts Are Enriching Drug Companies, Leaving Workers and Patients Behind*. Americans for Tax Fairness (online). Available at: https://americansfortaxfairness.org/wp-content/uploads/Pharma-Tax-Cut-Report-4.26.18-FINAL-.pdf.

59 McFarlane, L. (2018). 'Why is the NHS in crisis'? *Open Democracy* (online). (4 January). Available at: https://neweconomics.opendemocracy.net/why-is-the-nhs-in-crisis/; NHS Support Federation (2019). *Fund Our NHS: Is the NHS Under-Funded?* Available at: https://nhsfunding.info/underfunded/is-the-nhs-underfunded/.

60 Triggle, N. (2018). '10 charts that show why the NHS is in trouble'. *BBC News.* (24 May).

61 Dearlove and Saunders (2000), p. 588.

62 Triggle (2018).

63 McFarlane (2018).

64 Papanicolas, I., Mosialos, E., Abel-Smith, B., Gunderson, A., Woskie, L., Kjha, A. and Li, K.T. (2019). 'Performance of UK National Health Service compared with other high income countries: observational study'. *British Medical Journal* (online). (27 November). Available at: www.bmj.com/content/367/bmj.l6326.

65 NHS Support Federation (2019).

66 Triggle, N. and Butcher, B. (2019). '11 charts on the problems facing the NHS'. *BBC News.* (9 January); The Health Foundation (2019). *Health Spending as a Share of GDP Remains at Lowest Level in a Decade.* (30 July). Available at: https://www.health.org.uk/news-and-comment/charts-and-infographics/health-spending-as-a-share-of-gdp-remains-at-lowest-level-in#:~:text=However%2C%20over%20the%20last%20decade,7.6%25%20in%202009%2F10.

67 Papanicolas et al. (2019).

68 Nuffield Trust, Health Foundations, King's Fund (2017). *The Autumn Budget: Joint Statement on Health and Social Care.* (November). Available at: www.kingsfund.org.uk/sites/default/files/2017-11/The%20Autumn%20Budget%20-%20joint%20statement%20on%20health%20and%20social%20care%2C%20Nov%202017.pdf.

69 Triggle, N. (2018). 'NHS funding: Theresa May unveils £20bn boost'. *BBC News.* (17 June).

70 Charlesworth, A., Gershlick, B., Firth, Z., Kraindler, J. and Watt, T. (2019). *Investing in the NHS Long Term Plan.* Health Foundation (online). (June). Available at: https://reader.health.org.uk/investing-in-the-NHS-long-term-plan.

71 The King's Fund (2020). *NHS Funding: Our Position.* (22 October). Available at: www.kingsfund.org.uk/projects/positions/nhs-funding?gclid=EAIaIQobChMIpsK74pXi7QIVDrrtCh0eJwcqEAAYAiAAEgLnJfD_BwE.

72 NHS Support Federation (2019).

73 McFarlane (2018). See also: King's Fund (2019). *Key Facts and Figures About the NHS.* (8 November). Available at: www.kingsfund.org.uk/audio-video/key-facts-figures-nhs.

74 NHS Support Federation (2019).

75 Anandaciva, S. (2020). *Financial Debts and Loans in the NHS.* King's Fund (online). (2 July). Available at: www.kingsfund.org.uk/publications/financial-debts-and-loans-nhs#nhs-debt.

76 Street, R. (2017). 'Haemorrhaging cash: assessing the long-term costs of PFI hospitals'. *Journal of Construction Research and Innovation,* 8 (4), pp. 113–16.

77 NHS Support Federation (2019).

78 Papanicolas et al. (2019).

79 Titheradge, N. (2020). Coronavirus: imaging equipment "woefully underfunded"'. *BBC News.* (16 May).

80 Campbell, D. (2018). 'Shock figures from top thinktank reveal extent of NHS crisis'. *Guardian.* (5 May). Based on OECD data presented by the King's Fund.

81 Ewbank, L., Thompson, J., McKenna, H. and Anandaciva, S. (2020). *NHS Hospital Bed Numbers: Past, Present, Future*. King's Fund (online). (26 March). Available at: www.kingsfund.org.uk/publications/nhs-hospital-bed-numbers

82 Matthews-King, A. (2019). 'NHS hospitals forced to use emergency beds all year round to cope with demand, BMA warns'. *Independent*. (21 June).

83 McCarthy, N. (2020). 'The countries with the most critical care beds per capita'. *Forbes Magazine* (online). (12 March). Available at: www.forbes.com/sites/niallmccarthy/2020/03/12/the-countries-with-the-most-critical-care-beds-per-capita-infographic/?sh=426a48727f86

84 WHO (2020). *Acute Care Hospital Beds per 100,000*. Available at: https://gateway.euro.who.int/en/indicators/hfa_478-5060-acute-care-hospital-beds-per-100-000/

85 Morris, P. (2018). *NHS Hot Topics – NHS Bed Shortage*. MSAG (online). (14 December). Available at: https://themsag.com/blogs/nhs-hot-topics/nhs-hot-topics-nhs-bed-shortage.

86 Triggle and Butcher (2019).

87 King's Fund (2020). 'What's going on with A&E waiting times'? (25 March). Available at: www.kingsfund.org.uk/projects/urgent-emergency-care/urgent-and-emergency-care-mythbusters?gclid=EAIaIQobChMIhfOazdjo7QIVmKztCh1huQRFEAAYAiAAEgIvX_D_BwE

88 King's Fund (25 March, 2020).

89 King's Fund (25 March, 2020).

90 Campbell, D. (2015). 'A&E faces worst winter ever, top doctor warns'. *Guardian*. (31 October); Campbell, D. (2016). 'NHS hospitals facing toughest winter yet, say health experts'. *Guardian*. (21 December); Matthews-King, A. (2018a). 'NHS winter crisis officially worst on record and patients still suffering, final figures show'. *Independent*. (16 March); Campbell, D. (2018). 'Hospitals in race to combat "toughest ever" winter crisis for NHS'. *Guardian*. (8 December).

91 Matthews-King (2018a).

92 Matthews-King, A. (2018b). 'Government told to "urgently investigate 10,000 additional deaths" in the first weeks of 2018'. *Independent*. (15 March).

93 Papanicolas et al. (2019).

94 Campbell (5 May, 2018).

95 Buchan, J., Charlesworth, A., Gershlick, B. and Seccombe, I. (2019). *A Critical Moment: NHS Staffing Trends, Retention and Attrition*. Health Foundation (online). (February). Available at: www.health.org.uk/sites/default/files/upload/publications/2019/A%20Critical%20Moment_1.pdf; Royal College of Midwives (2019). *Senior Midwives Without Enough Staff to Meet Demand on Services Says New Survey*. Available at: www.rcm.org.uk/media-releases/2019/march/senior-midwives-without-enough-staff-to-meet-demands-on-services-says-new-survey/

96 Buchan et al. (2019), p. 2.

97 King's Fund (2020). *NHS Workforce: Our Position*. (26 October). Available at: www.kingsfund.org.uk/projects/positions/nhs-workforce

98 Lay, K. (2018). 'Medical school numbers must double to combat NHS doctor shortage'. *Times*. (25 June). This is a report on a study conducted by the Royal College of Physicians.

99 Buchan et al. (2019); Health Foundation, King's Fund and Nuffield Trust (2019). *Closing the Gap: Key Areas for Action on the Health and Care Workforce*. (March). Available at: www.kingsfund.org.uk/sites/default/files/2019-03/closing-the-gap-health-care-workforce-overview_0.pdf

100 The Open University (2018). *Tackling the Nursing Shortage*. (April), p. 8. Available at: https://cdn.ps.emap.com/wp-content/uploads/sites/3/2018/05/The_Open_University_Tackling_the_nursing_shortage_Report_2018.pdf.

101 HF, KF, NT (2019), p. 9.

102 HF, KF, NT (2019), p. 10.

103 Ford, S. (2018). 'NHS nurse pay set to rise by 6.5% over three years under new deal'. *Nursing Times* (online). (21 March). Available at: www.nursingtimes.net/news/workforce/nhs-nurse-pay-set-to-rise-by-6-5-over-three-years-under-new-deal-21-03-2018/.

104 BMA (2020). *Memorandum of Evidence to the Review Body on Doctors' and Dentists' Remuneration.* BMA (online). (January), p. 13. Available at: www.bma.org.uk/media/2123/bma-ddrb-submission-2020.pdf.

105 HF, KF, NT (2019), p. 13.

106 UNISON (2014). *UNISON Survey Shows That NHS Workers Are Overworked and Underpaid.* (22 November). Available at: www.unison.org.uk/news/article/2014/11/unison-survey-shows-nhs-staff-are-overworked-and-underpaid/. The sample size was 18,000 and 40 percent of respondents were nurses.

107 OU (2018), p. 10, 11.

108 BMA (2021). *How NHS Doctors' Pay Is Decided.* (8 July). Available at: www.bma.org.uk/pay-and-contracts/pay/how-doctors-pay-is-decided/how-nhs-doctors-pay-is-decided.

109 Ginsburg, N. (1979). *Class, Capital and Social Policy.* Basingstoke: Palgrave; Gough, I. (1979). *The Political Economy of the Welfare State.* Houndmills: Macmillan; Gough, I. (2000). *Global Capital, Human Needs and Social Policies.* Basingstoke: Palgrave; Standing, G. (2002). *Beyond the New Paternalism: Basic Security as Equality.* London: Verso.

110 Bowles, H. and Gintis, S. (1976). *Schooling in Capitalist America: Educational Reform and the Contradictions of Economic Life.* New York: Routledge and Kegan Paul; Cole, M., Hill, D., McLaren, P. and Rikowski, G. (2001). *Red Chalk: On Schooling, Capitalism and Politics.* Brighton: Institute for Education Policy Studies.

111 New Labour sought to repair the Tories relative neglect of education (which was not exempted from the general funding squeezes of the New Right years) because it was committed to a vision of a "knowledge-based" economy that would secure the international competitiveness of British capitalism. DTI (1998). See Callinicos, A. (2006). *Universities in a Neoliberal World.* London: Bookmarks.

112 Grubb, W.N. and Lazerson, M. (2006). 'The globalisation of rhetoric and practice: the education gospel and vocationalism'. H. Lauder, P. Brown, J. Dillabaugh and A.H. Halsey (Eds). *Education, Globalization, and Social Change.* Oxford: Oxford University Press.

113 Tomlinson, S. (2005). *Education in a Post-Welfare Society*, 2nd edition. Maidenhead: Open University Press, p. 216.

114 Doyal, L. (1979). *The Political Economy of Health.* London: Pluto Press.

115 Even though spending on healthcare did not increase significantly as a proportion of GDP under Conservative rule from 1979 until 1997, so in that sense it was retrenched, it did increase in real terms, by an average annual rate of 3.1 percent, which was marginally higher than the level needed (2.2 percent) to merely preserve the NHS at the same level. See Dearlove and Saunders (2000), p. 588.

116 Marx, K. (1967). *Capital: A Critique of Political Economy*, vol. 1. [1867]. Harmondsworth: Penguin, ch. 25; Marx, K. 'Wages'. K. Marx and F. Engels (Eds). *Collected Works*, vol. 6. London: Lawrence and Wishart.

117 Consequently, the vulnerability of elements of the working-age "surplus population" to turn to crime to make ends meet or to delinquency as an expression of social estrangement or to rioting as acts of protest. Spitzer refers to this part of the surplus population as "social dynamite". See: Spitzer, S. (1975). 'Towards a Marxian theory of deviance'. *Social Problems*, 22 (5), pp. 638–51. This part of the surplus population may be pacified either by welfare safety nets or by state repression (law and order politics, get tough criminal justice, and carceral expansion), or by a combination of both. Typically, in recent decades, neoliberal states, such as those in the UK and the USA, have placed growing emphasis and investment on repressive rather than welfarist controls, as has been evidenced by swelling correctional populations in both countries, just as crime rates have fallen. See Wacquant, L. (2009). *Punishing the Poor: The Neoliberal*

Government of Social Insecurity. Durham, NC: Duke University Press; Chambliss, W. (1994). 'Policing the ghetto underclass'. *Social Problems*, 41 (2), pp. 177–94); Parenti, C. (2000). *Lockdown America: Police and Prisons in an Age of Crisis.* London: Pluto Press.

118 See Murray. C. (1990). *The Emerging British Underclass.* London: Institute of Economic Affairs. This promulgated a moral underclass discourse as explanation of unemployment. For a debunking of the notion of a culture of welfare dependency, see Taylor-Gooby, P. (1992). *Dependency Culture: The Explosion of a Myth.* London: Routledge.

119 Albertson, K. and Stepney, P. (2020). '1979 and all that: a 40-year reassessment of Margaret Thatcher's legacy on her own terms'. *Cambridge Journal of Economics*, 44 (2), pp. 319–42; Jessop, B. (2005). *From Thatcherism to New Labour: Neoliberalism, Workfarism, and Labour Market Regulation.* Department of Sociology, Lancaster University. Available at: https://www.lancaster.ac.uk/fass/resources/sociology-online-papers/papers/jessop-from-thatcherism-to-new-labour.pdf.

120 Jessop (2005), p. 12.

121 Age UK (2020). *Later Life in the UK Today 2019.* Age UK Factsheet. Available at: www.ageuk.org.uk/globalassets/age-uk/documents/reports-and-publications/later_life_uk_factsheet.pdf.

122 Joseph Rowntree Foundation (2020a). *UK Poverty 2019–20: The Leading Independent Report.* York: JRF, p. 12; Joseph Rowntree Foundation (2020b). *UK Poverty 2019/20: Summary.* York: JRF.

123 O'Leary, J. (2019). 'Poverty in the UK: a guide to the facts and figures.' *Full Fact* (online). Available at: https://fullfact.org/economy/poverty-uk-guide-facts-and-figures/

124 Joseph Rowntree Foundation (2019). *Working Age Poverty.* Available at: www.jrf.org.uk/data/working-age-poverty

125 Wintour, P. (2014). 'George Osborne aims at tax credits and benefits in new squeeze on working poor'. *Guardian.* (30 September); Elliott, L. (2015). 'Fresh spending freeze has already begun, says George Osborne'. *Guardian.* (20 May).

126 *BBC News* (2012). 'Benefits squeeze to save £3.7bn in 2015–16, Osborne says'. (5 December); Booth, J. and Lucero, M. (2012). 'How it unfolded: Osborne raids benefits and pensions to plug deficit'. *Sunday Times.* (5 December).

127 Resolution Foundation (2019a). *The Benefit Freeze has Ended, but Erosion of the Social Security Safety Net Continues.* (16 October). Available at: www.resolutionfoundation.org/publications/the-benefit-freeze-has-ended-but-erosion-of-the-social-security-safety-net-continues/. This motivated the publication of a range of social policy texts in the 1970s, 1980s, and 1990s diagnosing the crisis of the welfare state and its retrenchment. For example: Mishra, R. (1984). *The Welfare State in Crisis: Social Thought and Social Change.* Brighton: Harvester Wheatsheaf; Mishra, M. (1991). *Welfare State in Capitalist Society: Policies of Retrenchment and Maintenance in Europe, North America and Australia.* London: Harvester Press; Offe, C. (1984). *Contradictions of the Welfare State.* London: Hutchinson; Ginsburg, N. (1992). *Divisions of Welfare: A Critical Introduction to Comparative Social Policy.* Thousand Oaks: Sage; Gough, I. and Therborn, G. (1991). *Can the Welfare State Compete? A Comparative Analysis of Five Advanced Capitalist Countries.* London: Macmillan.

128 Resolution Foundation (2019b). *The Generation of Poverty: Poverty Over the Life Course for Different Generations.* Available at: www.resolutionfoundation.org/publications/the-generation-of-poverty-poverty-over-the-life-course-for-different-generations/.

129 Atkinson, A.B. (2015). *Inequality.* Cambridge, MA: Harvard University Press.

130 Hills (1998), p. 4.

131 Resolution Foundation (2019b).

132 Scripps, T. (2019). 'UK pensioners suffer massive increase in poverty'. *World Socialist Web Site* (SSWS). Available at: www.wsws.org/en/articles/2019/09/06/pens-s06.html

133 Ebbinghaus, B. (2019). *Pension Reforms and Old Age Inequalities in Europe: From Old to New Social Risks.* European Sociological Association. Manchester Conference,

2019. Available at: www.researchgate.net/publication/335228524_Pension_reforms_and_old_age_inequalities_in_Europe_From_old_to_new_social_risks

134 Doward, J. (2019). 'UK elderly suffer worst poverty rate in western Europe'. *Guardian*. (18 August).

135 Teather, D. (2007). 'George Osborne restores pension link to earnings'. *Guardian*. (22 June).

136 Pension Wise (2020). *What Will My Total Income in Retirement Be?* GOV.UK (online). Available at: www.pensionwise.gov.uk/en/work-out-income

137 ONS (2020). *Employee Earnings in the UK: 2020*. GOV.UK (online). Available at: www.ons.gov.uk/employmentandlabourmarket/peopleinwork/earningsandworkinghours/bulletins/annualsurveyofhoursandearnings/2020

138 Ebbinghaus (2019).

139 Ebbinghaus (2019), p. 12.

140 Philp cited in Hall, J. (2017). *UK Pension Performance Among Worst in the Developed World*. Intelligent Partnership (online). Available at: https://intelligent-partnership.com/uk-pension-performance-among-worst-in-developed-world/. Accessed: 23/06/21.

141 OECD report on private pensions cited in Hall (2017).

142 Philp cited in Hall (2017).

143 See JRF (2020a); O'Leary, J. (2017). 'Are most Working Age People in Poverty also in Work'? *Full Fact* (online). (19 July). Available at: https://fullfact.org/economy/are-most-working-age-people-poverty-also-work/; Partington, J. (2018). 'Four Million British Workers Live in Poverty, Charity Says'. *Guardian*. (4 December).

144 Griffiths, D., Fenton, W., Polzin, G., Price, R., Arkesden, J. and McCaffrey, R. (2018). *The State of the Adult Social Care Sector and Workforce in England*. Leeds: Workforce Intelligence, Skills For Care, pp. 61–63.

145 Griffiths et al. (2018), p. 69.

146 Griffiths et al. (2018), pp. 31–32.

147 Chakelian, A., Grylss, G. and Calcia, N. (2020). 'How the UK's care homes were abandoned to coronavirus'. *New Statesman*. (24 April).

148 Griffiths et al. (2018), p. 34.

4

PREMATURE UNLOCKINGS
AND THE LATER LOCKDOWNS

Barely more than one-and-half calendar months after the start of the March 2020 lockdown, and with the first wave of the virus having only just began to recede from its mid-April peak, the PM announced plans (on Sunday, 10 May) to start unlocking the restrictions and reopening the economy.[1] From this point, it was clear that the more gung-ho MPs had the PM's ear over those urging caution, so that rapid easing of physical distancing rules (in comparison with other European countries such as Italy, Germany, Spain, and France) was exactly the course that the Government was set on. The plan for moving the UK back to normality (elaborated further by Johnson in parliament on 11 May and in the Government's *Our Plan to Rebuild* roadmap document released on the same day)[2] could not be described as cautious. Far from it. This was fast-track in its ambitions.

The unlocking of restrictions (under "Phase 1") was for immediate implementation. The first restrictions were relaxed the day after the PM's 10 May address to the nation. Others would be eased by mid-week. "Phase 2" would begin as soon as 1 June, barely three weeks later. "Phase 3" would, all going well (i.e. if the "data" allowed), be rolled-out bit by bit starting on 4 July. Phase 2 (starting 1 June) included the goal of a staggered re-opening schools – starting with Reception Year, Year 1 and Year 6 students. Phase 2 also planned for the re-opening of non-essential shops. Phase 3 (starting 4 July) appeared to entail the rapid albeit phased scaling down of all remaining lockdown measures, so that virtual normality would be restored within three months, by the start of August.[3]

The Phase 1 roll-out included a number of expectations/permissions. Starting from 13 May, people who cannot work at home should return to work so long as it was "safe" to do so, just as employers were required to ensure that workplaces were safe. Indeed, employees were to be "actively encouraged" to return to their workplaces, just as employers should actively encourage them to do so.[4] This applied to all employees who could not work at home, not those of particular branches

DOI: 10.4324/9781003275039-5

or sectors of industry, so as much to non-essential as to essential workers.[5] Yet the Government drafted its new rules for reopening workplaces only in the week prior to the lockdown being relaxed. This hardly provided employers with sufficient notice to plan for changes, let alone introduce them.

The guidance stated that

> businesses and workplaces should make every possible effort to enable working from home as a first option. Where working from home is not possible, workplaces should make every effort to comply with the social distancing guidelines set out by the Government.

Under these circumstances, "workplaces should keep employees socially distanced – and so two metres apart – from each other *wherever possible*". But "where this isn't possible, other measures should be taken to minimise risk", which may include "curtailing hot desking, keeping staff canteens closed and limiting the number of workers allowed in lifts at any one time". Employers should consider "finding more car parking and bike spaces and to provide changing rooms so staff can change clothes for work". Employees should opt for walking or cycling to work or for using a private car rather than public transport.[6]

Again, just like the general physical distancing guidance that led up to and accompanied the lockdown, none of this appeared terribly prescriptive or directive. Discretion for what constituted appropriate distancing measures was to be left to employers to determine, including on what was possible to implement and what was not. If physical distancing was not deemed possible, this was no barrier to reopening the workplace. Indeed, if alternative safety measures were considered impractical, nor would this rule out re-openings. As Frances O'Grady, General Secretary of the TUC, rightly pointed out, "this guidance fails to provide clear direction to those employers who want to act responsibly, and is an open goal to the worst of employers who want to return to business as usual".[7] Previously, during the lockdown, government guidance on physical distancing for those employers in workplaces that remained open had raised concerns owing to its permissiveness. This guidance included that where it was not practical for employees to be kept two metres apart employers may instead "permit" (i.e. instruct) them to work "side by side, or facing away from each other, rather than face to face, *if possible*".[8]

Employers, not employees, would determine whether or not workplaces were indeed safe, so workers who declined to return owing to health and safety concerns would not to be entitled to recompense under the furlough scheme – not unless their refusal was "reasonable" As UNISON's guidance puts it, "an employee cannot automatically refuse . . . return to work without a good reason".[9] A good reason would *not* be that workers considered that the general situation of COVID-19 was such that this would pose themselves or their colleagues a significant health and safety risk. A belief that a general return to work was wrong because premature would not be considered reasonable. This was even though the Government instructed only those workers unable to work at home to return, which of course was suggestive that on–site working was indeed considered risky by ministers up to a point. Moreover, since employers were required to ensure workplaces were safe, they too would risk being cut off from the various forms of government pandemic support for business (loans, tax relief, grants, etc.) if they declined to invite or instruct those of their employees who could not home-work to return. Therefore, under Phase 1, systematic economic pressure was being exerted on both employers and employees to acquiesce to a rapid return to work, irrespective of the prepared-ness of employers to implement or enforce physical distancing rules. The risks this posed to public health hardly need stating.

Starting immediately, from 13 May, people were permitted to engage in unlim-ited leisure and exercise in outdoor spaces (excluding in playgrounds or outdoor gyms). Being outdoors for purposes of unlimited recreation became included among the "reasonable excuses" for doing so – and doing that anywhere you wanted. Travel restrictions were ended. People were, as Johnson said, to be encouraged "to take more and even unlimited amounts of outdoor exercise, sit in the sun in your local park, drive to other destinations . . . [and] . . . play sports with members of your own household". They were also permitted to associate when outdoors with a single person from outside their own household.[10] However, whether or not this "associational other" should be the same person each or any time or may be some-one different was unstated. The fuzziness of the "meet with one person outside your household" rule obviously opened up the option of people associating freely with the full range of others who are part of their kin group or friendship network, albeit not at the same time. But, of particular concern was the lifting of travel restrictions, since placed alongside the general fuzziness of government safety mes-saging, this could easily lead to floods of people heading for the parks and coasts.

Naturally, the greatest concern was over the Government's plan to reopen schools, with parents and teachers voicing their opposition. Survey data indicated that a majority of parents disagreed with this, regarding a 1 June reopening as premature. This plan was also opposed for the same reason by the National Educa-tion Union (NEU) and National Association of Schoolmasters/Union of Women Teachers (NASUWT) teaching unions, by the head-teacher's union National Asso-ciation of Head Teachers (NAHT) and by UNISON – with NEU and UNISON both instructing their members not to engage with it and to abstain from preparing for the 1 June start. BMA publicly stated that it was "completely aligned" with the opposition of teachers, parents and unions. Certain local councils also declared that they would not reopen schools on 1 June.[11]

The opposition to this aspect of Phase 2 planning in particular was wholly sensi-ble. COVID-19 infection numbers were then still high and increasing (albeit more slowly and on a downward rate), whereas the curve of the UK outbreak was much less flattened or depressed than in other countries where lockdown easing had taken place (see later). There were also major regional variations in transmission rates, with some areas still reporting big increases. Children – especially primary-school-age children, who have little comprehension of personal space, would not be vigilant in following physical distancing rules, and enforcing these would be prohibitively difficult for teachers – especially given constraints of room space and number.

The governments of most European countries were at the same time (the spring of 2020) already starting to re-open schools, bit by bit, in a staggered approach. But this was also contrary to scientific advice and the concerns of teachers and parents in their own countries.[12] This showed that the UK government did not, of course, have a monopoly on playing politics (or political economy) with public health. But it was clear that, at the start of the Government's unlocking of controls, the COVID-19 outbreak was much more suppressed on the continent than it was in the UK. Moreover, it was then quite feasible that the UK outlook would not have improved substantially before the start of June. Re-opening schools from the start of June 2020 therefore posed a particularly high risk of triggering the start of another major spike.

This action plan taken as a whole certainly ran a severe risk of being premature and of generating a resurgence of the outbreak. This was made clear enough by the timeframes and numbers. Italy's full lockdown began on 9 March 2020 and was partially lifted on 4 May – hence spanning a total of 56 days.[13] Spain's started on 16 March 2020 and started to be eased on 9 May – hence spanning a total of 54 days. France's was implemented on 17 March 2020 and partially relaxed on 11 May – hence spanning a total of 55 days.[14] Germany's was introduced on 17 March 2020 and partially released on 6 May – hence spanning a total of 50 days.[15] By contrast, the UK did not operationalize its own (incomplete compared to these other countries) lockdown until 24 March 2020 and was already beginning to phase it out from 11 May, 48 days after it was implemented.

Thus, the UK started unlocking its lockdown at an earlier stage than the other leading European countries (and more than a week in advance of the worse-hit ones of Italy, Spain, and France). Even Germany – which fared much better in the first wave than virtually all of the other EU countries – had a longer lockdown than did the UK. This was despite the fact that the UK was, by the end of the first wave's peak in mid-May 2020 the European leader for COVID-19 fatalities, in fourth place internationally for the number of infections, and was less well prepared than any of the leading EU countries for the pandemic. In Germany, in the week prior to the partial unlocking of lockdown, there were 7,095 new recorded cases of COVID-19 infection and 679 deaths from the virus. In France, in the week prior, there were 8,277 new recorded cases and 1,485 deaths. In Spain, there were 17,013 new cases and 1,475 deaths, whereas in Italy the figures were 13,033 and 2,240, respectively. The UK, in stark contrast with these others, recorded 32,538 new cases of COVID-19 infection and 3,409 deaths in the week preceding the partial easing of its own lockdown.[16] This was almost twice as many infections as for second-placed Italy and more than four-and-a-half times more than for last (and best) placed Germany. This was also a rate of infection almost six times higher than for when the UK lockdown was introduced.

The Government's roadmap plan to scale down the March 2020 lockdown was delivered pretty much on schedule. Apparently, the proposed "data-led" unlockings just happened to coincide almost exactly with the planned dates, in sharp contrast to the reverse moves towards lockdown, which trailed the "data". This was unsurprising given that, despite policy supposedly being data-led, the

Government would (said Johnson) be "sticking to the roadmap like glue".[17] Garden centres, outside sports courts and pitches, and recycling plants opened on 13 May. House viewings also were restarted on 13 May.[18] On 31 May – in a particularly gratuitous move – the Government pretty much withdrew the force of sanction from the vestiges of those lockdown rules that applied to the household by dismantling the relevant police powers for dealing with breaches. The police no longer had the "authority to remove people who [were] contravening the requirement to stay overnight in their home from where they are staying". Nor could they "use force to break up a prohibited gathering taking place in private".[19]

On 1 June, outdoor food markets, automobile showrooms, and other outdoor sports amenities were re-opened. On the same day, outdoor gatherings of people from more than one household of up to six people were legalized along with the scrapping of the ban on people leaving home except when necessary (but with overnight stay away from home still prohibited).[20] On 11 June, outdoor public swimming pools and waterparks reopened.[21] One-person households were permitted to associate with another household of any size on 13 June, just as persons from one household were permitted an overnight stay in the house of the other. This was the start of the "support bubble" system. On 13 June as well, people were permitted to visit people in hospital or in hospices or care homes, just as people attending births and medical appointments were permitted to have a companion along.[22]

Two days later, most retail and other public-facing businesses were re-opened (apart from indoor sports and leisure centres, restaurants, pubs, nightclubs, bingo halls, casinos, cinemas, theatres, hairdressers, and libraries) as well as outdoor animal-centred leisure attractions. So too were betting shops and auction premises.[23] Before mid-July 2020, a range of other lifestyle and leisure venues had been re-opened – including tanning booths, beauty salons, tattoo parlours, body piercing centres, health spas, manicure and pedicure services, massage parlours, and so on.[24] By mid-July, Johnson was suggesting that advice to employees should change from "work home if you can" to "go back to work if you can".[25]

On 17 July, the (fairly loose and unenforced) prohibition on people using public transport for non-essential purposes was lifted.[26] The final unlockings were more-or-less rolled out before the start of August – and these included the re-openings of gyms, cinemas, pubs, clubs, restaurants and (on 25 July) indoor public swimming pools and other indoor sports facilities.[27] Starting from 1 August, the Government ditched altogether its work-from-home "if possible" guidance in favour of asking employers, as Johnson put it, "to make decisions about how their staff can work safely".[28] This was just two weeks after Patrick Vallance, the UK's Chief Scientific Officer, briefed the Parliamentary Science and Technology Committee that working from home remained a "perfectly good option" and that "there was absolutely no reason" to advise people any differently.[29]

The only exceptions to the pattern of unlockings were delays in the reopening of schools, casinos and bowling alleys, and in permitting wedding receptions of up to 30 persons. Casinos and bowling alleys due to reopen on 31 July were put back to 15 August. This was also the (deferred by two weeks) date that larger wedding gatherings would be allowed.[30] These interruptions to the unlockings were motivated by an upsurge in caseloads towards the end of July, which were sufficient to elicit a warning from Chris Whitty that "we have probably reached near the limit, or the limits, of what we can do in terms of opening up society".[31] This period coincided with the gestation period of the second wave of the virus. Caseloads had stopped declining by early July. After plateauing for a short while, they began to rise again in July, with the rate of increase quickening through August.[32] By mid-August, the number of new daily infections was higher than that in mid-June.[33] By the end of August, the number of daily new infections was higher than that in mid-May.[34]

Whitty's warning was not heeded. The Government's delays in implementing a narrow range of re-openings were simply tokenistic in the wider context of the great unlocking – and these were in any case momentary pauses. Eat Out to Help Out was launched from the start of August in order to entice people back into the newly reopened restaurants, cafes and bars. The Government forked out £849 million to finance the scheme, which subsidized 160 million meals.[35] August also saw repeated government advertising campaigns to encourage people to shift from homeworking to on-site working on the grounds that it was low risk to do so – with the latest one launched towards the end of the month.[36]

At the same time, Matt Hancock, who by early September 2020 was voicing his "serious concern" over the rising pandemic caseload (especially among young adults), and who insisted that ministers were vigilant in monitoring the situation,[37] resisted calls from scientists and public health experts to counterbalance office returns by making face masks mandatory in most workplaces.[38] By early September, the Government was instructing its own departmental heads to order employees back to their desks, irrespective of whether or not they could do their jobs from home.[39] This coincided with ministerial efforts to scapegoat the young for the rise in COVID-19 cases whose supposed disregard of physical distancing rules was blamed for the unfolding crisis.[40] Towards the end of the month, the PM's default was that the new wave of infections was attributable to "too many breaches" of the remaining restrictions by "freedom-loving Brits" (as Johnson put it) rather than the fact there were insufficient controls remaining in place.[41]

Ministers certainly received plenty of advice from scientific experts in the summer and autumn of 2020 urging caution on unlockings and further unlockings and pushing for the restoration of some controls. On 28 June, SAGE member Sir Jeremy Farr cautioned the Government that, with the re-opening of pubs, bars, restaurants, hotels and other businesses, the country was placed "on a knife edge". Since the decline in caseloads was slowing and nearing standstill, this made the situation "precarious . . . particularly in England". The all-in-one-go reopening of hospitalities could risk, he said, giving a major boost to the virus and store up "a very nasty rebound" in the run-up to winter, as people respond to the unlocking of a rafter of leisure and social venues by releasing their "pent-up energies" (as the

West Midlands police commissioner David Jamieson put it), that is, "letting their hair down", as the saying goes.[42]

On 5 September, epidemiologist Anne Johnson of University College London (UCL) voiced concern over the impending re-opening of university campuses. This would be, she said, a "critical moment" in the struggle to contain the pandemic, since the rising caseload since August was being driven by an upsurge of infections among the 20–29 age group.[43] Two days earlier, on 3 September, the Government's SAGE group released a report acknowledging that campus returns would generate "significant risk" of amplifying "local and national transmission". It was "highly likely" that there would be "significant outbreak associated with higher education", concluded the report's authors. Moreover, the report opined, "asymptomatic transmission" would make outbreaks originating on campuses "harder to detect".[44]

Professor Mark Walport, a former chief scientific adviser, warned the Government, on 12 September, that the UK was "on the edge of losing control" of the pandemic. As he put it: "It's a very, very fine balancing act, it's very important to get youngsters back to school, people to university, but it means we're going to have to hold back our contacts in other areas". If school, college and university re-openings were to proceed, there would need to be a tightening up of physical distancing elsewhere. But this, of course, was not happening. With the lifting of restrictions over the summer, people, especially young people, were not "behaving responsibly" by voluntarily acquiescing to distancing self-controls. Later, on 21 September, the Government's Chief Scientific Officer, Patrick Vallance, issued an even blunter warning. Unless urgent action was taken, he instructed ministers, there would be calamity:

> At the moment we think the epidemic is doubling roughly every seven days. If . . . that continues unabated . . . you would end up with something like 50,000 cases in the middle of October per day. Fifty-thousand cases per day would be expected to lead a month later, so the middle of November say, to 200-plus deaths per day. The challenge, therefore, is to make sure the doubling time does not stay at seven days. That requires speed, it requires action and it requires enough in order to be able to bring that down.[45]

Two days earlier, a number of non-aligned experts had urged the Government to re-impose certain of the restrictions that had been lifted as well as bring in some new ones. Former SAGE adviser, Professor Neil Ferguson, for example, warned that the UK faced a "perfect storm" owing to the summer unlockings, and that restoration of controls was needed "sooner rather than later" to mitigate against the harms to come. BMA chairperson, Dr Chaand Nagpaul, for example, spoke for his colleagues when he urged ministers to tighten up the recently re-introduced (on 14 September) "rule of six", since this was significantly looser than its predecessor.[46] This permitted indoor social gatherings of up to six people from as many households on unlimited occasions in a single day. (The previous version, introduced in the spring, permitted groups of no more than six persons from two households to meet in outdoor settings, including private gardens).[47] Nagpaul also urged the Government to reverse its get back to work if possible steer in favour of restoring the work from home if you can guidance that preceded it. Other recommendations included providing incentives for the public to use takeaway services rather than on-site dining, discouraging non-essential travel or commuting, and requiring hospitality venues to provide customers with face coverings at the door.[48] These all fell on deaf ministerial ears.

Eventually, on 19 September, Boris Johnson conceded that the second pandemic wave was real.[49] Three days later, he found reason to declare in the House of Commons that the UK faced a "perilous turning point" in the battle to control this (for him) newly discovered second wave. This was the occasion for announcing a range of "stringent" measures that could be in place for up to six months, and which would become law on 24 September. As might be expected, based on precedent, these were rather less impressive than the fanfare that greeted their introduction, and much less stringent than the peril of the moment appeared to warrant. Hospitality businesses would not be permitted to serve customers after 10 pm or before 5 am. Face coverings would become mandatory for employees working in shops. Wedding gatherings would be restricted to 15 persons. The Government would cease urging everyone to return to work, instead re-emphasizing that they may home-work if feasible. These "carefully judged" new rules would, Johnson said, reduce the transmission rate to manageable levels whilst minimizing "damage to lives and livelihoods".[50] The exercise of neither "stringency" nor "judgement" warranted any tightening of nationwide physical distancing regulations.

Whatever the impact of the new rules on livelihoods, they were never going to be enough to save lives or exert downward pressure on rising caseloads. Rather, with university returns kicking in, the situation could only get very much worse. Naturally, SAGE, in its report of 3 September, declined to draw the logical conclusion from its own concerns over the riskiness of a return to on-campus courses, or at least apparently not. Independent SAGE, by contrast, grasped the mettle. There should be no return to on-campus face-to-face teaching or learning at the start of the new academic year other than for courses where this was strictly necessary on practical grounds, the group cautioned.[51]

> We recommend that to protect the safety of students and staff, and prevent community infections, all University courses should be offered remotely and online, unless they are practice or laboratory based, with termly review points. Universities should focus on providing excellent quality remote learning by default, with regular review points, rather than deliver in-person teaching on campuses that are likely to close again.[52]

The feasibility of catering for on-site classes later on would need to be assessed based on careful analysis of the data. Independent SAGE also recommended: "Mitigations in classrooms and other spaces (e.g. corridors where social distancing is reduced) including face coverings, social distancing of two meters as the norm, ventilation, PPE provision, and regular cleaning", residential bubbling, and avoidance of "constantly changing in-person class compositions". Collective agreement on "Covid-safe behaviours on campus for students and university staff" should also be sought, whereas university leaders should consult fully with university staff with regard to "rigorous health and safety procedures".[53]

Towards the end of September 2020, as the second wave of the virus began to engulf the population as a whole, as local lockdowns came into play, and with "multiple and increasing outbreaks across university campuses", Independent SAGE reiterated these recommendations with greater urgency. Universities should immediately switch "all teaching and learning online by default" and render "essential in-person teaching and learning (e.g., components of laboratory or practice-based courses) contingent on the regular testing of students and staff . . . and with stringent adherence to face coverings, handwashing, social distancing, and ventilation mitigations".[54] By and large, universities did not respond to these recommendations, either in whole or in part. Nor did the Government, other than by expressing its confidence that the health and safety measures in place on campuses were sufficient to hold the line against the virus and ensure that campus life remained feasible.

Universities should also, opined Independent SAGE, offer "students the choice whether to live on campus/in their university accommodation or at home elsewhere (e.g., with parents and caregivers) and review at the end of the calendar year (i.e., December), and avoid numerous journeys between home and university". They must also "ensure that students who choose to remain at university while learning online maintain the right to return home for the rest of the term at any point, with accommodation fees refunded, and with testing before doing so". Moreover, those students needing to "self-isolate and to access online learning resources, including practical needs (e.g., food, laundry), learning (e.g., IT, connectivity), and social and emotional needs (e.g., buddy systems, regular wellbeing checks, online events)", must be fully and generously supported in these multiple aspects. Independent SAGE expressed its awareness that these measures had major resource implications for universities, so that government financial support for the sector was urgently needed. Alas, neither the Government nor university executives were ready to suspend on-site teaching and learning, let alone advise or support or resource students in alternative arrangements.

Jo Grady, President of University Colleges Union (UCU), was naturally less circumspect than government scientists in warning of the dangers of allowing perhaps as many as two million students to travel across the country *en route* to university campuses and in expressing scepticism over the claims of university bosses to have basically designed "Covid-secure" campuses for the students.[55] This was, she opined, a "recipe for disaster" inasmuch as this risked a "silent avalanche of infections". Campus returns for on-site classes would be "far more of a risk than perhaps the general public has appreciated", threatening "untold damage to people's health and exacerbating the worst public health crisis of our lifetimes".[56] This was not least because many if not most universities were insufficiently prepared or equipped to guarantee on-campus health security for either students or staff. The sheer number of students gathering within close confines (in access points – corridors and stairwells; in classrooms – including large lecture halls; in cafeterias and eateries; and in densely-populated student halls of residence) would also undermine the prospects of Covid-secure campuses.

But university bosses had lively corporate interests in acting in the manner of the child-catcher from *Chitty Chitty Bang Bang* by promulgating myths of the potential for risk-free studies. They were, of course, keen on campus returns. This was in order to fill lucrative halls of residence, to bring business to on-campus hospitality services, as well as to protect against students deciding to delay or defer their studies until the pandemic's end (since even partially virtual courses would be seen as potentially unpopular with students), hence reducing profits from student fees and rents.[57] Naturally, a government committed to fast-tracking "normality" everywhere was not going to resist these imperatives. Indeed, it was committed to reinforcing them.

These interests were institutionalized by the neoliberalization of HE in the UK. Initially, under New Right governance in the 1980s, this took the form of massively expanding the number of students going to university whilst allowing the value of the state grant per head to fall and offering students top-up loans to plug the gap. Then, under New Labour, this entailed ditching the student grant altogether in favour of student loans.[58] Thereafter, drastic reduction of public funding for universities in the austerity decade, along with the marketization of funding via the student loan scheme, has rendered universities dependent on revenues from room rentals and tuition fees in order to survive or prosper. This has incentivized university bosses to push up tuition fees along with student rents and of governments to acquiesce to or even encourage this commodification of students as cash cows.

Tuition fees were set at £1,000 per head when Tony Blair's government introduced them in 1997.[59] They were increased to £3,000 in 2004, also under New Labour.[60] In 2010, under the Lib-Con Coalition government, universities were permitted to raise fees up to £9,000.[61] Even this was not enough for the Russell Group of elite British universities, however. They had urged the Government to "liberalize" the financing of HE in the interests of "fairness" and "viability" (i.e. scrap any cap on tuition fees, in order to ensure that HE in the UK was globally competitive).[62] Inevitably, as tuition fees and accommodation charges have increased, so too has competition among universities for student enrolments. This has been accompanied by the hard-sell of a university education as indispensable to career success in the high-skills "knowledge" economy. The result has been, since the start of the 2000s, a relentless expansion of student numbers, leading to jam-packed campuses and halls of residence.

In this context, the only way university executives could have been motivated to avoid cramming the campuses just as COVID-19 cases began to escalate in the autumn was by means of financial grants from the Government – such as were being provided to other businesses to pull them through the pandemic. But these were not forthcoming, so that pressures on universities to capitulate to market forces and the dictates of economic self-interest were not alleviated. Indeed, the lack of government financial assistance ensured that universities would have to go it alone in planning and resourcing on-campus health and safety measures, with predictably uneven results. Students were destined to enter campuses at the start of the second pandemic wave in the autumn of 2020 where there were little or no provisions for COVID-19 testing or distribution of face coverings and where physical distancing guidelines were poorly enforced and did not extend beyond the "formal" campus to student halls of residence.[63]

The contrast with the official ideology legitimizing and incentivizing campus return could hardly have been greater. Ministers expressed their confidence

that universities . . . [were] . . . well prepared for the return of students by taking measures such as introducing social distancing on campus, limiting travel requirement for classes and staggering teaching across extended days to reduce numbers on site.

Health and safety guidance for universities was, they said, "under constant review". University bosses insisted that they had "robust" plans in place to ensure that students would enjoy safely all (or at least most) aspects of a normal university experience. The issue of on-campus health safety and security was, it was said, being taken "seriously". There would be clear rules and guidelines for students. There would be one-way people-flow systems in corridors and stairways. There would be restrictions on the number of students permitted to congregate in cafes or canteens or coffee bars and in libraries. There would be safety messaging and hand-sanitizer stations everywhere. There would be limits on the number of students in lecture halls and seminar classrooms so that physical distancing was possible. Perhaps virtual office hours with academic staff may replace face-to-face meetings. "Almost all institutions . . . [would] . . . be making greater use of online teaching methods for students studying non-practical subjects".[64]

As it transpired, universities would make efforts to deliver on these commitments (or at least many of them), to a greater or lesser extent. But their capacity to do so was dependent on the resources at their disposal, which in the absence of government financial support was highly uneven. For many, if not most, given the reality of mass recruitment, there were major constraints on the degree to which socially distanced spaces could be delivered or policed. Students were also hardly incentivized by the general lifting of physical distancing restrictions in society at large to be scrupulously adhering to on-campus regulations. There was also little appetite for alienating students by enforcing the rules since that could lead to students demanding reductions in fees or suspending their studies.

In the "unofficial" campus, in halls of residence, students were mostly left unsupervised, so that they could congregate and party as they wished. In any case, much student accommodation was shared occupancy, so that several students would occupy the same shared living space.[65] UCU's and Independent SAGE's sensible recommendation that campuses should cater for face-to-face classrooms only in those practice-oriented or vocational subjects that specifically required them (whereas academic subjects should be taught in online classes) was predictably set aside by many universities, despite them mooting this as a policy under consideration. By and large, university leaders across the sector committed all faculties and departments to delivering at least some on-site classes for all students, across the board, irrespective of whether or not it was feasible to deliver certain courses wholly virtually.

The results were as lamentable as they were predictable. By the end of September 2020, 50 UK universities were facing on-campus outbreaks. October was not older than a week before this had increased to 90. By October's end, the number had grown to 119. Thousands of students were confined to halls where they were often cooped up with others who were infected, joining long queues of those waiting to be tested. By 29 October, the number of officially logged cases of infection on university campuses across the country stood at 32,701, of which 31,860 were of students and 841 were of staff.[66] Owing to the general issues with reporting and recording – including the lack of basic functionality with the test-and-trace system – these numbers would be huge underestimates of real caseloads, especially since young adults are more likely to register mild symptoms or to be asymptomatic than older people. Under-recording would also be a function of the lack of capacity of many universities for on-site testing. Research conducted by PHE later estimated that almost one-fifth of university students had been infected by the virus during the autumn term (on my count around 360,000 students in total), including half of those living in on-campus halls of residence.[67]

The Government eventually responded to the crisis with an about-face. The advice to universities at the end of September was now to switch courses wherever possible to virtual learning. This would be to facilitate the return home of students for Christmas, so that two million or so travelling students would not ramp up infection rates right across the country. Students were also warned that some (e.g. on practice-oriented courses) could face compulsory quarantining before they would be permitted to return home.[68] The ignominious end of on-campus teaching quickly followed by virtue of the Government's impending November circuit-breaker lockdown. A week in advance of its implementation, ministers declared that it was on the way and set a date for it. This provided students with a window of opportunity (indeed impelling motive) to evade the risk of finding themselves locked down on campus over the seasonal period by making an immediate exodus from universities up and down the land. Now, in all likelihood, a large number of them – perhaps a majority – would have seized this opportunity, ignoring the appeals of university bosses to stay put until further notice.[69] The opportunity for a cautious, staggered return of students to their homeplaces was thereby squandered. It would be miraculous if this mass exodus prior to the second lockdown did not seed a rafter of new infection spirals across the UK.

Finally, on 11 November, six days after the circuit-breaker was rolled out, the Government got round to announcing a plan to offer students a six-day window to return home "safely" between 3 and 9 December for the start of the Christmas break. At the same time, ministers for the first time instructed (rather than advised) universities to switch to fully virtual delivery except where on-site teaching and learning was essential. The six-day returns window would supposedly be preceded by the week of pre-departure mass testing of students, with those failing a test being required to self-isolate for ten days. It was the responsibility of universities to organize and administer the plan.[70] Such imposed huge logistical demands on universities without the provision of central funding to support it. This was a recipe for inconsistency and inefficiency of delivery. This also rendered universities vulnerable to legal challenges from students over being compelled to be tested or having on-site learning commitments replaced by online ones, which as far as mass testing was concerned was a disincentive to compliance. This was also, to some degree at least, fastening the stable door after the horse had bolted.

But what of schools and colleges? The Government never once acknowledged the wisdom of putting the brakes on the phased reopening of schools starting with the return of primary children to the classroom at the start of June 2020. Rather, this was abandoned owing to resistance that made it untenable. Most parents simply refused to return their children and teachers voted with their feet by staying at home. Only 25 percent of children were returned in that first week. The plan was also shelved because school premises lacked the room size and the number of rooms to implement smaller classes that were required for physical distancing – as the teaching unions had been instructing the Government since the re-opening plans had been announced.[71] The full return of students to schools and colleges (along of course as we have seen with the return of students to university campuses) was postponed until September.[72] Schools continued to cater only for the children of essential keyworkers as they had done since the start of the 24 March lockdown.

This wholly justifiable caution of teachers and parents (supported by the medical profession) most likely played a major role in depressing the virus over the summer, so that NHS frontliners had some opportunity to recover from the first wave. But these gains would be undone in the autumn by government policy. Despite supposedly being informed by a "data-not-dates-led" policy, the September reopening of schools, colleges (and, as we have seen, universities) went ahead just as the calamitous second wave began to accelerate in earnest. The seven-day daily average caseload increased from 2,178 on 1 September to 15,299 by 5 October and to 24,677 by 10 November.[73] This undoubtedly gave the virus the impetus to spiral out of control which forced the Government into its second and third lockdowns. Schools and other educational settings would not reopen again until March 2021.

The second unlocking (from early March through to mid-July 2021) was destined to repeat the errors of the first, albeit in a social and political context reshaped by the vaccination roll-out programme and its success in getting jabs into the arms of the masses. This is explored in Chapter 8 on "Freedom Day". This changed context was not simply that the vaccine programme was highly successful in depressing hospitalizations and deaths. It was also that this gave renewed confidence to the Government's default prioritization of economic restoration and abstract consumerist-oriented liberties over safeguarding public health that may otherwise have been tempered by its negative prior consequences. This resulted in an "all eggs in one basket" pandemic defence policy that would depend entirely on the bio-technical fix of vaccine efficacy since the summer of 2021 and thereafter.

Local lockdowns and the tier system

The Government's premature and fast-track winding down of lockdown restrictions over the spring and summer of 2020 inevitably ran into its self-imposed limits. This was as the roll-back was confronted by rising caseloads from mid-July having declined steadily since the spring. As we have seen, the crux of the problem was that the lockdown was simply too short and was rather too loose to suppress the virus enough to prevent it from rebounding robustly as restrictions were eased. The ministerial response, beginning in July, was to attempt to control the resurgence by means of targeted tightening and relaxation of restrictions at the local level under a system of alerts. Locales that were classified as "areas of concern" owing to high rates of infection or sharply rising caseloads may then be made into "areas of intervention" or "areas of enhanced support". Such localized responses may be either a partial or fuller restoration of lockdown restrictions to stem the spread of the virus in a particular place or delaying or slowing the easing of restrictions locally that were going ahead elsewhere.[74]

Under this system, local lockdowns would be triggered by those spikes of cases that were considered high enough to escape controllability. This was in the sense that healthcare services in these areas were being placed under undue strain by a spiral of hospital admissions that threatened to exceed the capacity to manage them. Localized lockdowns would then, in theory, prevent local upsurges spreading out into region-wide or nation-wide outbreaks. The resort to localized lockdowns was thus intended to suppress the virus sufficiently so that the Government's dates-led roadmap to full economic normalcy would not be derailed. If the virus could be ring-fenced in a specific place, and brought under control in that place, the need to resort to the nationwide tightening of distancing rules would be avoided. PM Boris Johnson expressed his confidence that this system would indeed secure that goal. This, along with the test-and-trace system, would allow the UK to avoid the "nuclear deterrent" (as he called it) of another national lockdown.

> I certainly don't want to use it. And nor do I think we will be in that position again . . . We're genuinely able now to look at what's happening in much closer to real time, to isolate outbreaks and to address them on the spot, and to work with local authorities to contain the problem locally and regionally if we have to.[75]

Over the summer and autumn of 2020, local lockdowns were imposed right across the Midlands and the North of England, including: Leicester, Luton, Birmingham, Wolverhampton, Blackburn, Manchester, Bury, Bolton, Oldham, Salford,

Stockport, Rochdale, Burnley, Kirklees, Newcastle, Sunderland, and Durham. These were a conspicuous failure. Virtually every place in which they were implemented experienced rapidly escalating infection rates from mid-September onwards.[76] Local restrictions also did not stem the rising caseload nationally starting in mid-July 2020 and the ever-quickening acceleration of the rate of increase in August and especially in September. The seven-day average of new infections on 8 July was 614. By 26 July, it had risen to 769. By mid-August, it was 1,022. On 1 September, it had more than doubled, up to 2,178. By mid-September, the seven-day average new caseload had reached 3,659 – an increase of more than 40 percent since the start of the month. By September's end, the rate of infection had more than trebled again, in little more than two weeks, where a seven-day average of 11,148 new cases was recorded.[77]

This was an unsurprising result. The Government's strategy of local containment had little prospect of achieving its stated goals, for a number of reasons. First, the local lockdowns were of course wholly reactive. This was inasmuch as such responses were not intended to stamp out local surges, preventing these from growing into local crises, but rather to address these after they had assumed crisis magnitudes, or after they had escaped controllability. This was in order to prevent them spiralling into a national crisis, thereby triggering clamour for another national lockdown.

Second, as we will see (Chapter 6), the test-and-trace system simply was not up to the job of supporting the policy. Any rapid upsurge of cases anywhere tended to undermine the system, so that contacts of infected persons were not advised to self-isolate in a timely way or not contacted at all, and nor were test results processed quickly enough to prevent infected people passing on the virus. Researchers at UCL and the London School of Hygiene and Tropical Medicine estimated that, in order to suppress a second wave, in the context of school re-openings, test-and-trace would need to deliver certain outcomes. These were, *either* three-quarters of infected people had to be located and 68 percent of their contacts traced and isolated, *or* 87 percent of infected people had to be located and 40 percent of their contacts traced and isolated. However, the system was barely reaching 50 percent of contacts of infected persons, and levels of prior testing of infected persons were apparently low as well.[78]

Third, local lockdowns undermined the sense of national togetherness (i.e. of a population or people who were in the same boat in terms of privations and who were united in a common struggle against the virus and in defence of lives and the NHS) that was necessary to avoid fracturing and diluting adherence to physical distancing regulations. Indeed, local lockdowns may even elicit among some people subject to their restrictions outright disregard of the rules. A SAGE report of 23 April 2020 cautioned the Government to avoid local lockdowns on exactly those grounds.

> A consensus has evolved in the UK over the last weeks concerning the need
> for restrictive measures which suggests that support for restrictive measures

is contingent upon a sense of equality of sacrifice. . . . The proposed scheme undermines this core proposition. . . . Restrictions imposed in the UK during the epidemic have not led to conflict thus far because they have been perceived as fair (for the most part).[79]

Local lockdowns threatened to nurture the grievances of locals who could imagine themselves as being singled out unfairly or illegitimately by having restrictions re-imposed or preserved as people elsewhere were being freed or had been freed from them. Such feelings of being discriminated against or of being a victim of injustice may even be felt especially among the poor and minorities in lockdown areas owing to the fact that

> lower socio-economic positions are more susceptible to the virus and therefore "lockdown" will be more likely in areas of poverty relative to wealth. Even if an area cuts across ethnic residential and economic divides, this could lead to perceptions of inequality and stigmatisation of particular ethnic groups.

Such could only weaken the moral force of physical distancing norms in lockdown places and incentivize higher rates of non-compliance among people in these places. Indeed, localized lockdowns could even "lead to civil disorder" (including confrontations with the police) owing to the "sense of inequality" they may provoke.[80]

As it happened, the local lockdowns (including under the tier system) actually generated considerable dissonance as well between central government and local authorities in places that were placed under special restrictions. Local leaders would experience (and give vent to) the sense of injustice and discrimination felt by their constituents, questioning or disputing the data evidence that had led to the imposition of tighter controls on their own areas of jurisdiction. Such disputations over "why us specifically?" or "why are we being blamed?" were exacerbated by government officials' lack of transparency over how lockdown decisions were actually made. Ministers were also prepared to use bribes and threats to secure compliance. Local authorities that consented to lockdowns would receive central funds to support businesses whereas those which resisted would not. The result was either resentful acquiescence (as was the case for the Liverpool City Region and Lancashire authorities) or tense stand-offs between ministers and local authorities (e.g. in Greater Manchester and parts of the North East) that threatened to spiral into the latter's refusal to implement the new regulations.[81]

The Government's lack of transparency and clarity over these matters may have been a reflection of the fact that it was aware that it viewed the goals of local lockdowns differently to how local authorities would view them – and ministers did not consider it politick to publicize these differences. For local leaders, the only legitimate purpose of a local lockdown was to bring under control escalating caseloads in that specific area that could not be contained by other measures.

For ministers (and seemingly government-appointed health officials), by contrast, the main purpose of local lockdowns was to avoid tighter social restrictions across the whole country and head-off the threat of a national lockdown. Such divisions and strains between national government and local leaderships were built into the local lockdowns policy. These could only further fuel public antipathy towards the restrictions (and hence encourage their disregard by many people) in those areas under special measures.

Fourth, the local lockdowns were for the most part less stringent in the controls they imposed on people than those mandated under the original nationwide lockdown framework of March 2020 – and the first lockdown was hardly as stringent as many on the continent. These restored a lesser version of the controls of 24 March in keeping with earlier stages of the unlocking process. There were no time restrictions on spending time outdoors and no requirement that time spent outdoors must be only for purpose of exercise rather than leisure, socializing or recreation more generally. There were more exemptions of non-essential businesses from closures (e.g. garden centres and vehicle showrooms). Outdoor sports facilities remained open. Household bubbles (linking one adult households with another of any number of adults and children) were retained. Overnight stay in a linked household in the lockdown area was prohibited only if this was without good reason or "reasonable excuse". The "rule of six" for outdoor gatherings was preserved or reinstated.[82]

Finally, the prospect of corralling the virus was in any case quite simply unpractical owing to soft local and regional borders. This was because there were no outright travel bans (or restrictions on people from outside the lockdown area entering and then exiting it) and owing to the lack of regulatory surveillance of people flows across local borders from city to city within a regional centre and across regional boundaries. It is improbable that staff on public transport (or the transport police) would be proactive in checking if people's reasons for travel were essential ones or that the latter would be incentivized to sanction rule-breakers.[83] This was also owing to the sheer volume of commuter traffic within regions and between regions. In a situation where the virus is transmitting everywhere, albeit at different rates and volumes, lockdowns can work only as a united front, since only a common approach nationally to restrictions would cut off the continual export and import of cases back and forth across county lines.

The local lockdowns strategy of virus control committed public health policy to something resembling the amusement arcade game of "whack-a-mole" (as Raphael Hogarth memorably described it).[84] But this was perpetually and with little prospect of success. This was yet another run-out of the Government's default of avoiding dealing with problems until its own inactivity turned these into emergencies that would force it into last-ditch reversals, albeit too late to avert calamity.

The Government announced the termination of the local lockdowns policy on 12 October 2020, at which point its failure could no longer be denied. However, it was apparent that this was little more than a rhetorical change, for what replaced local lockdowns was really no more than a more complex and systematized version of the same thing. This was, of course, the three-tier "traffic-light" system of local alerts, which was rolled out on 14 October.[85] For that reason, its chances of success were scarcely any better than for its predecessor. Under the three-tier system, different areas of the country that were of particular pandemic concern would be placed under either "medium" (Tier 1) or "high" (Tier 2) or "very high" (Tier 3) alert. These different alert listings or flags would determine the nature and extent of the local measures to deal with the pandemic.

Medium-alerted areas (most of the country) would have minimal restrictions. Pubs and bars and restaurants would close at 10 pm. Indoor and outdoor gatherings would be based on the "rule of six". High-alerted places would have tighter restrictions. Here the "rule of six" would apply only to outdoor gatherings, with members of more than one household not permitted to mix indoors. There would also be the 10 pm curfew on hospitality venues. Very high-alerted places would have the tightest restrictions. In these areas, there would be no inter-household mixing either indoors or outdoors – except in public places such as parks or beaches, where the "rule of six" would apply. Here as well bars and pubs that were not serving "substantial" meals would be closed, but otherwise would stay open. So too would gyms, casinos, bookies, leisure and sports centres be shut. But in even the highest-alert areas, the restrictions were far short of a full community lockdown. Schools, colleges and universities would not be closed. Restaurants and retailers would remain open.[86]

It is difficult to countenance that ministers were not aware of the slimness of the odds that the three-tier system would control the virus, and of the appalling impact that non-control would have on public health in the autumn of 2020. This is because they were forewarned by their own scientific advisers. Chris Whitty, for example, spoke for SAGE when he voiced his lack of confidence in the efficacy of the system. Tiers would not, he said, be enough "to get on top of the virus" – not in the highest ones. In these, he opined, the "base will not be sufficient – I think that's very clearly the professional view".[87] Another SAGE member, Whitty's deputy, Professor Jonathan Van Tam, pointed out that the second COVID-19 wave was now a nationwide phenomenon, not one that mapped onto tiers or locales, which was at least suggestive that tougher nationwide measures were needed.[88] Not only that, but several weeks before, on 21 September, the SAGE committee had recommended that, in place of the failed local lockdowns, ministers should instead institute with immediate effect a circuit-breaker national lockdown to interrupt the rising tide of infections and hospitalizations.[89]

All of this was dismissed by a government that has always insisted that its policies were always "based on the science" and "data-led", with predictable results. Communities Secretary Robert Jenrick expressed ministerial scepticism over the notion of a national circuit-breaker on the grounds that infection rates and case numbers were not the same everywhere, for example:

> The argument for a national circuit-breaker is not one that I, personally, find, at all persuasive. This is to apply on a blanket level – the same approach in

Nottingham, the city which my constituency is next to, where the number of cases today is well over 700, to Somerset or Herefordshire, where the number of cases per 100,000 is below 40.[90]

This rather lost sight of the fact that cases were rising overall and in more places than not, so that the game of whack-a-mole was becoming untenable. When the tier system was introduced, on 14 October 2020, the average seven-day caseload of new cases was 17,266, By the end of the month, this stood at 22,696, and by 10 November it was 24,677.[91] Moreover, those places that went into local lockdowns in the autumn were simply transferred into the higher risk tiers under the new system, where they then remained.[92] The problem with Jenrick's reasoning was that, without a mechanism that would prevent areas with high rates of infection spilling over into neighbouring ones with lower rates, the second wave would continue to increase exponentially. But not even the first lockdown was justifiable, on Jenrick's logic, since nor did the first pandemic wave manifest on the same scale and at the same rate in all places. Well, of course not. That is not how pandemics work.

Delayed lockdown repeated

This grim determination of ministers to press ahead with the tier system reflected the desperation of a government which had turned the spectre of a second nation-wide lockdown into something that was diabolical. This rendered inevitable a repetition of the catastrophic error of deferred lockdown in response to the first wave that caused tens of thousands of unnecessary deaths in the spring. The second circuit-breaker lockdown (from 5 November to 2 December 2020) was introduced far too late and lifted far too soon to prevent a repetition of the heavy toll of human lives in the second and third waves. The premature lifting of the second lockdown ensured not only that the third lockdown was unavoidable but that this too was too late to prevent the virus again escaping control to wreak havoc in the population and generate huge pressures on the NHS.

The explanation for this is clear enough. Having taken a bigger economic hit on the first COVID-19 wave than every other developed (G7) country,[93] the incentive of the Government to take a lesser hit than the others on the second wave was radicalized almost to the point of obsession. (This imperative also meant that ministers were coming under increasing pressure from vociferous "libertarian" lockdown sceptics among its own MPs and party members who were set against any mandatory physical distancing controls on the grounds that these were stifling economic recovery). Such is the logic of inter-capitalist competition, where relative or comparative performance is more important than actual or real performance in measuring national economic success or maintaining a country's economic status in the world *vis-à-vis* the others. This *competitive* success (a success of rates and ratios rather than volumes or magnitudes) is what will restore business and investment confidence at home and suck in revenues from overseas. However, COVID-19 has no regard for the logic of capital. The tiers were unsustainable, simply because they could not hold the line against the virus.

Finally, on 31 October, the Government conceded the reality that events had rendered inevitable: the case for at least a short nationwide lockdown.[94] Johnson himself remained opposed to it. He (and his chancellor Rishi Sunak) were reportedly dragooned into reluctant compliance by Michael Gove, Matt Hancock, SAGE advisers and others, during a protracted and acrimonious meeting at No. 10, this eliciting his infamous exclamation: "No more f★★★★★★ lockdowns –let the bodies pile high in their thousands".[95] The decisive spur may have been the publication of a SAGE report the day before and its publicization in the media. This document could hardly have stressed the urgency of the situation more: "There is complete consensus in SPI-M-O that the current outlook for the epidemic's trajectory is concerning, if there are no widespread decisive interventions or behavioural changes in the near term". This concern was informed by the fact that modelling showed that the virus was spreading at a rate four-times faster than would generate the Government's "worst-case scenario" of 85,000 deaths over the winter.

> We are breaching the number of infections and hospital admissions in the Reasonable Worst Case planning scenario . . . based on COVID's winter planning strategy. The number of daily deaths is now in line with the levels in the Reasonable Worst Case and is almost certain to exceed this within the next two weeks.

Infections were doubling every 10–15 days, causing "between 43,000 and 74,000 new infections per day in England". Such was "significantly above the profile of the reasonable worst-case scenario", which depended on the "number of daily infections in England . . . [remaining] . . . between 12,000–13,000 throughout October".[96] This SAGE report was produced two weeks before it was published and made accessible to the media – on 14 October 2020. Yet this did not motivate ministers to reconsider the tier policy that would roll out on the same day. SAGE, of course, had urged the Government to implement a circuit-breaker lockdown three weeks before the report was generated. This was when the caseload was 5,000 new infections per day.

The circuit-breaker was declared on 31 October – but for a 5 November start.[97] The delay between the declaration of policy intent and policy implementation was itself hardly unusual. This too was simply the most recent case of the general pattern of foot-dragging behaviours. But, given the precarity of the situation, it was perhaps the most baffling. The delay basically provided a window of opportunity for people to "make the most" of their recently-regained freedoms from physical distancing restrictions – to socialize, to attend clubs and pubs and restaurants, to hold house parties, and so on – before the lockdown extinguished these opportunities. Such behaviour – which would likely deliver a further pre-lockdown boost to the virus – would hardly be unexpected. This would be motivated by the memory of the privations of the first lockdown, the contrast of that with the brief period in which something resembling normality was restored, the uncertainty over how long the new lockdown would last (since this could be extended), and the possibility that the circuit-breaker would (as was forewarned by ministers) be replaced by a tougher tier system than before when it ended.[98]

But Johnson would not extend the circuit-breaker beyond its planned 28-day timeframe. On the day it was brought in he made a point of committing the Government to its termination "without a shred of doubt" exactly on 2 December, even though some of his ministers were suggesting it could be extended if this was strictly necessary.[99] This commitment was for exactly the same reasons and in response to exactly the same pressures as motivated the tardiness of the lockdown's implementation. This of course was primarily to "balance" the needs of public safety with business needs and secondarily to head off the threat of a backbench rebellion of disaffected Tory MPs.[100]

The circuit breaker did indeed end on 2 December, prematurely. This was premature in the sense that national caseloads were insufficiently depressed to prevent the virus quickly rebounding in what may be classed as its third wave – at exactly the worst time of the year (in the midst of winter) for such a resurgence. The tier system returned (albeit briefly and fruitlessly), in a form that was publicized as being much tougher than before, but which in fact was not much more so.[101] Predictably too, this was unable to prevent caseloads rising again, as they did in the run-up to Christmas 2020 – and, again, for exactly the same reasons as before, notwithstanding the special impact of the new Kent variant in exacerbating the problem.[102] (By then, the Alpha Kent variant was outcompeting earlier strains owing to its radically enhanced infectiousness and its greater agility in outflanking the existing controls, driving up caseloads at a faster rate than before).

The emergence of the Kent variant as the dynamic strain of the virus in the UK in December 2020 particularly exposed the limitations of the second lockdown (since controls under the circuit-breaker were significantly less stringent than under the first lockdown – which itself was far from watertight). This fatally exposed as well the weaknesses of the tier system (since, as we have seen, this implemented lesser controls in the higher tiers than were brought in under the second lockdown). Despite the circuit breaker, the new variant generated rising infections right across Kent in November and early December, just as caseloads dropped back elsewhere in the country under the impact of the lockdown controls. The new variant was first detected on 20 September. But, for reasons that are unclear, either it was not recognized by scientists as a variant of concern or it was not declared by government as one (which of these is uncertain) until three months later, in mid-December, at which point it had spread across the country, was dominant in the capital and Southeast, and had been become one of the UK's gifts to the world.[103]

Scientists had charted the progress of "Kentish exceptionalism" in terms of the new variant driving rising caseloads under the second lockdown. This was bucking the national pattern since caseloads elsewhere were beginning to fall under the impact of the nationwide restrictions. It ought to have been clear at that point that what was happening in Kent was a matter of national concern. Since this was so, it was remarkable from a public health point of view that this did not motivate ministers to at least reconsider the wisdom of ditching the circuit-breaker on 2 December. But there is no evidence that the unfolding crisis in the Southeast impinged on their deliberations at all. Worse was to follow, however. Having terminated the lockdown in favour of a return to local tiers, the Government then itself acted to decisively undermine any remote chance of the revamped tier system succeeding. This was by basically declaring its intention (in complete disregard of the recommendations of its scientific advisers) to permit everyone, irrespective of whatever tier they were in, to travel up and down the country to join wider kin and gather together indoors in extended family "bubbles" of up to three households for several days over the festive season.[104]

Whether or not this remarkable decision was motivated by mere sentiment ("we cannot cancel Christmas") or by the electoral calculus and with an eye on the opinion polls ("we cannot be *seen* to cancel Christmas"), or more likely by a combination of both, can only be guessed at. Of greater certainty was that this was from a public health and safety perspective a recklessly cavalier decision, given that the second wave was resurging or was being overtaken by a third wave that was threatening to dwarf its predecessor. In the run-up to the Christmas holiday, scientists and public health experts and medics (both those aligned to the Government and those who were independent) urged ministers to abandon or at least moderate the plan. Simultaneously, they sought to protect the public from the negative health and safety impacts of acting on it by urging them to exercise caution during the festive season – to respect physical distancing and consider avoiding multi-household gatherings.[105] This was as more and more localities were forced into the higher tiers and placed under special measures. Even when the system was rolled out, 55 million people in England had already been placed in the two higher tiers.[106]

In the end, of course, the Government was forced by events into a U-turn – but as always far too late in the day to change the course of events. With less than a week's notice, on 19 December 2020, Johnson announced the introduction of a fourth tier of tighter restrictions from the next day in a last-ditch effort to save the tier system. This Tier 4 exceeded the restrictions of the circuit-breaker but were less strict than those under the first lockdown. Tier 4 required the closure of non-essential shops, leisure and entertainment venues and hairdressers. This also banned more than one person from a different household meeting in public. Indoor gatherings of people from two or more households were also prohibited. But, under Tier 4, people should still go to work if they could not work from home, whether or not their work was essential. Support bubbles were also preserved along with the right to take unlimited outdoor exercise or recreation. Schools and colleges would also re-open in Tier 4 areas at the close of the festive season as normal.[107]

London and much of Southeast were placed within the new tier. This meant that the Christmas "bubbles" could not go ahead for millions, after all, since that was ruled out for those under the new tier. Not only that, for everyone else, festive gatherings for members of three different households would be limited to

Christmas Day, not for the five days of the extended holiday period as was origi-nally mooted.[108] Now, 50 percent of the adult population, according to a survey by the ONS, said that they would take the opportunity provided by government to link up in bubbles of up to three households over the festive period, whereas only 38 percent said they would not.[109] And, at that late stage, by 19 December – that is, before Johnson's change of mind – most of them would have made their arrangements to do so. This too would have been encouraged by the Government's repeated reassurances that it would not renege on its Christmas undertakings.[110]

Under these circumstances, there was every prospect that plenty of people would neither abandon their holiday plans nor even scale these back. Nor did they. Matt Hancock upbraided Londoners as "totally irresponsible" for flocking to rail stations *en masse* and jam-packing trains in order to escape the capital in the few hours left to them before the restrictions kicked in. Many more left the Southeast by road – whether by car or by taxi.[111] This undoubtedly was the straw that broke the camel's back as far as the prospect of containing the resurgent second wave (or the rise of third wave that superseded it) was concerned. By 26 December, only small patches of the country were still under Tier 1, whereas the whole of the Southeast (with 24 million people and 40 percent of England's population) was under Tier 4, and virtually all of the Midlands and North was under either Tier 2 or Tier 3.[112] By New Year's Day (2021), 78 percent of England's population (44 million plus peo-ple) were under Tier 4, whereas 21 percent (12 million plus people) were under Tier 3. Tier 4 had now swallowed the North East and most of the North West, the Midlands, and the South West. Only 2,220 people (0.1 percent of the population) were under Tier 1.[113]

A third protracted national lockdown was hence made inevitable – and this necessity was made in Westminster. Its seeds and the health calamity that drove it were sown by the premature and incautious unlocking of restrictions since the spring and the failure to operationalize a functional test-and-trace system over the summer in readiness for the autumn and winter surges. These seeds were then cul-tivated by the tardiness and weaknesses of the local lockdowns and the tier system that were intended to "balance" the need for rapid economic recovery with the need to control the virus at least enough to prevent the NHS being undermined. The seeds were then brought to full bloom by ministers' reckless declaration of intent for extended Christmas bubbles, their tardy withdrawal from much of this commitment (which would incentivize non-compliance), and their refusal to lose face by restricting rather than terminating the bubbles altogether. If that was not enough, ministers then created the potential for super-spreading events by provid-ing a narrow window of opportunity for people to evade the Tier 4 restrictions by crowding into stations and on to the last trains and buses out of London, at the same time, *en route* to destinations up and down the land.

9 June 2021 (updated 22 December 2021)

Notes

1 Johnson, B. (2020). 'Boris Johnson's speech in full: "first, careful steps" to ease Covid-19 lockdown'. *Guardian*. (10 May).
2 Proctor, K. (2020). 'Point by point: the UK government's plan to leave lockdown'. *Guardian*. (11 May).
3 Cabinet Office (2020). *Our Plan to Rebuild: The UK Government's COVID-19 Recovery Strategy*. (11 May). Available at: www.gov.uk/government/publications/our-plan-to-rebuild-the-uk-governments-covid-19-recovery-strategy.
4 Brown, J. and Kirk-Wade, E. (2021). *Coronavirus: A History of English Lockdown Laws*. Briefing Paper No. 9068. (22 December). London: House of Commons Library, p. 6.
5 Proctor (11 May, 2020).
6 Cabinet Office (2020); Department for Business, Energy and Industrial Strategy and Department for Digital, Culture, Media and Sport (2020). *Working Safely During COVID-19*. GOV.UK (online). (14 May). Available at: www.gov.uk/guidance/working-safely-during-covid-19. A.
7 UNISON (2020). *Coronavirus: Your Rights at Work*. UNISON (online). (12 May). Available at: www.unison.org.uk/coronavirus-rights-work/covid-19-advice-reps/. Accessed: 15/05/2020.
8 Palmer, S. (2020). 'What are the government's new rules for reopening workplaces – and will they work'? *People Management* (online). (4 May). Available at: www.peoplemanagement.co.uk/news/articles/governments-new-rules-reopening-workplaces; Palmer, S. (2020). 'Thousands of workers raising workplace safety concerns, MPs reveal'. *People Management* (online). (24 April). Available at: www.peoplemanagement.co.uk/news/articles/thousands-workers-raising-workplace-safety-concerns-mps-reveal.
9 UNISON (12 May, 2020).
10 Brown and Kirk-Wade (2021), p. 7; Cabinet Office (11 May, 2020).
11 Andersson, J. (2020). ' "We are not safe or protected": UK schools reopening on 1 June would be "unsafe", teachers say'. *I-News*. (7 May); *BBC News* (2020). 'Coronavirus: doctors' union says it's too soon to reopen schools'. (15 May); Elvin, S. (2020). 'Another council defies Government and says it will not reopen schools on June 1'. *Metro*. (16 May); Weale, S. (2020). 'Unions tell staff "not to engage" with plan for 1 June school openings'. *Guardian*. (12 May).
12 Connolly, K. and Willsher, K. (2020). 'European schools get ready to reopen despite concern about pupils spreading Covid-19'. *Guardian* (online). (1 May).
13 *BBC News* (2020). 'Coronavirus: Italy's PM outlines lockdown easing measures'. (27 April).
14 *BBC News* (2020). 'Coronavirus: France eases lockdown after eight weeks'. (11 May).
15 *BBC News* (2020). 'Coronavirus: Germany reopens shops as lockdown is relaxed'. (6 May); *ITV News* (2020). 'Germans emerge from lockdown as strictest stay-at-home measures are eased'. (6 May).
16 Worldometer (2020). *Covid-19 Coronavirus Pandemic: Countries*. Available at: https://www.worldometers.info/coronavirus/#countries. Accessed: 12/05/2020.
17 *BBC News* (2020). 'Coronavirus: government to "bring forward proposals" on reducing 2m social distancing rule'. (21 June).
18 *BBC News* (2020). 'Coronavirus: house moves and viewings to resume in England'. (12 May).
19 Brown and Kirk-Wade (2021), p. 6.
20 Public Health England (2020). *The Health Protection (Coronavirus, Restrictions) (England) (Amendment) (No. 3) Regulations 2020*. GOV.UK (online). (1 June). Available at: www.legislation.gov.uk/uksi/2020/558/made.
21 *BBC News* (2020). 'Coronavirus: outdoor pools and lidos struggling to reopen'. (11 July).

22 DHSC (2020). *Meeting People From Outside Your Household*. GOV.UK (online). (10 June). Available at: https://web.archive.org/web/20200613131448/www.gov.uk/guidance/meeting-people-from-outside-your-household.

23 Public Health England (2020). *The Health Protection (Coronavirus, Restrictions) (England) (Amendment) (No. 4) Regulations 2020*. GOV.UK (online). (12 June). Available at: www.legislation.gov.uk/uksi/2020/588/made.

24 The National Archives (2020). *The Health Protection (Coronavirus, Restrictions) (England) (Amendment) Regulations 2020 (Revoked)*. GOV.UK (online). (13 July). Available at: www.legislation.gov.uk/uksi/2020/447/contents/data.htm.

25 *BBC News* (2020). 'Coronavirus: no reason to change working from home advice – Vallance'. (16 July).

26 *BBC News* (2020). 'Coronavirus: Boris Johnson sets out plan for "significant normality" by Christmas'. (17 July).

27 Department for Digital, Culture, Media and Sport (2020). *Government Announces Gyms and Pools to Reopen Safely*. Press Release. GOV.UK (online). (9 July). Available at: www.gov.uk/government/news/government-announces-gyms-and-pools-to-reopen-safely.

28 *BBC News* (17 July, 2020).

29 *BBC News* (16 July, 2020).

30 *BBC News* (31 July, 2020).

31 *BBC News* (31 July, 2020).

32 GOV.UK (2020). *Cases in United Kingdom: Cases by Specimen Date*. Available at: https://coronavirus.data.gov.uk/details/cases. Accessed: 12/08/2020.

33 Hockaway, J. (2020). 'UK records highest number of new cases in two months as 1,441 test positive'. *Metro*. (14 August).

34 Bland, A. (2020). 'UK records 1,715 Covid cases in largest weekend figure since mid-May'. *Guardian*. (30 August).

35 Hutton, G. (2020). *Eat Out to Help Out Scheme*. London: House of Commons library. Briefing Paper Number CBP 8978. (22 December).

36 *BBC News* (2020). 'Coronavirus: campaign to encourage workers back to offices'. (28 August).

37 *BBC News* (2020). 'Coronavirus: further 2,988 cases confirmed in UK'. (6 September); *BBC News* (2020). 'Coronavirus: Hancock concern over "sharp rise" in cases'. (8 September). Available at: www.bbc.co.uk/news/uk-54066831.

38 *BBC News* (2020). 'Coronavirus: UK "not considering" compulsory face masks in workplaces'. (19 August).

39 Parkinson, J. (2020). Coronavirus: civil servants "must get back to offices quickly"'. *BBC News*. (5 September).

40 *BBC News* (6 September, 8 September, 2020). See also: Rosney, D. (2020). 'Coronavirus: young people breaking rules risk "second wave"'. Interview with Matt Hancock. *BBC News*. (7 September).

41 Murray, J. and Sparrow, A. (2020). 'UK coronavirus: Boris Johnson says, "there have been too many breaches" and warns restrictions could go further'. *Guardian*. (22 September).

42 *BBC News* (2020). 'Coronavirus: UK "on knife edge" ahead of lockdown easing, scientist warns'. (28 June).

43 *BBC News* (2020). 'Coronavirus: "critical moment" as students return to university'. (5 September).

44 SAGE (2020). *Principles for Managing SARS-CoV-2 Transmission Associated With Higher Education*. (3 September). Available at: https://assets.publishing.service.gov.uk/government/uploads/system/uploads/attachment_data/file/914978/S0728_Principles_for_Managing_SARS-CoV-2_Transmission_Associated_with_Higher_Education_.pdf.

45 *BBC News* (2020). 'Covid-19: UK could face 50,000 cases a day by October without action – Vallance'. (21 September).

46 *BBC News* (2020). 'Coronavirus: report "rule of six" breaches, minister urges'. (14 September).

47 Johnson, B. (PM). (2020). *Speech: Prime Minister's Statement on Coronavirus (COVID-19): 28 May 2020.* The Prime Minister's Office. GOV.UK (online). (28 May). Available at: www.gov.uk/government/speeches/pm-press-conference-statement-on-the-five-tests-28-may-2020.

48 Walawalkar, A. (2020). 'Experts call for stronger measures as UK daily coronavirus cases hit four-month high'. *BBC News*. (19 September).

49 *BBC News* (2020). 'Covid: PM considering new restrictions amid second coronavirus wave'. (19 September).

50 *BBC News* (2020). 'Coronavirus: new covid restrictions could last six months, says Boris Johnson'. (22 September).

51 McKie, A. (2020). 'University teaching should stay remote, says Independent Sage'. *Times Higher Education*. (21 August).

52 The Independent Scientific Advisory Group for Emergencies (2020). *Independent SAGE Statement on Universities in the Context of SARS-CoV-2.* Independent SAGE (online). (3 September). Available at: www.independentsage.org/university_final_sept/.

53 Independent SAGE (3 September, 2020).

54 Independent SAGE (2020). *Independent SAGE Emergency Statement on Universities in the Context of Rising SARS-CoV-2 Cases in Late September 2020.* (28 September). Available at: www.independentsage.org/wp-content/uploads/2020/09/Universities-late-Sept-statement-28-9-20-final.pdf.

55 2019/20 saw a total of 2.53 million students studying at university in the UK. Applicant numbers were higher for 20/21 than for 19/20. See: Clark, D. (2021). *Number of Students Enrolled in Higher Education in the United Kingdom from 2009/10 to 2019/20.* Statista (online). (12 June). Available at: www.statista.com/statistics/875015/students-enrolled-in-higher-education-in-the-uk/; UCAS (2021). *Rise in Number of Students Planning to Start University This Autumn.* UCAS (online). (25 June). Available at: www.ucas.com/corporate/news-and-key-documents/news/rise-number-students-planning-start-university-autumn.

56 *BBC News* (2020). 'Coronavirus: university return "could spark Covid avalanche". (30 August).

57 Thus, Professor Carl Heneghan, Director of the Centre for Evidence-Based Medicine at the University of Oxford, was happy to report to the BBC that "right now it is as safe as it ever has been" to go back to campuses (*BBC News*, 30 August, 2020).

58 Hall, R. (2003). 'From student grants to tuition fees'. *Guardian*. (23 January).

59 *BBC News* (1999). 'Teaching and higher education act'. (6 May).

60 *BBC News* (2004). 'Blair wins key top-up fees vote'. (27 January). Available at: http://news.bbc.co.uk/1/hi/uk_politics/3434329.stm.

61 The Public Whip (2010). *University Tuition Fee Cap – Raise Upper Limit to £9,000 Per Year.* The Public Whip (online). (9 December). Available at: www.publicwhip.org.uk/division.php?date=2010-12-09&number=150.

62 Attwood, R. (2010). 'Russell group: if you want the best, the cap must go'. *Times Higher Education*. (18 March).

63 Mueller, B. (2020). 'It really was abandonment: virus crisis grips British universities'. *New York Times*. (6 October).

64 *BBC News* (30 August, 2020).

65 Mueller (2020).

66 UniCovid UK (2020). *Tracking Covid-19 at U.K. Universities.* UniCovid UK (online). Available at: https://unicovid.uk/. Accessed: 24/01/2021.

67 Vusirikala, A., Whitaker, H., Jones, S., Tessier, E., Borrow, R., Linley, E., Hoschler, K., Baawuah, F., Ahmad, S., Andrews, N., Ramsay, M., Ladhani, S.N., Brown, K.E. and Amirthalingam, G. (2021). *Seroprevalence of SARS-CoV-2 Antibodies in University Students: Cross-Sectional Study, December 2020, England.* Public Health England (online). Available at: https://papers.ssrn.com/sol3/papers.cfm?abstract_id=3787684. https://deliverypdf.

ssrn.com/delivery.php?ID=15511902106907411211711511500510901100005604100407903401112012309108311302508901010600502602403011706304408910408007808202301802905904306405512008211906710410810901904902005302312311408110200106912410309301000010812112611401910400300507710412309412600880EXT=pdf&INDEX=TRUE

68 Adams, R. (2020). 'Williamson sets out plan to allow students in England home for Christmas'. *Guardian.* (29 September).

69 Oddly, there does not seem to be any research conducted that estimates the number of students who deserted campuses before the November 5 month-long lockdown.

70 Merrick, R. and Tidman, Z. (2020). 'University students to go home for Christmas as soon as lockdown ends'. *Independent.* (11 November); Quinne, B. and Weale, S. (2020). 'Covid: England students to get six-day window to get home before Christmas'. *Guardian.* (11 November).

71 Weale, S. (2020). 'Reopening schools: what is happening in England'? *Guardian.* (9 June).

72 DfE (2020). *Schools and Colleges to Reopen in Full in September.* Press release. (2 July). Available at: www.gov.uk/government/news/schools-and-colleges-to-reopen-in-full-in-september.

73 GOV.UK (2020), Accessed: 15/11/2020.

74 National Archives (2020). *The Health Protection (Coronavirus, Restrictions) (Leicester) Regulations 2020.* Legislation.GOV.UK (online). (4 July). Available at: www.legislation.gov.uk/uksi/2020/685/contents/made.

75 *BBC News* (2020). 'Coronavirus: Boris Johnson "does not want second national lockdown"'. (19 July).

76 Halliday, J. and Pidd, H. (2020). 'Local lockdowns failing to stop Covid spread in England, experts warn'. *Guardian.* (22 September).

77 Public Health England (2021). *Coronavirus (COVID-19) in the UK.* GOV.UK (online). Available at: https://coronavirus.data.gov.uk/. See data under "Cases" and "Deaths". Accessed: 09/06/2021.

78 Gallagher, J. (2020). 'Testing and tracing "key to schools returning", scientists say'. *BBC News.* (4 August).

79 Stott, C. (2020). *Localised Lifting.* SAGE report (0235). [Redacted]. (23 April). Available at: https://assets.publishing.service.gov.uk/government/uploads/system/uploads/attachment_data/file/888746/6b._Localised_lifting_S0235_Redacted.pdf.

80 Stott (2020).

81 McCoid, S. (2020). 'Refusing Tier 3 restrictions is "not an option" says Mayor Steve Rotherham'. *Liverpool Echo.* (13 October); Pidd, H. and Halliday, J. (2020). '"It's all about putting the blame on us": Lancashire's reluctant path to tier 3 deal'. *Guardian.* (16 October).

82 Smith, C. (2020). *Local Lockdowns: The Legislative Framework in England.* UK Parliament: House of Commons Library. Available at: https://lordslibrary.parliament.uk/local-lockdowns-the-legislative-framework-in-england/

83 *BBC News* (2020). 'Covid-19: fewer than 0.1% fined for no masks on trains'. (26 September).

84 Nice, A. and Hogarth, R. (2020). *Coronavirus: Local Lockdowns.* Institute for Government (online). (5 October). Available at: www.instituteforgovernment.org.uk/explainers/coronavirus-local-lockdowns.

85 *BBC News* (2020). 'Covid: Boris Johnson tells of "dashboard warnings" over rise in cases'. (12 October); Heffer, G. (2020). 'Coronavirus: Boris Johnson confirms new three-tier system of local lockdowns for England'. *Sky News.* (12 October); Walker, P., Elgot, J. and Pidd, H. (2020). 'Boris Johnson unveils three-tier Covid restrictions for England'. *Guardian.* (12 October).

86 Walker et al. (2020).

87 Heffer, G. (2020). 'Coronavirus: Professor Chris Whitty says Tier 3 rules 'not sufficient' on their own to limit COVID-19'. *Sky News.* (12 October).

88 Campbell, L. and Sparrow, A. (2020). 'UK coronavirus: Chris Whitty warns tier 3 measures alone "not enough to get on top" of spread'. *Guardian*. (12 October).

89 SAGE (2020). *SAGE 58 Minutes: Coronavirus (COVID-19) Response, 21 September 2020*. GOV.UK (online). (12 October). Available at: www.gov.uk/government/publications/fifty-eighth-sage-meeting-on-covid-19-21-september-2020.

90 Jagger, D. (2020). 'Government rejects Covid "circuit breaker" lockdown'. *Telegraph and Argus*. (19 October).

91 Public Health England (2021), Accessed: 04/04/2021.

92 Merseyside was placed from the outset in the highest tier. Scott, E. (2020). *Covid-19 Local Alert Levels: Three-Tier System for England*. London: UK Parliament, House of Lords Library.

93 Thompson, M., Liakos, C. and Ziady, H. (2020). 'UK crashes into deepest recession of any major economy'. *CNN News*. (12 August).

94 *BBC News* (2020). 'Covid-19: PM announces four-week England lockdown'. (31 October).

95 *BBC News* (2021). 'Covid: Boris Johnson's "bodies pile high" comments prompt criticism'. (26 April); Colson, T. (2021). 'Boris Johnson witnesses say they will swear on oath he said he'd "let the bodies pile high in their thousands"'. *Business Insider*. (27 April); Walters, S. (2021). 'Boris Johnson: "let the bodies pile high in their thousands". PM's incendiary remark during fight over lockdowns is latest claim in No10 drama – amid spectacular row with Cummings'. *Mail*. (25 April); Parsley, D. (2021). 'Boris Johnson made "bodies pile high" comment after "finally" backing second lockdown Dominic Cummings claims'. *I-News*. (26 May).

96 SAGE (2020). *SPI-M-O: Consensus Statement on COVID-19*. SAGE. GOV.UK (online). (14 October). Available at: https://assets.publishing.service.gov.uk/government/uploads/system/uploads/attachment_data/file/931162/S0808_SAGE62_201014_SPI-M-O_Consensus_Statement.pdf.

97 *BBC News* (31 October, 2020).

98 *BBC News* (2020). 'Covid-19: PM sets out "tougher" post-lockdown tiers for England'. (23 November).

99 Elgot, J. (2020). 'The many U-turns on the road to England's third lockdown'. *Guardian*. (4 January).

100 Rayner, T. (2020). 'Coronavirus: Boris Johnson to insist lockdown is time limited as Tory backbench rebellion grows'. *Sky News*. (2 November).

101 Walker, P. (2020). 'Boris Johnson sets out new three-tier system of Covid restrictions for England'. *Guardian*. (23 December).

102 Public Health England (2021), Accessed: 09/06/2021. In fact, caseloads nationally began to rise again before the circuit-breaker ended.

103 Chowdhury, J., Scarr, S., MacAskill, A. and Marshall, A.R.C. (2021). 'Variant of concern'. *Reuters*. (26 March).

104 *BBC News* (2020). 'Covid-19: Three households can mix over Christmas in UK'. (25 November). This decision was apparently brokered between Johnson and the devolved governments in Scotland, Wales, and Northern Ireland.

105 *AOL News* (2020). 'Scientists warn of third wave risk over Christmas bubble plan'. (25 November); *BBC News* (2020). 'Covid Christmas rules: caution urged over household mixing'. (25 November); Davis, N., McIntyre, N. and Duncan, P. (2020). 'Scientists warn against Christmas gatherings in UK despite relaxed rules'. *Guardian*. (11 December); Elgot, J. and Davis, N. (2020). 'UK medical journals call for Christmas Covid rules to be reversed'. *Guardian*. (15 December); Whitehead, J. (2020). 'We may "pay for" Christmas parties with January and February lockdowns, scientists warn'. *I-News*. (12 December).

106 *BBC News* (2020). 'Covid-19: shoppers return to stores under England's new tier system'. (2 December).

107 Blackall, M. (2020). 'Tier 4 Covid rules in England: latest restrictions explained'. *Guardian*. (4 January).

108 Stewart, H. (2020). 'PM announces "tier 4" Covid curbs and curtails Christmas mixing in England'. *Guardian*. (19 December).

109 Duncan, P., Davis, N. and Geddes, L. (2020). 'Half of Britons say they will form a Christmas Covid bubble'. *Guardian*. (18 December).

110 These assurances were given virtually right up until the point they were withdrawn, so that people would have no inkling of what was coming (Elgot, J. (2021). 'Losing "freedom day" is galling for Boris Johnson, but things could get worse'. *The Guardian*. (14 June)).

111 *BBC News* (2020). 'Covid-19: St Pancras crowds "totally irresponsible"'. (20 December); Edmonds, L. (2020). 'Londoners who fled capital ahead of Tier 4 restrictions were "totally irresponsible" says Matt Hancock'. *Evening Standard*. (20 December).

112 *BBC News* (2020). 'Covid-19: tougher Covid rules begin for millions in UK'. (26 December).

113 *BBC News* (2020). 'Covid-19: twenty million in England added to toughest tier of restrictions'. (31 December); Marris, S. (2020). 'COVID-19: three quarters of England will be in Tier 4 from tomorrow as rules extended'. *Sky News*. (31 December).

5
BORDER INSECURITIES

As COVID-19 spread across the borders of China's neighbours in January of 2020, with community outbreaks in Hong Kong, Macau, Taiwan, South Korea, and Singapore, and as the death toll began to mount during February, the UK government placed no border restrictions (let alone travel bans) on foreign travellers from the worst affected zones. This was not even to and from Wuhan in Hubei province in China, from where the virus originated.[1] As for British returnees, the prudent safety-first course was to test and quarantine them on arrival. Not only did this not happen, but there was very little debate or discussion on whether or not it should happen.

This inactivity was almost certainly legitimized by the remarkably tepid response of the Government's scientific advisers to the issue of border defence. SAGE did not hold its first discussion meeting on the pandemic until 22 January. This placed on the agenda discussion of advice from NERVTAG on border security. The minutes indicated that SAGE did not approve or recommend quarantining people from Hubei. Nor did they (or NERVTAG) see any useful purpose in airport screening arrivals from China or anywhere else. This was "irrespective of the current limited understanding of the epidemiology". Why not? "Temperature and other forms of screening are unlikely to be of value and have high false positive and negative rates".[2] This was neither an auspicious start nor an impressive logic. The negatives here were over-emphasized and the benefits were under-played.

In the same vein, the next SAGE gathering of 28 January endorsed the advice of NERVTAG that there was no case for providing border-control personnel who were in close contact with entrees from high-risk countries with basic PPE. This was even though it was accepted that on a "reasonable worst-case scenario" some inbound travellers from China would be infected.[3] The reason for this guidance was unstated, but it was likely to be that any health benefits would be outweighed by the economic costs. There was also, of course, a chronic shortage of PPE,

DOI: 10.4324/9781003275039-6

which may have simply deterred the Government's advisers from recommending its deployment at the border (since the NHS would be prioritized). Perhaps if PPE had been stockpiled, so that there was confidence in the sufficiency of supply, NERVTAG would have advised SAGE differently, and perhaps this advice would have been endorsed.

Border policy January–June 2020

As for the Government's response, this unfolded tardily. It took the FCO until 25 January to change its travel advice for Britons travelling to or from Wuhan. This was from cautioning people against all travel except that which was essential in favour of recommending that they eschew all travel whether essential or not.[4] Nor did the Government instruct border officers to screen inbound people from Wuhan. Two articles in the *Mail* of 23 January drew attention to this. This was more than one-and-a-half months after the first confirmed cases in Hubei province, long after the WHO noted the seriousness and possible international impact of the outbreak, following on from China's Wuhan lockdown. The first of these stated:

> Passengers arriving at Heathrow from the virus-hit Chinese city of Wuhan last night told the *Mail* they had not been subject to any screening. Instead, they were given a Public Health England leaflet, advising them to contact doctors if they felt ill. By contrast, countries including the US, Malaysia and Singapore have introduced more rigorous checks, with all passengers arriving from Wuhan having their temperature taken, regardless of whether they have any symptoms.[5]

The second article reported that the Government was "accused of not doing enough to screen people arriving from infection-hit Wuhan – with Heathrow officials simply handing out one-page leaflets to passengers". This noted that, despite the Government's newly announced intention to conduct airport checks, "there was little sign of these".[6] This piece could also have drawn attention to the fact that the "checking" (i.e. self-reporting and leafleting) was only for arrivals at Heathrow, not other UK airports.

A piece published in the *Telegraph* on 27 January 2020 reported the experience of "Mr. Marland", a returnee from Wuhan, who was, he said, "at no point . . . checked or tested for signs of coronavirus". Having contacted the NHS helpline, Mr Marland was surprised by the response. "Instead of being called in immediately for a test, he says he was asked only if he had 'the sniffles'". When he replied in the negative, "the specialist . . . told him to call back if he started feeling unwell. With that, the conversation was over". Marland resided within five minutes' walk of the Wuhan wet market from where the virus probably originated. Even though it was already known that the incubation period of COVID-19 was at least a week and it was suspected that carriers could be asymptomatic, he was not advised to do any form of physical distancing. As Marland said: "It feels like they are leaving the door open to this thing".[7] Marland was not alone. Hundreds of Britons were at this juncture returning to the UK from Wuhan and passing through the national turnstiles without any checking or monitoring or self-isolation guidance. Indeed, between 10 and 27 January, it was estimated that 1,561 people had entered the UK from Wuhan, of whom only 10 percent were asked to provide an email address or contacted with advice on what they should do if they experienced symptoms.[8]

The Health Secretary, Matt Hancock, eventually announced an update of government guidance for inbound travellers from Wuhan on 27 January.[9] Now returnees were asked to self-isolate even if they showed no symptoms of the virus. This was hardly a quarantine, however, since incoming travellers were not compulsorily detained in special centres or legally required to self-isolate at another location, but were instead asked to voluntarily self-isolate in the community. Only those who said they were unable to self-isolate at home would have access to quarantine facilities on request.[10] Despite the fact that by then the virus had spread right across mainland China, the FCO at that point (28 January) saw fit only to warn UK travellers that they should not travel to China unless this was for essential purposes.[11]

As most other countries started bringing in travel restrictions, starting from January 2020, the UK government requested only that inbound travellers from mainland China call the 111 NHS hotline if they felt unwell. By contrast,

> on 22 January Singapore began to require the 14-day quarantine of all symptomatic arrivals from China. By 29 January it had begun to temperature check all incoming flights, and to deny entry to all arrivals from Hubei province. On 1 February these measures extended to deny entry to anybody who had been in China in the previous 14 days. The following day, the USA similarly banned the arrival of anybody who had been in China during the previous 14 days apart from returning US residents. New Zealand took the same measure on 3 February.[12]

It was not until 7 February that this FCO guidance was amended, so that inbound travellers from other virus hotspots in South Asia were also advised to call in and self-isolate, albeit only if they were experiencing symptoms.[13] This was despite the fact that authorities in Thailand, Japan, South Korea, Hong Kong, Taiwan, Malaysia, and Macau were reporting community outbreaks and were themselves closing their borders to slow the importation of cases to and from their neighbours.

Minutes of the SAGE meeting of 3 February revealed that there was no discussion of the potential efficacy of travel restrictions in lowering infection rates or reducing the number of people who may become ill or die. Instead, discussion was "on how travel restrictions might help give the NHS time to prepare". Since introducing some (unspecified) border controls would likely reduce rather than eliminate imported infections, these were deemed of little value. This was on the grounds that these would be "draconian" and would require "co-ordination", yet would likely delay the pandemic by less than a month, unless these cut imported cases by up to 95 percent.

According to SAGE, "only a month of additional preparation time for the NHS would be meaningful".[14] Although the next SAGE meeting of 4 February acknowledged that "a delay now in the arrival and spread . . . [of COVID-19] . . . would be beneficial for improving NHS readiness and ability to handle cases", the committee nonetheless could not quite agree to recommend the border controls that would deliver the beneficial outcome. Instead, they declared themselves "content with the validity of the statement (issued on 3 February)".[15] SAGE had agreed in the meeting of 3 February to request of the Department of Transport and the Home Office "wide-ranging estimates on people entering the UK from China" to consider at the next meeting.[16] But, if these requests were made, or were actioned, the results were not discussed at the 4 February meeting.

Even FCO guidance on its travel webpage that people should consider avoiding those South Asian countries experiencing community outbreaks, reconsidering their travel plans, was tepid, conveying no sense of urgency, and certainly no element of prescription. All should *consider* changing their plans was the guidance. To travel or not to travel, that was a matter for individuals to decide, based on their own good reasons, or how important they considered their own reasons to be.[17] Nor was there, as we have seen, any routine airport screening or temperature testing of arrivals at UK airports, not from Hubei, or from mainland China, or from neighbouring South Asian countries that were experiencing spikes of community transmissions.[18] So, there could be no quarantining of any inbound travellers who were carrying the virus from any of the then high-risk countries.

On 13 February SAGE was invited to consider new research on the impact of travel restrictions in curbing the transmission of the virus in and from China to overseas in the earlier stages of the outbreak. The conclusions drawn by the authors were that the restrictions had led to a 77 percent "reduction in cases imported from mainland China to other countries" up until mid-February and had restricted most imported cases to "neighbouring countries such as Japan (13.8%), Thailand (13%), and South Korea (11.3%)". Thereafter, the research data showed, "sustained . . . travel restrictions to and from mainland China only modestly affect the epidemic unless combined with a 50% or higher reduction of transmission in the community", at which point "early detection . . . [i.e. track and trace] . . ., hand washing, self-isolation and household quarantine will likely be more effective than travel restrictions at mitigating this pandemic".[19]

What SAGE made of the research is unclear. But there was no modification of its position on border defence. Perhaps this was because the "modest" later benefits impressed the group as more important than the "major" earlier ones. If so, the logic remained elusive. Even modest benefits are real and of significance. And, *of course*, once community transmissions are consolidated anywhere they (rather than imported cases) will account for the bulk of new infections. The point, of course, is that border defence is a way of curtailing the import of infection as far as possible *in the first place*, whereas later community outbreaks if these spiral out of control reflect the failure of these border controls as well as the failure of *other* within-border measures. There is no record of SAGE discussing borders any further from between 6 and 27 February 2020.[20] Therefore, for exactly the period during which research suggested that border and travel restrictions would be most efficacious in reducing the importation of cases, these seemingly became a non-issue for SAGE, just as it was for the Government.

SAGE returned to the matter of border defence in its meeting of 3 March. Its members perused a research paper examining the impact of travel restrictions on the within-borders spread of the virus within China. This found that "measures implemented pre-emptively could reduce cases in the first week of introduction by 37%". Moreover, "had interventions been applied earlier, for example by 3 weeks, the effects would have been greater, leading to a 95% reduction in cases", the study concluded. This SAGE paper referred to other research which

> estimated that earlier pre-emptive measures could have reduced the number of Chinese cities affected from 308 to 61. The paper also referenced a study led by Asami Anzai of Hokkaido University in Japan, which estimated that travel restrictions out of Wuhan prevented 226 cases being exported . . . a reduction in exported cases of 70%.[21]

But this was to no avail. SAGE was apparently unmoved. Minutes from this meeting did not record recommendations relevant to border defence policy, even though the research under scrutiny warranted reappraisal of the UK's open borders.

Thus, as the virus struck Europe in February 2020 – leading to the unfolding human tragedy in Italy, followed by those in Spain and France – the Government stuck doggedly with this open-borders policy. From 25 February, only arrivals from Wuhan, the rest of Hubei in China, from Iran, and from two regions of South Korea (Daegu and Cheongdo) were advised, not legally required, to self-isolate, even if asymptomatic, and to call 111 if they had symptoms. Arrivals from a much larger number of often hard-hit COVID-19 countries (the rest of China beyond Hubei, Hong Kong, Macau, Thailand, Malaysia, Singapore, Vietnam, Taiwan, Cambodia, Laos, Myanmar, Japan, South Korea except Daegu and Cheongdo, and Northern Italy) were advised they should not "undertake any special measures, but if they develop symptoms they should self-isolate and call NHS 111".[22] As reported by the Home Affairs Select Committee:

> These measures focused on the same countries/areas as those taken by other national governments, although the nature of the measures differed: for example, from 28 February Germany required all arrivals from China, South Korea, Japan, Italy and Iran to report their health status before entry. Singapore banned all arrivals from Cheongdo and Daegu in South Korea on 26 February, and New Zealand banned arrivals from Iran on 28 February. South Korea, which had begun screening and quarantining arrivals from Wuhan from 3 January, had by the end of January established 288 screening clinics offering tests and required arrivals from China to undertake quarantine.[23]

These controls were of greater or lesser scope and rigour – but everywhere these were much tighter and tougher than in the UK. Most remarkably, no border restrictions or controls were brought in even to curb people flow back and forth from Italy, the then centre of the European crisis. "In the first three months of the year there were nearly 25 million arrivals into the UK".[24] The vast bulk of these arrivals would be accounted for by the tourist trade, of Britons returning from the EU, with Italy and Spain being especially popular destinations, as well as tourist visitors arriving from the EU, including from Italy and Spain.

Yet the FCO saw it as necessary only to advise Britons travelling to Italy that they should do so only for essential purposes, having failed to raise a concern with the high volumes of tourist traffic between the two countries. This was on 9 March.[25] By then, local community quarantines were in place in many Italian towns (since February's end), whereas schools and universities had been shut down since 4 March. Indeed, the whole of the north of Italy went into lockdown on 8 March.[26] In the same vein, FCO travel advice for Britons bound for Spain was not upgraded to warn against all but essential travel until 15 March.[27] This, again, was lagging far behind the spiralling pandemic in that country, and it was subsequent to the Spanish national lockdown of 14 March 2020.[28]

Nor still was there any policy in evidence of passenger screening or monitoring, not even random or episodic, and not even for incoming passengers from Italy or Spain. It took until 26 February for Hancock to recommend that inbound travellers from the locked-down north of Italy should self-isolate even if they were not feeling unwell, even though it was established that asymptomatic transmission was real.[29] Whereas the WHO was sceptical about the efficacy of travel restrictions, on the grounds that these could deflect governments from other protective measures, and owing to their economic ill-effects, their guidance was clear that governments of affected countries must uphold rigorous airport checks, screen international arrivals, contact-trace, and apply strict quarantine policies. The WHO reiterated this throughout January and February.[30] Yet, according to hundreds of testimonies gathered by Otto English, arrivals to the UK in the first few months of 2020 reported a radical difference between border entry to the UK in comparison with their own countries and others they had visited. This was inasmuch as the UK unlike the others had no temperature checking, or mandatory quarantining, or even guidance on physical distancing. When visitors inquired of border guards if they needed to self-isolate, the reply was that they should do so only if experiencing symptoms. This was the case, according to visitor testimonies, throughout February, March, and into April.[31]

On 26 February Matt Hancock claimed: "We have put in place enhanced monitoring measures at UK airports, and health information is available at all international airports, ports and international train stations".[32] These "enhanced measures" were not in place and nor did they appear thereafter. On 2 March, the Government declared that border controls were pointless, and its *Coronavirus Action Plan* of 3 March made no mention of border defence through travel restrictions. Rather, the March Action Plan simply spoke the language of within-border delay and mitigation. Britain's political leaders remained resolute in their determination to keep the country fully "open for business". By contrast, a dozen EU countries had closed their borders by mid-March 2020, effectively suspending the Schengen visa zone,[33] whereas the EU as a whole closed its borders to all visitors from outside except those on essential business on 17 March.[34]

The UK was, again, out on a limb internationally. The Government simply never did restrict its borders, nor control them, either in the run up to the crisis, or as it unfolded, in those crucial early months of 2020. By contrast, by mid-April, according to research carried out by the Pew Research Center in the USA and by Oxford-based analysts in the UK,[35]

> 130 countries had introduced some sort of travel restrictions since the . . . outbreak began. . . . These include screening, quarantine and bans on travel from high risk areas. As a result, at least 90 per cent of the global population lives in countries with restrictions on non-citizens and non-residents arriving from abroad, while 39 per cent live behind borders that are entirely closed to foreigners. Since then authorities in Japan, China, Germany and elsewhere have tightened or extended travel controls, while many require passengers to be tested.[36]

As Professor of Epidemiology and Public Health at the Royal Society of Medicine, Gabriel Scally, observed: "The UK is an outlier. It is very hard to understand why it persists in having this open border policy. It is most peculiar".[37] Scally was not alone amongst public health experts in his puzzlement. Professor Ian Jones, a leading virologist based at the University of Reading, urged the Government to introduce travel restrictions from China without delay early in February. This was on the grounds that this was a "simple" and "proactive" step to slow the import of the disease to these shores. This message was reiterated in a statement released soon after by several scientists following a meeting convened by the Science Medical Centre.[38]

Officially, the Government's reason for setting itself against such interventions was that these would make no more than an "extremely limited contribution" to limiting the spread of the virus.[39] This was informed by a certain body of scientific opinion and research evidence,[40] though hardly unanimously. Hardly unanimously, not only because this judgement of efficacy was contested, but also because there is a paucity of historical research examining the impact of travel restrictions and other border-protection measures (such as quarantining inbound travellers) on cross-border transmission of infectious diseases. Indeed, the scepticism of certain public health experts about the effectiveness of border defence may reflect an assumption that so-called globalization cannot be reigned in (or should not be reigned in), rather than the odd belief that pandemics can somehow magically cross borders without people carrying them over. This is owing to the economic harms and civil rights restrictions that obstructing "globalization" would generate, so that borders are always porous (or should always be).

Since such controls are antithetical to the sensibilities of neoliberal individualism, or of a consumerist rights culture, certain experts are led by confirmation bias to discover in the ambivalence of the evidence reasons to reject these controls. Sceptical expertise (where this is informed by specific studies) tends to lose sight of something that is hardly hiding in plain sight. This is the fact that where travel restrictions have previously been brought in to deal with the spread of infectious diseases (such as novel influenza) these have been applied with variable stringency and are usually cases of bolting the stable door after the horse has bolted. Travel restrictions, for example, are not as stringent as outright travel bans or closed borders. Quarantining of inbound travellers, for example, will work only if the quarantined are prevented from infecting health staff or are not released prematurely into the community.

On the ministerial logic, because border restrictions and airport temperature screening would not *solve* the crisis (given that these could not *guarantee* against a community outbreak), they were rejected. This was the same rationale for the Government's corresponding refusal to impose internal bans on large-scale gatherings. These were also dismissed by ministers (and apparently by government scientific advisers) because the benefits were seen as moderate ones.[41] According to SAGE's scientific assessment (as PHE told it) of 22 January 2020, temperature screening at the border would be imperfect, since this would detect "only" up to 50 percent of exported cases.[42] This legitimized the Government's inaction thereafter on the basis of supposedly scientific guidance, as ministers chose to interpret the inefficiencies of the practice as simply rendering it as "not effective" (as Emma Moore, Chief Operating Officer of UK Border Force, put it).[43]

As for border defence policies generally, the Government's reading of SAGE's guidance was that because "the number of imported cases was about 0.5% of domestic cases . . . stricter border restrictions earlier on would not have had an impact" on the course or magnitude of the UK pandemic.[44] The problem with this reasoning ought to be obvious. But to state the obvious: *everything counts*.

However, at least some scientific experts close to the Government did not reject border defence policies. Temperature screening and testing of arrivals, for example, were regarded by some as useful. Professor Neil Ferguson of Imperial College London, and also of the SAGE group, described border temperature screening as having "a degree of effectiveness", although "it should not be seen as a panacea". The reason it should not be seen as a panacea, he said, was that temperature screening would not necessarily identify people who were incubating the disease or who were asymptomatic. Nonetheless, it may, he said, pick out some of these, as well as those who were symptomatic – hardly a negligible benefit. The same basic point was made by Professor David Heymann of the London School of Hygiene and Tropical Medicine.[45] Similarly, according to Professor Gabriel Leung of the University of Hong Kong's Ki Ka Shing Faculty of Medicine, although temperature screening was "leaky", it had significantly reduced importations of cases in those countries that introduced it early on in the pandemic. Temperature screening, he said, was effective inasmuch as it operated in the manner of "sentinels to warn us to step up further measures at the border".[46]

The point these experts wished to affirm was not that border defence was pointless but that this would not alone suffice to vanquish the virus. As Scally put it: "Travel restriction is not of course by itself going to do the job . . . But all of these things are additive".[47] In other words, COVID-19 needs to be tackled not by a "magic bullet", but by a rafter of protective measures, layered onto each other, which would include border protections. Even if the benefits of a thoroughgoing and timely border-control policy were small, in relation to the whole package of measures, they would still be benefits. The strength or efficacy of public health defence policy hinges not on single policies but on the whole package of measures.

A meta-review of 23 different studies of the effect of travel restrictions on the cross-border transmission of influenza has found that these did reduce its spread, albeit by only 3 percent. But a study of the impact of travel restrictions in damping down on the cross-border spread of the Ebola outbreak originating in West Africa in 2014 found that these did slow its progress by several weeks.[48] This was even though in most of these cases the border controls were neither timely nor thoroughgoing and consequently were less impactful than was possible. Such may be considered a major gain since this would allow significantly longer time for public health authorities to prepare for an outbreak. Of more immediate relevance, a study of the Chinese government's Wuhan travel ban found that this slowed COVID-19's spread to mainland China by 3–5 days, even though by then "most Chinese cities had already received many infected travellers", so that its effectiveness was diminished by virtue of lateness. The Wuhan lockdown also reduced the international importation of cases by almost 80 percent up until mid-February 2020.[49]

The UK was particularly well placed to implement a border-control policy owing to its paucity of land borders (excepting the one between the Irish Republic and Northern Ireland) with other countries. The countries of the EU did not have this advantage. By contrast, after the Wuhan outbreak spiralled, another island country, the Philippines, moved swiftly to bring in air travel lockdowns – not only for travel to and from China, but also to and from other virus hotspots, such as Hong Kong, Macau, Taiwan, and South Korea. Indeed, it was one of the first to do so. Not only were aggressive border restrictions brought in, but also systematic airport screening and quarantining. Consequently, for six weeks after the first confirmed case in the Philippines (on 20 January 2020),[50] the number of infections in the country scarcely moved, just as transmission escalated rapidly in neighbouring countries that did not act as swiftly, with the first fatality not occurring until 2 February.[51] The number of confirmed cases in the Philippines was, right up until 6 March, almost static, just three in total, with each of these rooted out by energetic contact-tracing and quarantining, despite the fact that the government could draw only on limited resources for testing and tracing.[52] In the end, there was a community breakout in the country, the source of which was a traveller from Japan – a country which was not added to the list of countries on the travel-ban list.[53] Nonetheless, the Philippines' example showed that a border-defence policy was perfectly feasible.

The Philippines' example was not any kind of international anomaly. In June, the Home Affairs Select Committee, when reviewing the Government's first-wave pandemic performance, "took evidence from experts from Hong Kong, Singapore and New Zealand on measures taken in their respective countries, all of which adopted stricter approaches to the border than the UK, and much earlier".[54] These public health experts reported to the committee that the timely implementation of compulsory quarantining and travel restrictions would have been effective in protecting the UK from importing the virus, since these policies had undoubtedly protected their own countries.

Confronted with the Home Office's claim that only half a percent of the UK's pandemic caseload could be traced to overseas sources, thereby invalidating a border defence policy, Professor Ying (of the Hock School of Public Health based at the National University of Singapore) was incredulous:

> In a country like Singapore, essentially all our cases are the result of importations. Be it secondary, tertiary or subsequent chains, I see this as crucial. When we start thinking of figures like 0.5% it grossly underestimates the impact of importation risk because everyone who comes in will seed additional clusters, and each member within that cluster will go on, and then it's the dangerous nature of Covid-19 being so infectious. . . . I would hesitate to put much faith in that figure of 0.5% – is it the only primary chain of infections? All the infections will be attributed to importations.[55]

These judgements were endorsed by the other public health experts reporting to the Select Committee. According to Professor Leung,

> around the world, the places that have imposed border restrictions earlier on have tended to come out much better with local outbreaks. . . . If you had imposed border restrictions earlier on that picture would have looked quite different.

Similarly, epidemiologist Professor David Skegg (of the University of Otago in New Zealand) reported to the MPs that

> border measures would be most effective if they had been done very early. As with New Zealand, all these [UK] cases were imported. This disease did not originate in the UK. It would have been much more effective if you'd done this in February.[56]

Reviewing this evidence, the Select Committee concluded that the Government had "in the early phase" of the pandemic placed "insufficient emphasis . . . on the importance of controlling importation from overseas as a method for containing the virus or delaying its spread". Moreover, its chief scientific advisers had effectively sanctioned this particular case of British exceptionalism by dismissing as "draconian" the border control policies that were being phased in by other countries. As the committee put it:

> The decision by SAGE only to consider measures that could deliver a full month's delay to the spread of the virus was a mistake and it is very hard to understand why that approach was taken. Additive measures that could have contributed to more effective containment should have been considered, and delays even of a few days alongside the introduction of other domestic measures such as social distancing and lockdown could have had a significant impact on the scale of the outbreak in the UK.[57]

Remarkably, SAGE's dismissal of border defence (or at least of those border defence measures that it discussed) was not based on scientific facts. There is no evidence from the minutes of SAGE meetings that the group took upon itself the task of collating and analysing research data that would illuminate the efficacy of the border defence measures being introduced in vanguard territories or countries such as Hong Kong, New Zealand, Singapore, or the Philippines. Just three papers exploring the impact of travel restrictions were considered and none were relevant to these countries.

Nor indeed is there evidence from the record that SAGE was drawing on the knowledge of pandemic management of those countries that have experience of successfully suppressing major viral outbreaks of life-threatening diseases (e.g. MERS, SARS), nor indeed drawing on knowledge of COVID-19 itself from those countries that had experienced outbreaks before the UK and which were developing policies based on this knowledge. This peculiar insularity would explain why SAGE appears to have assumed (erroneously) that COVID-19 would unfold in the manner of an influenza pandemic.[58] This in turn likely informed the committee's judgement that delay and mitigation rather than suppression (including by radical border defence) was the preferable course of action.

The crucial failing of the ministerial response, however, was not delays in protecting the UK's borders from arrivals from the South Asian hotspots, or indeed in maintaining weak border defences generally throughout the period from the start of the pandemic up until June 2020. Rather, the crucial mistake was its failure to limit or monitor access to the UK from the worst-hit EU countries since February of that year. It was this aspect of the open borders that was destined to be the major importer of the virus to these shores. Even though, as we have seen, arrivals from Hubei and from hard-hit parts of South Korea were eventually requested to self-isolate starting in February, the Government acted as if it was oblivious to the threat of importing the virus from visiting nationals of European countries (or from returning Britons infected in these countries) – initially from Italy and Spain, latterly from France and Germany. Yet it was these countries that posed the greater threat of virus importation owing to the sheer volume of cross-border travel between them.

Italy was not placed on the quarantine list (whereby arrivals would be asked to self-quarantine for 14 days) until far too late. Spain never was placed on that list at all throughout the first wave. Nor, indeed, was France, even though the country followed hot on the heels of Spain in seeing caseloads spill out of control, forcing the country into nationwide lockdown. And so, during a period when arrivals from Vietnam, Taiwan, Thailand, and Singapore were subject to non-mandatory restrictions,

> arrivals from Spain, France and Germany remained subject to no specific precautionary guidance despite the clearly significant and increasing numbers of infections in those countries. Furthermore, while data is not publicly available on a daily or weekly basis, Civil Aviation Authority figures show that, during February and March 2020, 3,482,702 people travelled between UK and Spanish airports, 1,305,441 between the UK and France and 1,401,837 between the UK and Germany. By comparison, 190,170 people travelled between the UK and Singapore, 136,068 between the UK and Thailand, and 23,861 between the UK and Vietnam.[59]

As if to compound the error, the UK government then, on 13 March, retracted the limited self-isolation advice it had been offering to arrivals from all high-risk countries – including from Italy.[60] Consequently, the prospect that arrivals from the new European hotspots (especially Spain and France) would be subject to guidance in some shape or form evaporated. This peculiar decision (which was not apparently informed by SAGE advice since there are no minutes referring to discussion of the matter between 3 and 23 March 2020) meant that there were no border defence controls at all from anywhere in operation from that date right up until 8 June. Screening and testing of arrivals, and self-isolation of asymptomatic arrivals from high-risk destinations, having hardly got started, was ditched. The Government offered no explanation for this "highly unusual" U-turn (as the sub-committee put it).[61] This was implemented just as other countries were radically tightening their borders.[62]

Retrospectively, the Government's rationale was justified by the Health Secretary on the grounds that escalating virus transmission within the UK rendered border defence from outsider infections inefficacious, especially in the context of falling numbers of entrees from overseas.[63] This was claimed to be based on scientific advice that was updated almost daily. Yet several requests by the Select Committee (nine in total from 23 March up until 1 July 2020) for ministers to release for scrutiny this scientific guidance that informed the decision were ignored.[64] This is strongly indicative that there was no such guidance. Instead, bizarrely, ministers presented SAGE's deliberations of 23 March as support for the Government's reversion to "borderless Britain". This was even though this was ten days after the Government's decision was made and was not about the efficacy of border protections *per se*.[65] Rather, in that meeting, SAGE opined that restricting flights from France, Italy, and Germany at that point would have very little impact on the UK pandemic because these countries did not have higher caseloads than the UK and importations from overseas would be just a fraction of the UK caseload.[66]

This was a remarkable rendition of the numbers game in the service of the misuse of statistics to support a do-nothing policy. As Priti Patel, the Home Secretary explained,

> there is no need to enforce additional self-isolation requirements on those entering the UK. The scientific advice is very clear that doing so at this time would not have any significant impact on epidemic progression in the UK. The same social distancing rules apply to new arrivals into the UK as apply to the population as a whole, and, in particular, anyone developing symptoms will be required to self-isolate. The number of imported cases is a very small percentage of current cases in the UK, and incoming travellers from other countries which are also experiencing Covid-19 epidemics do not present a significant additional risk.[67]

The peculiar "logic" deployed here may be summarized as follows. Since caseloads in the UK from domestic transmission were high and increasing rapidly, so that the proportion of total cases attributable to importation from overseas was declining sharply relative to the total caseload, there was simply no point in border protection measures. But, of course, even if the percentage of total cases attributable to importations was low, this may add up to thousands of new cases being brought in from overseas, especially from virus hotspots. Such was a likely scenario owing to the high number of entrees. Despite a major drop in the number of arrivals, owing to travel restrictions elsewhere, there were still a million people entering the UK in the ten days before the 24 March 2020 lockdown. Hundreds of thousands more would enter the UK before mid-April.

With health services struggling to cope with rising domestically generated caseloads, the importation of additional cases could only add to the burden and worsen the impact of the pandemic. The Government's major stated goal of its March Action Plan was at that point (before mid-March) to delay the spread of the virus in order to ease pressure on the NHS in advance of the spring. Obviously, tightening up the UK's borders would have been consistent with this strategy whereas abolishing entry restrictions manifestly was not. Not only that, by eschewing all border controls, the Government also ran the risk of importing potentially more infectious new variants into the UK. This danger did not appear to register on ministerial thinking at all.

Now, suppose it were true that only 0.5 percent of total UK cases up to that point (before 13 March 2020) were attributable directly to importations. This figure was presented by SAGE and it was used to legitimize the Government's laissez-faire approach to border security. But, even if the 0.5 percent figure were correct, these were still cases that needed to be dealt with by the NHS, and which the service would have avoided dealing with if protective measures at the border were in place. As Professor David Skegg of the University of Toronto pointed out, policymakers ought to consider the actual *number* of imported cases as a matter of importance when considering the efficacy of border restrictions, not simply the *proportion* of imported cases relative to total infections.[68] And what of all the domestic cases that were attributable *indirectly* to importation? This happened to be all of them. COVID-19 did not originate in the UK.

It is also important to note that the 0.5 percent figure is highly contentious and scientifically disputed for four good reasons at least. First, this was seemingly linked to estimates of the median population prevalence rate worldwide rather than the prevalence rate for hotspots.[69] Second, as the Select Committee pointed out, this 0.5 percent figure "was not calculated until 22 March".[70] This is significant because before then the percentage of the UK caseload that was directly attributable to importations would have been considerably higher. Between 13 and 22 March, the UK pandemic took off, with a huge spike of domestically transmitted infections. During that period, the proportion of importations in the caseload total would have fallen sharply very quickly.

Thirdly, and more tellingly, the 0.5 percent calculation of the relative contribution of imported cases to the UK pandemic's first wave appears almost scientifically meaningless. This is because it is unclear what should be counted as among infections from importations. As Professor Teo Yik Ying explains,

> if I enter the UK today and I am infected I could spread it on to perhaps five other contacts around me, and those five other contacts could go and spread on to other people, perhaps another five each, so that will be 25 or 30 people in total. Are all 30 people attributed to me or is it only the first initial five? . . . I see this to be absolutely crucial because when we start to think about figures like 0.5% it will grossly underestimate the impact of importation risk, because [for] everyone that comes in we will perhaps see additional clusters.[71]

Finally, the 0.5 percent figure is simply arbitrary in another sense. This is because it can be related only to a specific date in the course of the pandemic beyond which border (and indeed within-border) defences were undone, so that local infections rapidly outstripped imported ones. But it was precisely the inadequacy of border defences that led to this situation. Hence, the 0.5 percent "argument" is merely tautological. As Professor Scally elucidates:

> the figure of 0.5% is used quite widely – and I must admit that I get quite confused, because it seems to me to be quite imprecise as to what exactly people are talking about. Clearly, at some point in this epidemic, it was 100% of cases that had been imported. That, for me, is the important thing. We should not regard it as, because we failed to contain it inside the country, there is no point in stopping new cases. . . . In my view, every single opportunity should have been taken to detect cases and stop transmission. That includes border control and the importation of fresh cases from abroad.[72]

The Government's other retrospective justification for ditching border defence altogether from 13 March 2020 was that border controls were superseded by the piecemeal phasing in from mid-March of within-border measures in accordance with the March Action Plan as it shifted the UK's response from its contain stage to its delay and mitigate stages.[73] Yet these within-border restrictions were even less stringent than the cross-border ones placing requirements on arrivals that they replaced. The UK lockdown was still ten days away. Prior to that, physical distancing guidance was tardy, weak and ambivalent. "Advice to stay at home applied only to those households with a suspected case . . . and was not legally enforceable for another 13 days".[74] The wholly predictable result was that

> thousands of new infections were brought in from Europe in the ten days between the withdrawal of guidance and the introduction of lockdown on 23 March [2020] . . . even though the overall number of people arriving in the UK was decreasing. . . . Evidence shows it is highly likely that uncontrolled importations of the virus from European countries contributed to the rapid increase in the spread of the virus in mid-March, and the overall scale of the outbreak in the UK. . . . Border measures in the UK were lifted rather than extended on 13 March at a time when the number of infections being imported from abroad was still rising. . . . The . . . failure to have any special border measures during this period was a serious mistake that significantly increased both the pace and the scale of the epidemic in the UK.[75]

Reflecting on the impact of the UK's open-border policy from the start of the pandemic until the introduction of more stringent controls after 8 June 2020, Neil Ferguson estimated there was a high likelihood that nine-tenths of case importations of the virus into the UK in this period were not picked up owing to the absence of checking or screening controls at the border or self-isolation of arrivals.[76] These were largely importations from the EU.

A genome sequencing study conducted by epidemiologists from Oxford University, Edinburgh University and the COVID-19 Genomics UK Consortium (COG.UK) examined the origin of case importations from the start of the pandemic up until 8 June 2020. This calculated "that nearly a third of importation lineages were from Spain, with a further 43% from Italy and France". By contrast, only 0.008 percent of imported cases were from China. The study also found that most importations of the disease took place in March, this peaking at 900 a day on 15 March after border restrictions were abolished.[77] Professor Annelies Wilder-Smith, of the London School of Hygiene and Tropical Medicine, estimated that at least 1,000 infected persons and likely as many as 10,000 (from a million entrees overall) crossed into the UK between 13–23 March 2020.[78] The bulk of these were from Spain, since Italy by then was in lockdown.[79]

Border policy June 2020–July 2021

Johnson's government eventually enacted a border defence policy of some stringency in the summer of 2020. The PM gave advance notice of this in his address to the nation of 10 May.[80] On 8 June compulsory quarantining of virtually all international arrivals (for a period of 14 days) was introduced with £1,000 fines for quarantine violators.[81] From the perspective of the need for rational public health protection, this was a welcome, if radically overdue, response. Yet this policy shift was manifestly inconsistent with the Government's earlier rationalizations for eschewing border controls and its ditching of even the limited restrictions that were belatedly introduced. Earlier controls were rejected or abandoned on the grounds that indigenous transmission was outstripping imported cases. But, in the run-up to 8 June, caseloads, hospitalizations and deaths were also much higher in the UK than in the EU countries (which opted for earlier and longer lockdowns), just as they were in the majority of south Asian countries (including all of the former hotspots), and indeed in much of the developed and developing world generally.[82]

Moreover, although the new border controls were certainly far tougher than any of their predecessors, they remained far looser and therefore much less efficacious than those of other countries. The new restrictions would not apply to arrivals by sea or rail, it was initially proposed, though this was later revised.[83] This peculiar exemption was apparently agreed in a private telephone conversation between Johnson and French president Emmanuel Macron.[84] Travel bans or controls (except for returning nationals or residents) were rejected because these would stifle the recovery of the tourism and aviation industries. In the absence of such restrictions, there were no actual quarantine centres to cater for foreign nationals. And so entrees from any country irrespective of its pandemic situation would be free to use public transport to find their way from airports to their destinations – although government advice was that all arrivals should use private transport. Nor was there any systematic or rigorous monitoring of compliance with quarantine rules; random spot checks (by means of telephone calls) would cover just 1 percent of arrivals.[85]

This was hardly a robust disincentive for non-compliance as lockdown restrictions were downscaled in the summer of 2020 and as people were encouraged or pressurized to return to their workplaces. This was perhaps especially true of tourists from overseas who were hardly likely to be motivated to travel to these shores in order to lock themselves away in a hotel or guest house for two weeks. Under such circumstances, the case for entry port screening and testing of arrivals ought to have been manifest. Other countries – such as Iceland, Singapore, Hong Kong, and South Korea – were at this time combining rigorous at-the-border testing with quarantine and other safeguards. But entrees to the UK were reportedly surprised to discover that no monitoring (not even temperature screening) was in place at the arrival ports. Not only that, although arrivals were required on entry to fill out passenger locator forms stating their UK addresses, they were not asked to provide evidence of their residential arrangements.[86] There were 194,900 arrivals in the UK during June 2020. This was a higher volume of entrees than in April or May.[87] It is probable that plenty of COVID-19-infected persons passed through the national turnstiles in the period from 8 June until the quarantine policy was phased out at the start of July.

Travel corridors

Compulsory quarantine was replaced by the policy of travel corridors on 6 July 2020,[88] having been announced by the Government on 29 June. Countries with lower rates of COVID-19 transmission than the UK and stable caseloads were to be classed as low-risk places and green-flagged. Those with comparable levels of COVID-19 transmission were to be classed as medium risk and amber-flagged. The placing of countries on the listings was to be determined by two factors: (1) the national infection prevalence rate and (2) the direction of travel in terms of caseload numbers, including at local levels.[89]

Red-flagged countries were those where infection rates were considered out of control because these were rising and were significantly higher than in the UK. People were permitted to travel to and from green-flagged countries (i.e. those which were deemed as lesser risk owing to having lower rates of infection than in the UK) without having to self-isolate on entry to the UK. Entrees from amber-flagged countries would still have to quarantine for two weeks. Travel to and from red-flagged countries was lawful but was subject to 14-day quarantine and was expected to be only for essential purposes. As before, it was a matter for the aspirant traveller to decide whether or not his or her travel was essential. Quarantine hotels were promised for those who could not organize their own self-isolation, but these did not materialize.

Travel corridors were intended to open up especially short-haul tourism (since most EU countries were green-flagged from 10 July, despite variable rates of transmission), though longer-haul travel to or from many destinations was possible. As such, these were not so much intended as a more nuanced or precise system of border protection than blanket quarantines, even though this was how ministers presented them, and these were welcomed as such by leisure and travel industry bosses. Rather, travel corridors were intended as a substantially weaker system of control, in order to incentivize cross-border commerce and consumerism.

This was implicit in Transport Secretary Grant Shapps's press briefing of 3 July 2020 explaining and commending the new policy. This was titled "Self-isolation lifted for lower risk countries in time for holidays this summer". Holidaying opportunities were extolled therein as "good news for the British people and great news for British business".[90] This incentivization of overseas travel was a success, with holiday bookings reported by operators as skyrocketing in response to the easing of restrictions.[91] Yet these travel corridors were introduced during a period when the pandemic was growing internationally – as it was from its December 2019 origins right up to July 2020's end, before briefly levelling out, then renewing its ascent. In mid-June, the daily new international caseload was 128,601 on the official count. By mid-July, this had almost doubled, to 254,165.[92]

Thus, all of the weaknesses of the previous policy and its implementation were preserved. To these weaknesses was added that of lack of transparency regarding decisions over which countries were to be green-listed, amber-listed or indeed red-listed. This was noted by the Parliamentary Select Committee in its fifth report (on border control measures) of 30 July 2020.[93] But this opacity of ministerial decision-making on the issue has remained right up to the time of writing of this chapter (17 July 2021) – and this was destined to further diminish the efficacy of border defence.

Now people could freely enter the UK without COVID-19 testing at the border (or indeed advance testing in the country of origin), and in the overwhelming majority of cases without any monitoring or checking for the virus thereafter. Given the Government's failure to operationalize a functioning contact track-and-trace system, this policy posed major risk of significant levels of importations of cases that would fuel within-border transmissions. The benefits of green-list travel corridors were, ostensibly, for entrees from any country with a lower rate of transmission than the UK. But, at the time, the UK had a higher transmission rate than most of the developed world, so that the risk of importing significant numbers of infected even from green-listed places was hardly negligible. As David Skegg pointed out, facilitating people congestion on commercial flights (where the air supply could only be recirculated internally) and in airports, ferry terminals and national public tourist hotspots was in any case at odds with physical distancing. For Gabriel Scally, swapping around imports and exports of the infectious did not "seem to be a great idea under any circumstances".[94]

In July 2020, 1,260,400 people travelled from overseas to the UK – either inbound tourists or returning holidaymakers. In August, this increased, by almost two-and-a-half times, to 3,106,500.[95] Public health experts and scientists had cautioned ministers against a speedy return to mass-market travel and tourism, for obvious reasons, to no avail.[96] Professors Leung and Ying for example, expressed their reservations in evidence they gave to the Select Committee on border controls. Mass-market international travel was "obviously" incompatible with a policy of trying to suppress the virus, they said. Singapore, Ying pointed out, had opened travel corridors only for business travellers, not for holidaymakers or those travelling for personal or family reasons.[97]

The Government was unmoved. In September 2020, Boris Johnson rejected at-the-border testing of arrivals on the grounds that this would provide a "false sense of security" that importations of the virus would be significantly reduced by such a measure. This would, he opined, detect only 7 percent of the incoming COVID-19 cases.[98] Also in September, Dominic Rabb, Foreign Secretary, was dismissive of Shadow Home Secretary Nick Thomas-Symonds' recommendation that ministers ought to introduce a "robust testing regime" for entrees from amber-listed or red-listed countries whereby they would be tested at the entry port prior to quarantining and then tested again five days later before being cleared for release.[99] Rabb's logic of dismissal was a familiar one – since this was deployed by ministers throughout the pandemic to gainsay virtually every public protection measure. Twice-testing was, he opined, "no silver bullet" for stopping the importation of new cases, since this would detect only 10 percent of cases of infection at the border. Rabb did not comment on how many cases of infection he thought would be picked up by the second test. Nor did he reveal the sources informing his radically negative judgement of the efficacy of merely on-arrival testing.

As for Johnson's "false security" claim, the sensible reply to that would be to simply question how such a claim could possibly be made with confidence. Why would not ramping up border defence encourage people to take more seriously the danger of cross-border importations? Why could not the public be educated that at-the-border testing was no magic bullet? The obvious riposte to Rabb's (and Johnson's) rationalizations would be to point out that making pre-departure testing a condition of entry to the UK, in addition to on-arrival screening and later follow-up testing, would majorly add to the robustness of the UK's border defences. And, in any case, why was it not worthwhile to prevent 7–10 percent of importations? Surely that was better than preventing none. Other countries were, of course, beginning to impose pre-departure testing requirements on would-be entrees. And, in due course, this was to become the international norm.

Infection rates in the UK had stopped falling and had levelled out by mid-June 2020 in the aftermath of the first wave. They were soon to renew their upward movement owing to the unlocking of restrictions.[100] Yet September and October combined saw almost 4.5 million international travellers enter the UK.[101] Importation of large numbers of infections from overseas was thus inevitable in this period, and this undoubtedly made a significant contribution to the second wave that would eventually force ministers to take the country back into lockdown in November of that year. Renewal of mass tourism travel was also high risk for the importation of new variants of concern – such as the more transmissible South African (Beta) variant. This variant was discovered in its country of origin in October 2020 but had been spreading locally since August. Although cases of the South African variant were not detected in the UK until 22 December 2020, it is entirely possible that it was exported to the UK before it was discovered in its place of origin.[102]

The Government implemented the second "circuit-breaker" lockdown starting on 5 November as caseloads spiralled and threatened again to overload the NHS. Remarkably, however, despite the gravity of the domestic situation, the Government persisted with its open travel corridors and traffic-light listing system rather than switching back to a mass quarantine policy. As Boris Johnson put it, come what may, "Britain should not cut itself off from the world".[103] In November 690,000 travellers entered UK borders, whereas in December it was 895,000. The brevity of the second lockdown (which was ended on 2 December) ensured that the virus was insufficiently suppressed to choke off the second wave, or to prevent this rapidly transitioning into a bigger third wave. Consequently, a third (this time prolonged) lockdown was inevitable, this one commencing on 5 January 2021, as ministers could no longer resist the conclusion that this was necessary in order to protect the NHS from unmanageable caseload volumes. Yet the travel corridors remained firmly intact, and there were a further 631,500 arrivals on UK shores in January 2021.[104]

The Government even attempted to further boost the volume of cross-border travel by introducing a scheme in mid-December 2020 whereby entrees from non-green listed countries could swap the 14-day quarantine for a five-day one by paying for a single test from a private provider on the fifth day of their stay in the UK.[105] This scheme was manifestly at odds with their earlier stated reasons for rejecting Thomas-Symonds' five-day quarantine plan. This also cast into doubt why ten- or 14-day quarantines and attendant testing (which were the international norm) were even necessary. As such, the scheme encouraged public scepticism over the utility of such restrictions, which travel industry bosses were happy to mobilize.

Not only that, the new scheme obviously discriminated against lower-income travellers, especially if these were in family groups, owing to the cost of the commercial testing (up to £120 per person). Such could only incentivize returnees to evade quarantine by making travel arrangements that masked red-listed or amber-listed destinations so that re-entry to the UK was via green-listed transit countries that could be presented as destination countries. Consequently, this period saw the import of another variant of concern, the Brazilian (Gamma) variant. This was seen as being as potentially dangerous as the locally grown Kent variant that was driving the UK's second and third waves owing to its higher levels of infectiousness compared to most strains.

Brazil, like the UK, was a country that was high risk for factory-producing dangerous variants, owing to the failure of its government to suppress caseloads. President Jair Bolsonara committed the country, virtually from the outset, to a radical herd immunity strategy of "managing" the virus, in order to keep the economy fully open for business. Bolsonara refused to endorse a national lockdown or local lockdowns, or to legally mandate physical distancing, or to close or limit borders, or to support internal or cross-border travel restrictions. At the same time, home-working, mask-wearing, and quarantining received no official government backing and was actively discouraged. Bolsonara himself refused to wear a mask and urged supporters not to do so on the grounds that masks offered no protection from the virus. Mask-wearing was, he said, the last taboo to be broken. He also declared that he would not get vaccinated.[106] Local state authorities were thus forced instead to introduce their own restrictions – including physical distancing, homeworking, circuit-breaker lockdowns, etc. But, without central backing or federal resourcing, and with these measures being actively undermined by Bolsonara's continual underplaying of the danger posed by the virus ("little flu", "media trick", etc.),[107] these were inevitably fragmented and of limited efficacy.[108]

Despite catastrophic levels of infection, hospitalizations and deaths in Brazil over several weeks from the start of November and throughout December 2020, Johnson's government was unresponsive. There were no moves to suspend direct flights to and from Brazil. This was, admittedly, before the Brazilian pandemic was linked to the associated new Gamma variant of concern, but nonetheless, the severity of the Brazilian crisis appeared to warrant a more urgent response. In the end, it was Bolsonara who stopped direct flights from the UK to Brazil, in order to protect the country against the Kent (Alpha) variant. This was effective starting on Christmas

Day.[109] By contrast, the UK government did not ban people coming to the UK from Brazil or people from Brazil flying in indirectly to the UK from neighbouring or travel-aligned countries until 14 January 2021.[110] This was several days after the new variant was flagged as one of concern.

Travel corridors were eventually terminated on 18 January 2021 in favour of a return to mass quarantining of arrivals. Travellers from overseas were for the first time required to take and pass a pre-departure COVID-19 test and to self-isolate on arrival for ten full days (this being reduced from 14 days).[111] This was, as Johnson put it, in a classic closing-the-stable-doors-after-the-horse-has-bolted type statement, to "protect against the risk of as yet unidentified new strains".[112] In practice, they had already been closed – by the decisions of more than 40 other national governments to suspend flights from the UK to prevent importation of the Alpha variant.[113] So, the termination of the corridors, like the lockdown decision of 23 March the year before, was a case of government policy being dragged, slowly and reluctantly, into alignment with a health and safety agenda by the decisions of others (formerly: those of the public, employers, and business owners; latterly, those of foreign governments).

As for mass quarantining, this was, as before, a deeply flawed system for containing importations of the virus, and for exactly the same reasons as before. Arrivals from high-risk countries were not tested on entry; nor was their compliance with the quarantine rules monitored. There were, of course, no government quarantine facilities where entrees from hotspots would be compulsorily detained. Consequently, cases of the Brazilian Gamma variant of concern were imported into the UK in February 2021, provoking frantic efforts to track and trace the carriers in order to break transmission chains. The infected entrees arrived from between one and five days before quarantine hotels were introduced.[114]

Whatever protection was offered by mass quarantine was short-lived, however. On 15 February, with the UK still firmly trapped in the grip of its third pandemic wave, and barely six weeks into the latest lockdown, the Government restored a revamped version of the traffic-light-led travel corridors policy.[115] The prospect of such a move appears to have provoked some disquiet amongst government scientific advisers, though whether this motivated them to caution ministers is unknown. In its deliberations of 21 January, in response to recent importations of the Beta and Gamma variants, SAGE concluded that only the "complete, pre-emptive closure of borders or the mandatory quarantine of all visitors upon arrival in designated facilities, irrespective of testing history, can get close to fully preventing the importation of cases or new variants".[116]

As for the travel corridors policy itself, this was basically the same scheme as before, with two modifications. First, travellers from red-listed countries were barred from UK entry unless these were returning residents. "Non-British or Irish nationals and non-UK residents from red list countries were not allowed to enter the UK at all". Second, returnees from red-listed countries were required to self-isolate in government-approved quarantine hotels whereas travellers from amber-listed countries should make their own self-isolation arrangements. British and

Irish nationals and people from overseas with residency entitlements were also required to make their own advance reservations at one of these government-approved isolation facilities before travelling to the UK. At first, on the reopening of travel corridors, aside from the red list, there were no other lists. Rather, all countries not on the red list were treated as equivalents in terms of COVID-19 risk. The amber and green lists were introduced on 17 May 2021, tailing such developments in other countries.[117]

The hotel quarantine aspect of the system was, predictably, shambolic, with the hallmarks of it being a rushed and ill-thought job. The scheme was confirmed only on 5 February 2021 – ten days before it would start.[118] Only five airports servicing quarantine hotels were included in it, one of which was Farnborough, a small facility catering for privately-owned aircraft or privately-charted flights. The north of the country was virtually uncatered for, since none of the largest airports apart from Birmingham International and London Heathrow and London Gatwick were included in the scheme.[119] Consequently, thousands of returnees would have to endure not simply the inconvenience and financial costs of compulsory quarantine but also the added inconvenience and cost of lengthy commutes back to their homeplaces after release.

Other "teething troubles" included a dysfunctional quarantine hotel reservations website that crashed within hours of its launch.[120] The problem here was delays in awarding contracts to hotels that would participate in the scheme. These, according to the PM, were unsigned ten days before the first red-list arrivals were due back in the UK on the travel corridor system's launch day.[121] When exactly they were signed has not been disclosed. They were reportedly still unsigned less than a week in advance of the scheme's launch.[122] This may explain why the hotel bookings site was launched just four days before the scheme went live – only to be immediately overwhelmed by the high volume of users logging on simultaneously.

The Government's infatuation with preserving the freedom of mass commercial travel to and from "safe" countries even across and during successive national lockdowns ensured that (by mid-July 2021) the Kent variant was internationalized, becoming the most "globalized" of them all to date, having been exported to more than 50 other countries. By contrast, the South African variant had by then been identified as being present in 20 countries, including the UK, whereas the Brazilian variant was discovered in ten.[123] British exceptionalism thus manifested as membership of a very exclusive club of countries by the summer of 2021. That is, a membership of one. This was inasmuch as the UK had managed by then not only to incubate one of the most transmissible variants (the Kent Alpha) but also to draw inside its borders every one of the other variants of biggest concern (South African, Brazilian, plus the Indian Delta).

Such was the consequence of the inadequacies of the Government's at-the-border defences, of the prematurity of its border re-openings following or even during domestic lockdowns, and of its incentivizing ordinary Britons to travel overseas at the first opportunity. Following the re-opening of travel corridors in February 2021, the volume of entrees into the UK rose inexorably, month by month, and accelerating sharply in the summer season. In March of 2021, 386,600 travellers entered the UK. In April it was 447,300. In May, 527,000 travellers entered the country. In June it was 855,800, whereas in July it was 1,439,800. August – since this corresponds with school summer holidays – was predicted to see a doubling of these numbers.[124]

At the time of writing (17 July 2021), the importation of Delta is, of course, the latest one of concern to date, and under circumstances that are as predictable as they are lamentable. This was yet another tale of tardy and reactive border defence. This doubly mutated variant was detected in India on 25 March 2021. This was just as the country experienced major increases in community transmission rates as its second wave began to build, with recorded caseloads doubling from a seven-day average of 18,000 on 8 March to 36,000 on 21 March.[125] Much worse was to come. The subsequent public health catastrophe that rapidly enveloped the country was later acknowledged as being driven especially by the new strain, though India had also imported high numbers of cases of the Alpha variant from the UK.[126]

Yet ministers did not announce that India would be added to the UK's red list of high-risk countries (whereby all entrees except returning UK residents would be barred entry and returners would be required to quarantine in a government hotel) until 19 April 2021,[127] with the new restrictions taking effect on 23 April. This was more than a month after the discovery of the new variant of concern and almost three months into India's second wave.[128] And this was as India's daily new caseload rose from 81,444 on 1 April to 275,306 on 18 April.[129] By contrast, India's neighbours, Pakistan and Bangladesh, were added to the red list on 2 April, supposedly owing to fears over the import of new variants. These restrictions started on 9 April, even though caseloads were lower in these countries and were increasing much less sharply than in India.[130] Moreover, the delay between the announcement of India's addition to the red list and the operationalization of the change handed would-be travellers a three-day window to enter the UK without quarantine or on-entry testing that thousands would avail themselves of.[131]

Yvette Cooper, chair of the Parliamentary Select Committee, described Johnson's "catastrophic error of judgement" (as Layla Moran put it) in delaying adding India to the red list as "inexplicable".[132] Professor Christina Pagel, Director of Clinical Operational Research at UCL, and member of the Independent SAGE group of scientists, found the decision (or non-decision) "ridiculous".[133] Ridiculous it may have been (though I would say not if considered on the grounds of its likely motivation), but whether or not it will be catastrophic in its effects remains to be seen. High-risk it certainly was, however, since, in Pagel's words, the Delta variant "has several concerning mutations" that could render it not only more infectious but also better at evading the body's defences (even if these defences were boosted by vaccines). As Professor Paul Hunter explained:

> These two escape mutations [of Delta] working together could be a lot more problematic than the South African and Brazilian variants [which] have only got one escape mutation. . . . It might be even less controlled by vaccine than the Brazilian and South African variants.[134]

For sure, as well, the delay defied explanation from a moral standpoint. But perhaps it was at least less mysterious if it was considered from an economic standpoint. India is one of the UK's bigger trade partners outside the EU and developed world – the sixth largest, in fact.[135] Clearly, the Government was looking to extend that relationship in the post-Brexit world, by forging closer links with the second-largest economy in South Asia. Border closures are not especially good for business – and especially not for a country that, having abandoned the EU free-trade zone, was casting around for new commercial partnerships.

By 16 April 2021, the first cases of Delta importation into the UK were confirmed.[136] This was on the same day that Boris Johnson announced that he could see no reason why his planned visit to India to discuss a post-Brexit trade deal should not go ahead.[137] Three days later Johnson found it "only sensible" to cancel the trip.[138] By mid-May inter-community transmission of Delta was firmly established, as it began to outcompete the 50 percent (or so) less infectious Alpha variant.[139] By the start of June, Delta had become the dominant strain in the UK and was spreading rapidly, especially in primary and secondary schools.[140] By mid-June virtually all new cases of infection in the UK (98 percent or so) were attributable to Delta,[141] and this was responsible for such high caseloads that it was clear that the virus was outflanking existing physical distancing controls. This, in the end, of course, caused the PM to postpone his original "Freedom Day" of 21 June.

At the time of writing, 19 July's "Freedom Day" is imminent. If this goes ahead, as seems inevitable, the Government's current travel corridors policy (with its extensive and ever-growing red list), which it has no plans as of yet to ditch, and which it appears will persist, will be rendered anomalous. This is because the COVID-19-inspired restrictions that are imposed on foreign entrees and on returning travellers from red-listed places will be radically at odds with the virtual absence of controls or restrictions on the non-travelling locals.

Thus, vaccinated foreign nationals or residents from amber-listed countries would have to self-isolate for ten full days. Returning UK residents from amber-listed countries who had been vaccinated under the NHS programme would not – since this requirement was abolished by the Government on 8 June to oil the wheels of mass tourism overseas travel.[142] And, most radically, returning residents from red-listed countries with rates of COVID-19 infection typically much lower than in the UK, who have been negative-tested before departure, and who are also twice-vaccinated, will continue to be compulsorily detained in quarantine hotels at astronomical financial cost, where they will also be twice-tested. This is as everyone else is free to disregard physical distancing and mask-wearing, attend mass spectator events and bars and clubs without a vaccination "passport" or negative COVID-19 test result, refrain from providing contact information to the staff of leisure or hospitality venues for track and trace, and so on. This is indeed as twice-vaccinated people and under 18-year-olds are exempted from self-isolation unless they have actually failed a test, and as everyone is incentivized to disregard prompts from the test-trace system to self-isolate and take a test.

There is no way this inconsistency can be rationally explained on the grounds of a public safety agenda. This is undermined by double standards, pure and simple. The supposed grounds for "Freedom Day's" lifting of restrictions was that vaccination by itself was sufficient public health protection, so that mandatory physical distancing was dispensable. But, if so, why would vaccinated entrees and returners from non– green-listed places not also be permitted to dispense with these "unnecessary" restrictions? If the answer to this question is that the restrictions are actually necessary, after all, then how is "Freedom Day" even defensible?

There would be a semblance of reason to the Government's border policy if it was only those unvaccinated or untested foreign residents from amber-listed or red-listed countries or those returning UK residents from red-listed countries who were required to self-isolate in the community or submit to hotel incarceration. In the context of "Freedom Day", compelling the double-jabbed to do so was, under the Government's own rhetorical logic, senseless, if not disingenuous. But, of course, the rationale for "Freedom Day" was the real absurdity and disingenuity in the situation. Instead of relaxing border restrictions to match the dismantling of internal controls, the internal controls should have been preserved, if not tightened, as caseloads accelerated over the summer.

How might these double standards that appear paradoxical, if not illogical, be explained? The hidden function of the Government's anomalously quasi-strict border control policy post-19 July 2021 (which stands in sharp contrast to its weak, lax or absent border controls for much of the pandemic) will henceforth, for as long as it persists, be likely to be the ideological one of maintaining in the public eye the fiction of its commitment to protecting the population from the virus that in practice is to be cast to the winds. This rather more than the appeal of legally mandating the commercial exploitation of red-list travellers by corporate hoteliers (who are charged £1,700 for their quarantine) would be the main purpose of the policy. Carceral hotels to snuff out alien variants from overseas are emblematic of this "commitment". These demonstrate symbolically the greater danger posed to the public by these foreign imports *vis-à-vis* merely locally grown ones, which also dovetails with the phobias of the Brexit imagination. This is just as domestic conditions of uncontrolled spread of the virus fuel the production of new home-grown variants that pose potentially far bigger dangers.

All of this said, however, there are of course strong competing political motives for why the Government would wish to ditch border controls altogether, which hardly need spelling out. These would be the same reasons for why border controls were weak, tardy, or virtually non-existent for much of the pandemic. The incongruity between "Freedom Day" domestic freedoms and tight restrictions on overseas travel may also invite legal challenges in the courts. So, it is more than feasible that these "other" reasons may be considered more advantageous for ministers than those in favour of sticking with the travel corridors and country listings in the none-too-distant future. How long current policy with regard to placing tight restrictions on entrees and returnees from red-listed places and on foreign nationals visiting the UK from amber-listed places will survive post-19 July in today's "post-pandemic" Britain remains to be seen. My own view is that these will be done and dusted before winter (of 2021) is upon us. There is every prospect of the red list (and amber list) being scrapped altogether by then (along with the quarantine hotels). At this point, the risk of importing new variants of concern that may outdo even Delta in terms of their infectiousness and their potential capacity to outflank the vaccines would be greatly magnified.

17 July 2021 (updated 26 August 2021)

Notes

1 Matthews, S., Boyd, C. and Blanchard, S. (2020). 'UK government issues new travel advice warning Britons flying back from nine countries to phone NHS 111 if they feel even slightly ill – as pressure mounts on ministers to ban all travellers from coronavirus-hit China'. Mail. (7 February).

2 HCHAC (2020). *Home Office Preparedness for COVID-19 (Coronavirus): Management of the Borders*. Fifth Report of Session 2019–21. HC 503. London: House of Commons, p. 8.

3 HCHAC (2020), p. 9.

4 *Reuters* (2020). 'Britain advises against all travel to China's Hubei province'. (25 January).

5 Borland, S., Cachia, A. and Payne, T. (2020). 'UK on killer virus alert'. *Mail.* (January 23).

6 Fernandez, C. (2020). 'Temperature tests on jets from epicentre city'. *Mail.* (January 23).

7 Gardner, B. (2020). '"I could be spreading deadly virus in the UK"; coronavirus outbreak; British teacher who flew back to UK from Wuhan fears advice given to him by NHS may be wrong'. *Telegraph.* (27 January).

8 Clifton, K. (2020). 'Coronavirus latest: more than 1,400 travellers recently back in UK from Wuhan told to "self-isolate"'. *Independent.* (27 January).

9 Allegretti, A. (2020). 'Coronavirus: recent travellers from Wuhan to UK told to self-isolate'. *Sky News.* (28 January).

10 Clifton, K. (2020). 'Coronavirus: more than 1,400 travellers back in UK from Wuhan told to self-isolate'. *Evening Standard.* (27 January).

11 *BBC News* (2020). 'Coronavirus: foreign office warns against "all but essential travel" to China'. (28 January); Meechan, S. (2020). 'Is it safe to China and Hong Kong? UK Government updates coronavirus advice'. *Chronicle.* (1 February).

12 HCHAC (2020), p. 10.

13 Matthews et al. (2020).

14 HCHAC (2020), p. 9.

15 HCHAC (2020), p. 10.

16 HCHAC (2020), pp. 9–10.

17 Foreign and Commonwealth Office (2020). *Travel Advice: Coronavirus (COVID-19): Guidance for British People Travelling Overseas During the Coronavirus (COVID-19) Pandemic.* GOV.UK (online). (26 March). Available at: www.gov.uk/guidance/travel-advice-novel-coronavirus

18 English, O. (2020). '"No checks please, we're British": indefensible UK border policy'. *Byline Times.* (19 May).

19 HCHAC (2020), p. 11.

20 HCHAC (2020), p. 12.

21 HCHAC (2020), p. 13.

22 HCHAC (2020), p. 11.

23 HCHAC (2020), p. 12.

24 Grierson, J. (2020). 'UK coronavirus border controls more effective if done earlier, MPs told' *Guardian.* (10 June).

25 Quinn, B. and Robinson, G. (2020). 'Foreign office warns Britons against all but essential travel to Italy'. *Guardian*. (9 March).

26 Lawler, L. (2020). 'Timeline: how Italy's coronavirus crisis became the world's deadliest'. *Axios*. (23 March).

27 *ITV News* (2020). 'List of countries foreign office advises Britons not to travel to amid coronavirus outbreak'. (15 March).

28 Hernandez-Morales, A. (2020). 'Spain goes into lockdown'. *Politico*. (14 March).

29 DHSC (2020). *COVID-19: Health Secretary's Statement to Parliament*. GOV.UK (online). (26 February). Available at: www.gov.uk/government/speeches/covid-19-health-secretarys-statement-to-parliament

30 WHO (2020). *WHO Advice for International Travel and Trade in Relation to the Outbreak of Pneumonia Caused by a New Coronavirus in China*. (10 January). Available at: www. who.int/news-room/articles-detail/who-advice-for-international-travel-and-trade-in-relation-to-the-outbreak-of-pneumonia-caused-by-a-new-coronavirus-in-china; WHO (2020). *Updated WHO Advice for International Traffic in Relation to the Outbreak of the Novel Coronavirus 2019-nCoV*. (27 January); WHO (2020). *Key Considerations for Repatriation and Quarantine of Travellers in Relation to the Outbreak of Novel Coronavirus 2019-nCoV*. (11 February); WHO (2020). *Updated WHO Recommendations for International Traffic in Relation to COVID-19 Outbreak*. (29 February). Available at: www.who.int/news-room/articles-detail/updated-who-recommendations-for-international-traffic-in-relation-to-covid-19-outbreak

31 English (2020).

32 DHSC (26 February, 2020).

33 Thiessen, T. (2020). 'Coronavirus: some of these 24 European countries have closed their borders to tourists'. *Forbes*. (14 March).

34 European Council and Council of the European Union (2020). *Video Conference of the Members of the European Council, 17 March 2020*. Available at: www.consilium.europa. eu/en/meetings/european-council/2020/03/17/

35 Connor, P. (2020). 'More than nine-in-ten people worldwide live in countries with travel restrictions amid COVID 19'. *Pew Research Center* (online). (1 April). Available at: www.pewresearch.org/fact-tank/2020/04/01/more-than-nine-in-ten-people-world-wide-live-in-countries-with-travel-restrictions-amid-covid-19/

36 Clark, P., Harding, R., Chazan, G., Dombey, D., Shepherd, C., Hughes, L., Williams, A., Blood, D. and Haslett, B. (2020). 'Britain's open borders make it a global outlier in coronavirus fight'. *Financial Times*. (16 April).

37 Clark et al. (2020).

38 Knibbs, J. (2020). 'Coronavirus warning: travel ban could be issued 'imminently' as scientists demand action'. *Express* (online). (7 February).

39 Clark et al. (2020).

40 Rogers, A. (2020). 'Travel bans and quarantines won't stop virus'. *Wired*. (6 March).

41 Clark et al. (2020).

42 Grierson (2020).

43 HCHAC (2020), pp. 16–17.

44 Grierson (2020).

45 Fernandez (2020).

46 HCHAC (2020), p. 17.

47 Clark et al. (2020).

48 Cited in Rogers (2020).

49 Chinazzi, M., Davis, J.T., Ajelli, M., Gioannini, C., Litvinova, M., Merler, S. and Pastor, A. (2020). 'The effect of travel restrictions on the spread of the 2019 novel coronavirus (COVID-19) outbreak'. *Science*, 368 (6489) (April 24), pp. 395–400. Available at: https://science.sciencemag.org/content/368/6489/395

50 *ABS/CBN* (2020). 'Philippines confirms first case of new coronavirus'. (30 January).

51 *NBC News* (2020). 'First coronavirus death outside China reported in Philippines'. (2 February).

52 PH Department of Health (2020). *DOH Confirms 3rd COVID-19 Case in PH*. PHDOH (online). (5 February).

53 Punzalan, J. (2020). 'Philippines' new coronavirus cases now at 5, including potential local transmission'. *ABS/CBN News* (online). (6 March).

54 Grierson (2020).

55 Grierson (2020).

56 Grierson (2020).

57 HCHAC (2020), p. 3.

58 HCHAC (2020), p. 9.

59 HCHAC (2020), pp. 14–15.

60 HCHAC (2020), p. 15.

61 HCHAC (2020), p. 3.

62 For examples see HCHAC (2020), pp. 20–23.

63 Hancock, M. (2020). *Covid-19*. Vol. 673: debated on Monday 16 March 2020 (16 March). London: Hansard, UK Parliament, House of Commons.

64 HCHAC (2020), p. 33.

65 SAGE discussed instead the efficacy of introducing new *specific* restrictions – that is, curbing or reducing flights – not whether or not other border protection measures – that is, quarantining, advice to self-isolate even if asymptomatic, testing, etc. – would be of benefit.

66 HCHAC (2020), pp. 28–29.

67 Patel, P. (Home Secretary). (2020). *Letter to the Chair, Home Affairs Committee*. London: Home Office. (9 April). Available at: https://committees.parliament.uk/publications/663/documents/2956/default/.

68 Grierson (2020).

69 Aston, J. (Home Office Chief Scientific Officer). (2020). *Letter to the Chair, Home Affairs Committee*. London: Home Office. (4 May). Available at: https://committees.parliament.uk/publications/995/documents/7818/default/.

70 HCHAC (2020), p. 34.

71 HCHAC (2020), p. 37.

72 Scally quoted in HCHAC (2020), pp. 37–38.

73 DHSC (2020); Professor John Aston (Home Office Chief Scientific Adviser). *Letter to the Home Affairs Select Committee*. (3 May). Available at: https://committees.parliament.uk/publications/995/documents/7818/default/.

74 HCHAC (2020), p. 34.

75 HCHAC (2020), p. 3, 27.

76 HCHAC (2020), p. 27.

77 HCHAC (2020), p. 24, 25.

78 According to Border Force statistics, 1,174,700 people entered the UK in those ten days. Cited in HCHAC (2020), p. 29.

79 HCHAC (2020), p. 24.

80 Mason, R. (2020). 'Boris Johnson's lockdown release condemned as divisive, confusing and vague'. *Guardian*. (10 May); Grierson, J. (2020). 'UK quarantine plan: what will it mean for travellers'? *Guardian*. (22 May).

81 BBC News (2020). 'Coronavirus: UK quarantine plans and £1,000 penalties confirmed'. (3 June).

82 Worldometer (2020). *Covid-19 Coronavirus Pandemic: Reported Cases and Deaths by Country or Territory*. Available at: www.worldometers.info/coronavirus/#countries. Accessed: 22/06/2020.

83 Stewart, H., Grierson, J. and Proctor, K. (2020). 'Business groups brand UK's quarantine plan for arrivals "isolationist"'. *Guardian*. (22 May).

84 Mason (2020).

85 BBC News (3 June, 2020).

86 Murray, J. (2020). 'First arrivals under UK quarantine rules: "they didn't even check my temperature"'. *Guardian*. (8 June).

87 Home Office (2021). *Statistics Relating to Passenger Arrivals Since the COVID-19 Outbreak, February 2021*. GOV.UK (online). (25 February). Available at: www.gov.uk/government/statistics/statistics-relating-to-passenger-arrivals-since-the-covid-19-outbreak-february-2021/statistics-relating-to-passenger-arrivals-since-the-covid-19-outbreak-february-2021.

88 *BBC News* (2020). 'Coronavirus: England's quarantine-free list of countries published'. (3 July). *BBC News* (2020). 'Coronavirus: Quarantine rules end for dozens of destinations'. (10 July).

89 *BBC News* (2020). 'Coronavirus: UK to open up European holidays from 6 July'. (27 June); Calder, S. (2020). 'Government to introduce summer holiday "traffic light" quarantine system'. *Independent*. (27 June).

90 Shapps, G. (2020). *Self-Isolation Lifted for Lower Risk Countries in Time for Holidays This Summer*. Department for Transport, Foreign and Commonwealth Office. GOV.UK (online). (3 July). Available at: www.gov.uk/government/news/self-isolation-lifted-for-lower-risk-countries-in-time-for-holidays-this-summer.

91 *BBC News* (2020). 'Coronavirus: holiday bookings "explode" as travel restrictions ease'. (27 June).

92 Worldometer (2020).

93 HCHAC (2020), p. 4.

94 HCHAC (2020), p. 54.

95 Home Office (25 February, 2021).

96 HCHAC (2020), p. 4.

97 HCHAC (2020), pp. 54–55.

98 *BBC News* (2020). 'Coronavirus: airport tests "give false sense of security", says Johnson'. (4 September).

99 *ITV News* (2020). 'No silver bullet to deal with quarantine and Covid-19 at airports, insists Dominic Raab'. (6 September).

100 Worldometer (2020). *Countries – United Kingdom: Daily New Cases in the United Kingdom*. Available at: www.worldometers.info/coronavirus/country/uk/. Accessed: 15/10/2020.

101 Home Office (25 February, 2021).

102 PHE (2020). *Confirmed Cases of COVID-19 Variants Identified in UK*. GOV.UK. (23 December). Available at: www.gov.uk/government/news/confirmed-cases-of-covid-19-variants-identified-in-uk; *BBC News* (2021). 'Coronavirus: UK must "come down hard" on South African variant'. (1 February).

103 Stewart, H. (2020). 'UK government to ban travellers from Brazil amid new Covid variant, PM hints'. *Guardian*. (13 January).

104 Home Office (25 February, 2021).

105 Veselinovic, M. (2020). 'COVID-19: travellers can shorten quarantine on arrival from next month – but they'll have to pay for it'. *Sky News*. (24 November).

106 Savarese, M. (2020). 'Brazil's Bolsonaro rejects COVID-19 shot, calls masks taboo'. *Associated Press News* (online). (27 November). Available at: https://apnews.com/article/pandemics-brazil-health-coronavirus-pandemic-latin-america-0295d39d3032aa14c6675b-8b4080e8cc.

107 Phillips, T. (2020). 'Brazil's Jair Bolsonaro says coronavirus crisis is a media trick'. *Guardian* (online). (23 March). Available at: www.theguardian.com/world/2020/mar/23/brazils-jair-bolsonaro-says-coronavirus-crisis-is-a-media-trick; Phillips, T. (2020). 'Bolsonaro says he "wouldn't feel anything" if infected with Covid-19 and attacks state lockdowns'. *Guardian* (online). (25 March). Available at: www.theguardian.com/world/2020/mar/25/bolsonaro-brazil-wouldnt-feel-anything-covid-19-attack-state-lockdowns.

108 Barone, M., Chaudhury, N., de Oliveira, L.X., Chaluppe, M., Helman, B., Patricio, B., Weiselberg, R., Ngongo, B. and Giampaoli, V. (2021). 'Brazil, a country collapsing during the covid-19 pandemic'. *British Medical Journal*. (26 March). Available

at: https://blogs.bmj.com/bmj/2021/03/26/brazil-a-country-collapsing-during-the-covid-19-pandemic/; Ferigato, S., Michelle, F., Amorim, M., Ambrogi, I., Fernandes, M. and Pacheco, R. (2020). 'The Brazilian government's mistakes in responding to the COVID-19 pandemic'. *Lancet*, 396 (10263) (21 November), p. 1636. Available at: www.thelancet.com/journals/lancet/article/PIIS0140-6736(20)32164-4/fulltext.

109 GardaWorld (2020). 'Brazil: authorities ban direct flights from UK, effective December 25'. *GardaWorld* (online). (24 December). Available at: www.garda.com/crisis24/news-alerts/421156/brazil-authorities-ban-direct-flights-from-uk-effective-dec-25-update-22.

110 Stewart, H. (2021). 'UK government to ban travellers from Brazil amid new Covid variant, PM hints'. *Guardian*. (13 January); Stewart, H. and Weaver, M. (2021). 'UK bans arrivals from South America over Brazilian Covid strain'. *Guardian*. (14 January).

111 Home Office (2021). *Statistics Relating to Passenger Arrivals Since the COVID-19 Outbreak, August 2021*. GOV.UK (online). (26 August).

112 *BBC News* (2021). 'Covid: UK to close all travel corridors from Monday'. (15 January).

113 *CNN News* (2020). 'UK travel ban: these countries have imposed new restrictions'. (25 December); Sibthorpe, S. (2020). 'COVID-19: which countries have restricted travel to and from the UK over new variant'? *Sky News*. (25 December).

114 *BBC News* (2021). 'Covid-19: Brazil "variant of concern" detected in UK'. (28 February); *BBC News* (2021). 'Brazilian variant: Hancock denies quarantine delays put lives at risk'. (1 March); *BBC News* (2021). 'Brazil variant: search for mystery case narrows to 379 households'. (2 March); *BBC News* (2021). 'Covid: four more cases of Brazil variant found in England'. (18 March).

115 Gayle, D. (2021). 'UK minister defends delay over Covid quarantine hotels'. *Guardian*. (5 February).

116 Scientific Advisory Group for Emergencies (2021). *SAGE 77 Minutes: Coronavirus (COVID-19) Response, 21 January 2021* (5 February). GOV.UK (online). Available at: www.gov.uk/government/publications/sage-77-minutes-coronavirus-covid-19-response-21-january-2021.

117 Home Office (26 August, 2021).

118 DHSC (2021). *Press Release: Government Confirms Mandatory Hotel Quarantine to Be Introduced From 15 February. GOV.UK. (5 February)*. Available at: www.gov.uk/government/news/government-confirms-mandatory-hotel-quarantine-to-be-introduced-from-15-february.

119 Calder, S. (2021). 'Travel industry hits out at "clueless" launch for hotel quarantine scheme'. *Independent*. (12 February).

120 *Reuters* (2021). 'Britain's hotel quarantine booking system crashes after launch'. (11 February).

121 *BBC News* (2021). 'Covid: ministers risking lives over quarantine plan "delay", says labour'. (4 February); *BBC News* (2021). 'Covid-19: no contracts awarded yet for hotel quarantine plan'. (5 February).

122 Proctor, K. (2021). 'UK Government has not signed any "quarantine hotel" contracts a week before new travel rules begin'. *Holyrood*. (9 February); O'Reilly, L. (2021). 'Government yet to sign hotel quarantine contracts with one week to go'. *Evening Standard*. (8 February).

123 Roberts, M. (2021). 'What are the Delta, Gamma, Beta and Alpha Covid variants'? *BBC News*. (15 July). Available at: www.bbc.co.uk/news/health-55659820.

124 Home Office (26 August, 2021).

125 *BBC News* (2021). 'Coronavirus: "double mutant" Covid variant found in India'. (25 March).

126 *BBC News* (2021). 'India Covid: government says new variant linked to surge'. (6 May).

127 *BBC News* (2021). 'Covid-19: India added to coronavirus "red list" for travel'. (19 April).

128 *Sky News* (2021). 'COVID-19: Boris Johnson under fire over "delaying" India travel ban as experts warn against planned easing of lockdown'. (16 May).

129 Worldometer (2021). *Covid-19 Coronavirus Pandemic: Countries: India*. Worldometer (online). Available at: www.worldometers.info/coronavirus/country/india/. Accessed: 17/07/2021.

130 *BBC News* (2021). 'Covid 19: Pakistan among new countries added to England's travel ban list'. (2 April).

131 Allegretti, A. (2021). 'Thousands could fly to England from India before it joins Covid travel "red list"'. *Guardian*. (19 April).

132 *Sky News* (16 May, 2021).

133 Davies, N. (2021). 'Covid variant first detected in India is found in the UK'. *Guardian*. (15 April).

134 Davies (2021).

135 Trading Economics (2021). *United Kingdom: Exports by Country*. Available at: https:// tradingeconomics.com/united-kingdom/exports-by-country. Accessed: 16/07/2021; Trading Economics (2021). *United Kingdom: Imports by Country*. Available at: https:// tradingeconomics.com/united-kingdom/exports-by-country. Accessed: 16/07/2021.

136 Hockaday, J. (2021). 'First cases of "double mutant" Covid from India found in UK'. *Metro*. (16 April); *ITV News* (2021). 'Covid: cases of India coronavirus variant found in UK features two mutations that could be "of concern"'. (16 April).

137 *BBC News* (2021). 'Covid: Boris Johnson's India visit to go ahead despite rise in cases'. (16 April).

138 *BBC News* (2021). 'Coronavirus: "only sensible" to cancel India trip, says Johnson'. (19 April).

139 *Sky News* (2021). '"Catastrophic error of judgement": PM under fire over "delaying" India travel ban'. (16 May).

140 Torjesen, I. (2021). 'Covid-19: Delta variant is now UK's most dominant strain and spreading through schools'. *British Medical Journal*, 373 (8295) (4 June). Available at: www.bmj.com/content/373/bmj.n1445

141 Schraer, R. (2021). 'Covid: why has the Delta variant spread so quickly in UK'? *BBC News*. (13 June).

142 Home Office (26 August, 2021).

6

COMMUNICATIVE AMBIVALENCE AND TEST AND TRACE

Two aspects of the UK government's management of the pandemic will be addressed in this chapter. Firstly, the Government's communications strategy with regard to educating the public about how to keep themselves and others safe from the pandemic. Government pandemic and physical distancing messaging has been characterized by ambivalence throughout the pandemic. This is to such a degree that many would doubt that there has been a coherent strategy behind these communications at all. My contention, however, is that a strategy can be discerned, and this strategy would account for the apparent lack of clarity in the messaging. Secondly, the Government's much-heralded NHS Test and Trace system, which under-performed spectacularly at considerable cost to the public purse. The under-performance was to such a degree that the system was inefficacious in delivering on the primary goal that was set for it – of disrupting transmission chains where these occurred in order to avoid repeat lockdowns, local or national. These failings too may be considered as aspects of British exceptionalism for reasons that will be set out. This chapter will deal with events from the start of the British pandemic up until mid-July 2021.

Communicative ambivalence ("mixed messaging")

A striking feature of the Government's handling (or mishandling) of the UK pandemic has been a pattern of public health and safety messaging characterized by ambivalence, equivocation, obfuscation and downright misinformation. Cases of this phenomenon have been addressed elsewhere in the present enterprise. These include the contortions of ministers over face coverings and border controls over the course of the pandemic. These include the insistence that schoolchildren were very low risk to catch or transmit the virus (to justify school re-openings and

DOI: 10.4324/9781003275039-7

delayed closures) alongside PHE data reports showing that major school outbreaks were real. This includes constantly shifting estimates of the number of ventilators that were needed and were being procured during the first wave. And, most recently, this includes the hubris over "Freedom Day" in the run-up to July 2021. According to this, people were incentivized to return to "normality" (on the grounds that this was not only safe but was also virtue) alongside being advised to exercise caution and respect for others. Here too people were instructed that there was no going back to lockdowns because the vaccines had broken the capacity of the virus to drive up hospitalizations and deaths, just as they were advised that there may be "rough waters" ahead and social restrictions may return.

Another example of the phenomenon was the Government's ever-shifting explanations for why frontline staff in the first wave were not able to access the PPE they needed. Initially, this was attributed to distribution bottlenecks, then to staff "over-using" the kit, and only latterly and obliquely to insufficiency of procurement. A further example was the ministerial U-turn on testing policy – which of course was never acknowledged as being one. This was marked by the shift away from a policy of COVID-19 testing in just hospitals (in March 2020) to one of mass population testing in April of that same year. The former was justified on the grounds that it was the only sensible way of managing a pandemic. The latter was justified on exactly the same grounds.[1]

I will focus on two examples of the Government's penchant for "mixed" messaging. These are both cases where ambivalence of official health and safety messaging actually was potentially corrosive of physical distancing behaviour. The first case was discernible in the midst of the first national lockdown (commencing 24 March 2020), in advance of Johnson's roadmap that set out the winding down of restrictions over the summer. This was a period during which public information releases concerning physical distancing restrictions were notably lacking in clarity, and increasingly so in the latter stages, from mid-April 2020 onwards. This case was also instructive in that it was one in which the pattern of messaging would threaten to dilute or undermine the national lockdown that the Government was formally committed to.

This perhaps reflected behind-the-scenes disputes inside the Cabinet, and dissonance between ministers and the backbench – with some ministers (e.g. Rishi Sunak, Michael Gove and Liz Truss) reportedly agitating for a swift end to the lockdown as the economic costs piled up. The media reported the whisperings of anonymous government insiders of the imminence of easing of restrictions here and there – that is, of re-opening schools, libraries, rubbish tips and garden centres, and of allowing people to leave their homes for non-essential purposes (e.g. recreational pursuits other than once-daily exercise – sunbathing, picnicking).[2] This provoked banner headlines in the tabloids of an imminent road to normalcy (e.g. "First Steps to End of Lockdown" – *Mirror*; "Hurrah! Lockdown Freedom Beckons!" – *Mail*). Rumours were also circulated in the press about the upcoming curtailment of the furlough scheme (owing to the concern of ministers or officials that extending it beyond July would encourage "dependency") and of supposed plans to allow young people greater freedoms from physical distancing than the old (who would remain compulsorily housebound).[3]

Such messaging would only weaken the efficacy of physical distancing rules by encouraging the public to believe that the restrictions were of lesser importance than before, indeed that they were on their last legs, or on the brink of disappearing altogether. The rumours of the ending of furlough protections for stay-at-home workers could hardly avoid incentivizing people to head back to the offices. Equally, the whispering that freedoms from lockdown may be extended to young people but not the elderly would risk stoking up grievances among the latter, who would justly feel discriminated against. Such would for them undermine the legitimacy of the lockdown and weaken the sense of everyone sharing the same privations in a common battle against the virus, so that they were less motivated to stick to curfew rules.

Public compliance with physical distancing would also be diluted for the same reason by Johnson's own press releases in advance of the roadmap to the effect that government announcements on changes to lockdown restrictions were on the way. This was to be the pattern right across both the major nationwide lockdowns of 2020 and 2021 – where in advance of the roadmaps setting out the process of easing restrictions were press announcements suggestive of what was imminent. Of course, the "dates-led" approach to unlockings could itself hardly fail to deter people from imagining that the defeat of the virus was set in stone and was being quickly accomplished.

The Government's ditching of its "*Stay Home, Protect the NHS, Save Lives*" COVID-19 health and safety slogan in favour of "*Stay Alert, Control the Virus, Save Lives*" was perhaps the most striking example of the growing vagueness or fuzziness of its public messaging during the first lockdown. The new message was rolled out on 10 May 2020 in advance of Johnson's announcement of the roadmap plan of summer unlockings.[4] Now, the purpose of any such billboard-style messaging is supposedly to offer crystal-clear guidance in soundbite mode on how people should behave. But, unlike its predecessor, this one could hardly accomplish its goal. This was because its meaning, since this was open to interpretation, required clarification, which defeated its own purpose.

How exactly, according to this guidance, would people "control the virus"? Well, apparently by "staying alert", rather than by "staying home". "Stay alert" – but what exactly does that mean? Well, according to Housing and Communities Secretary, Robert Jenrick, this meant "staying at home *as much as possible* [my emphasis], but being alert when you do go out, by maintaining social distancing, washing your hands, respecting others in the workplace and the other settings that you'll go to".[5] This of course beggared the question. If the meaning of the new message was indeed "stay home", then why did it need to be changed to "stay alert"? Did people really need to be advised to be vigilant when outside given that physical distancing was necessary? Such considerations led to the devolved governments deciding to stick with the original health and safety message until the summer.

The danger of such mixed messaging (in truth, diluted, weakened, if not self-contradictory messaging) defusing or blunting public adherence to lockdown restrictions and physical distancing rules more generally ought to have been manifest – even to ministers. This being the case, such raises the possibility that such informational ambivalence could be artifice, a matter of strategy, rather than merely confusion or incompetence on the Government's part. This would be the strategy of deliberating undermining the first lockdown by seeking to erode public compliance with it. This certainly could have been the motive for the actions of those "anonymous insiders" who were cranking the media rumour-mill of easing-down measures in the pipeline. This was as they acted as proxies for ministers, MPs or party factions who would consider the economic price of the lockdown as too high to continue paying. Such whisperings in the ears of journalists not only put pressure on ministers to start rolling-back physical social distancing earlier rather than later, but this also may have the benefit of facilitating a drift towards non-compliance in the general public that would render the lockdown policy unworkable.

Such, alas, is a wholly feasible interpretation of the "confused" messaging of the Government as well. This is because the obvious reluctance of ministers to introduce the lockdown in the first place (in order to avoid harming businesses) would equally translate into their desire to lift it at the first opportunity (in order to restore businesses). But an obstacle to the rapid unwinding of lockdown controls would be a general public that was supportive of such restrictions, whether for the reason of fear of illness (to oneself or loved ones) or a sense of collective solidarity in seeing off a dangerous pandemic. Since ministers cannot afford to be seen as openly subordinating the goal of saving lives to the goal of freeing businesses, a more subtle way of doing that would be to formally support the lockdown whilst incentivizing the public to render it untenable. That way, ditching the lockdown would simply be legitimized by acknowledgement that Johnson's "freedom-loving Britons" were not prepared to abide by it. If or when hospitalizations and deaths then spiralled to levels that most people would consider unacceptable, ministers would then also be well-placed to deflect blame for this away from itself and on to the "irresponsible" citizens who undermined the rules by disregarding them.

The second example of ambivalent or "mixed" messaging I will address pertains to the pattern of ministerial advice and guidance that unfolded in the summer and autumn of 2020, as COVID-19 caseloads began to build up into the second wave. This attributed the developing crisis not to the incautious dismantling of restrictions, the insistence on full school returns, plus accompanying incitements of people to return to hospitality venues, but to the socially irresponsible behaviour of young adults. As Hancock explained:

> It's so important that everybody does their bit and follows the social distancing because it doesn't matter how old you are, how affected you might be by

this disease, you can pass the disease on to others. So don't pass the disease on to your grandparents if you're a young person, everybody needs to follow the social distancing.

Or, as Housing and Communities Minister Robert Jenrick, put it:

We have to keep hammering the message home. Of course the people in those age categories are unlikely to become extremely unwell as a result of having the virus. But they are able to pass it on to others. . . . There's a responsibility on younger people to not just stay at home, obviously to go out and go to work and to enjoy pubs and restaurants, but to do so in accordance with the guidelines.[6]

That such messaging was "mixed", or "confused" was noted by Professor Susan Michie, a behavioural scientist and member of SAGE. Michie rebuked the Government for "signalling" young people "to go out and about as usual", by lifting preventative restrictions, only to then tell them that "you are the problem" when they do just that.[7] But self-contradictory would be a better term for this messaging. So too would be disingenuous. For, according to Jenrick, young people have not only a right to go out and enjoy themselves in social settings but also a *responsibility* to exercise that right. This is alongside their responsibility not to! Strong clear safety guidance (e.g. avoid for now crowded leisure venues involving alcohol consumption where physical distancing would be difficult) was precluded by the simple fact that ministers did not actually want to deter anyone from using those venues and doing so freely and maximally.

If young people were utterly confused by all of this, it would not be surprising. As I have noted before, ambivalent or outrightly inconsistent messaging (along with messaging that is at odds with actual policy) can only weaken public adherence to physical distancing etiquette. In part, this is because this encourages scepticism (even cynicism) about the efficacy of sticking to these rules. As I have suggested earlier, the ambivalence or inconsistency of government messaging and guidance is unlikely to be a symptom of its own muddled thinking or confusion. This is owing to the *consistency of its inconsistency* of messaging over the course of the pandemic. Rather, the "mixed" or "confused" or "self-contradictory" messaging has more likely been a matter of intention. If so, this is in order to ensure that the public is not incentivized into becoming so overly risk-averse that the re-opening of the economy is frustrated by people opting to limit or trim their engagement with actual workplace and consumer opportunities other than virtual ones.

This is shown by the fact that government messaging has tended to be clearer on some things rather than on others. This has been one-sided inconsistency. As Hancock insisted, in the autumn of 2020, as caseloads expanded exponentially: "Covid-secure workplaces are safe", as are Covid-secure hospitality venues, so that virus spread could occur only if people flaunted rules that were "clear".[8] Therefore, there was no good reason why, according to the Health Minister, you would not abandon home-working or why you would think twice about frequenting busy clubs, pubs and restaurants. Yet, with regard to safety measures in these sorts of places, the Government itself had shown that it was hardly committed to rigorous physical distancing. Here guidance was looser and flakier.

Such was symbolized by its reduction of the "two metre rule" to the "one metre plus rule" or "one-to-two metre rule" (with caveats) earlier in the summer of 2020. This was following a review that foregrounded the economic deficits of the former in comparison with the latter, so that hospitality premises and workplaces could cater for higher numbers of workers and customers. As the authors of the review stated:

> With a 2 metre rule in place, it is not financially viable for many businesses to operate; industry bodies for example, have estimated that outlets in the hospitality sector could make only 30% of pre-COVID-19 revenues with 2m distancing, as opposed to 60–75% at 1m. In sectors that are currently closed (including in accommodation, food services and recreation), over 1.75 million jobs have been furloughed across the UK. Many of these are at risk if reopening is not viable at 2 metres.[9]

This was also revealed by the fact that the Government did not consider Covid-security in these sorts of venues (where physical distancing would always pose a challenge) as requiring mandatory mask-wearing, even though it was established that aerosol transmission was real.

Population testing and NHS Test-and-Trace

This lack of preparedness by government for the British pandemic extended as well into chronic under-investment in resources and facilities for testing for and tracking or tracing the virus. I will focus here especially (though not exclusively) on events during the first wave that began in the spring of 2020 and in the run-up to the second wave that began in earnest in September of that year. This is because having an effective national contact testing and tracing system in place was absolutely necessary if the lockdowns were to be avoided (or at least reduced in scope and duration) and as a fundamental condition for beginning to release them. The Government's failure to operationalize these systems ensured that the autumn 2020 circuit-breaker lockdown and the extended third lockdown that began at the start of January 2021 were inevitable and that the latter was protracted. This failure also ensured that the human costs of the second and third waves were much greater than they could or should have been.

Priority testing

On the cusp of the crisis, unlike in many other countries, which had stockpiled testing kits, the resources to carry out mass testing simply did not exist in the UK.

Not only that, at the start of the UK outbreak, there were only eight public health test facilities in the country that could process and interpret lab results. By contrast, in other countries, the tests could be processed by a far more extensive and developed laboratory network. For mass testing in the UK to be possible, a wider network of laboratories had to be set up – which, from a delayed and standing start, took several weeks to accomplish. This had to be done right in the eye of the pandemic storm. Consequently, as reported by the BBC, "as of 29 April [2020, as the first wave was ebbing], the UK had carried out 8.83 tests per 1,000 people, whereas Italy had conducted 31.6 per 1,000, Germany 30.4 (as of 26 April) and South Korea 11.98". This was according to data collated by online scientific publication *Our World in Data* from official sources.[10]

For these reasons, at the early stages of the UK outbreak, only hospital patients with symptoms were tested for the virus, alongside a little bit later NHS frontline workers,[11] owing to the scarcity of test kits and the lack of processing capacity in laboratories. Moreover, community tracking-and-tracing was suspended altogether for several weeks as hospital admissions escalated and testing capacity was overwhelmed.[12] Testing for all essential workers and their families was not introduced until 24 April 2020 when an online booking system went live on the UK government website.[13] Predictably, the booking system proved less than robust, crashing within hours of opening, and was taken offline owing to high demand.[14]

Testing was later extended to care homes, as the pandemic ran amok in the care sector in April and May of 2020, though weekly testing of care staff was not announced as government policy until the week starting 6 July, despite this being announced as a priority. By the end of the month, Care UK were reporting five-week delays in most homes acquiring tests, and prior to that, a weekly testing system that had "never really got off the ground with the scale we needed".[15] This problem, along with those of delayed or lost results, plus a growing backlog of tests, as infection rates began to rise again in care homes in the autumn of last year, remained pertinent throughout 2020.[16]

Even testing of frontline NHS staff hardly got started before April 2020, even though testing resources had been targeted on them, despite a government press statement (delivered by Michael Gove deputising for the virus-infected Matt Hancock) of 27 March that such testing would be rapidly up-scaled over the next few days.[17] By the start of April only 2,000 of 500,000 frontline NHS workers had been tested, just 0.4 percent of the total.[18] By mid-June, even though NHS testing had been majorly ramped-up, ongoing or regular (i.e. weekly testing of staff) was still not in place for NHS frontliners owing to a lack of testing capacity. Rather, from the start, testing was rationed, even on the COVID-19 front line, with this being allocated to staff with symptoms and those working in places where there was a heavy concentration of cases.[19] Estimates based on studies of London maternity wards are suggestive that up to 60 percent of frontline NHS workers who contracted COVID-19 during the rise and fall of the first wave were likely to have been asymptomatic.[20]

By the start of October 2020, on the cusp of the second wave's takeoff, the overall situation was unchanged. A Parliamentary Select Committee report published on 1 October found that, despite a policy of priority testing of NHS staff in virus hotspots, even here weekly testing was not being delivered. Testing of asymptomatic staff "appears not to have been introduced where the virus is surging in the North East and the North West".[21] This was despite the fact that weekly testing was known to be essential for protecting staff and patients given the dangers of asymptomatic spread and the unreliability of test results based on a single swab (with 30 percent of them being considered as yielding incorrect results).[22] The committee concluded, drawing on the testimony of scientific experts, including that of Chris Whitty, that there was a "compelling case" for weekly testing of all NHS staff, without which there was "significant risk . . . of higher levels of health-care associated infections in a second spike".[23] As Jeremy Hunt, a former health secretary, commented on the report's findings:

> Weekly testing of NHS staff has been repeatedly promised in hotspot areas – but is still not being delivered. . . . Failure to do so creates a real risk that the NHS will be forced to retreat into being a largely Covid-19–only service during a second spike.[24]

Community testing

As for community or population testing, this was for much of March 2020 virtually non-existent. By 11 March only 1,250 people had been tested, at which point eight people had already died from the virus.[25] This was then expanded from a standing start, albeit only incrementally. But this remained at a meagre level until the tail end of April, though accompanied by outlandish ministerial claims that mass testing was planned for an unspecified later date. Just 3,826 tests had been carried out by 16 March, for example, whereas a daily tally of 10,000 plus was not achieved until 2 April. Eventually, on 1 April, Public Health England declared itself for a policy of community or population testing. Yet nothing resembling this got started until the end of the month.[26] Hancock then announced (on 2 April) the Government's target of conducting 100,000 tests per day by the end of the month.[27] From that point, daily testing rates increased steadily, though for most of the month testing capacity was a fraction of the end-of-month goal. On 20 April, for example, only 18,206 tests were reported as being carried out.[28]

Thereafter, testing capacity began to accelerate. By 23 April, Matt Hancock claimed it had reached 51,000 tests on that day. This nonetheless was barely more than 50 percent of the end-of-month target.[29] Indeed, the 31 April target of 100,000 looked highly likely to be missed, since only 81,611 tests were supposedly carried out on the day before the deadline. But Hancock declared mission accomplished right on deadline day, with 122,347 tests supposedly carried out on that day. This was creative accounting to say the least. On closer inspection, the real figure was 83,347, because a full third of the supposed tests (39,000 of them) were unproven, since the swab samples had not been returned. Thousands of test kits that were mailed out on that same day (which could not possibly have been used) were included in the count. So too were re-tests (10,000 plus) where the results of the previous ones needed to be checked. The number of verifiable new tests on deadline day (31 April 2020) was, strictly speaking, only around 73,000.[30]

Having claimed success on its own arbitrarily self-imposed 31 April 100,000 headline target, with the assistance of a large dose of sleight-of-hand, these dizzy heights could not be matched for several days. This was a temporary hiatus though. Henceforth, the number of daily tests (or testing capacity) grew rapidly, reaching 350,000 by the start of July. Progress was hardly smooth and linear, however. Rather, this was interspersed with dips or falls, owing to the accumulation of shortages and bottlenecks. From July and through much of August, the number of daily tests fell back to less than 325,000. Nonetheless, by the start of September, a new high of 375,000 daily tests was reportedly conducted.[31] And so, from being an international outlier for relatively low levels of population testing throughout the spring of 2020, the UK from mid-summer 2020 had become a world leader, with 421,791 tests per million of the population reportedly carried out by 16 October.[32]

Even so, the initial response during the first wave was far too slow, so that the Government was forced to play catch-up for several months owing to its lack of advance preparations. Moreover, the objectivity of ministerial claims for the number of new tests that were carried out from the start of the process through to the autumn months is certainly questionable and has been contested by statisticians.[33] The main bone of contention was the inclusion in the testing statistics of the capacity to deliver tests (i.e. the number of test kits available for use), irrespective of whether these were administered or the results returned or processed, plus daily counts of repeat tests on the same persons. (Public Health England recommended repeat testing, for a number of reasons, including of borderline positives). This was basically the conjurer's trick of classing testing capacity as synonymous with actual testing and of encouraging a view that testing of the same persons was testing of new persons.[34] As David Norgrove, chairperson of the UK Statistics Authority, wryly commented:

> It is . . . hard to believe the statistics work to support the testing programme itself. The statistics and analysis serve neither purpose well. . . . The aim seems to be to show the largest possible number of tests, even at the expense of understanding.[35]

In fact, the Government did not over this period (from the start of population testing up until at least the end of September of 2020) publish statistics on the number of daily tests carried out, and nor did it publish figures on the number of repeat tests on average per person. Rather, statistics on the number of people "newly tested" in England each week were gleaned from the test-and-trace statistics. These indicated that in the first half of September, 82,000 such tests per day were being conducted. To this point may be added another. This is that statistics for testing capacity were typically overstated because they were based on ideal situations (e.g. optimal staff levels at testing facilities) that rarely existed in the real world. In a rational world, laboratory capacity would be measured by what can be practically accomplished given actual resources and operational constraints. Instead, ministers attributed any discrepancy between actual testing, on the one hand, and supposed capacity for testing, on the other hand, to laboratories that were performing under-capacity.[36]

These data weaknesses were the consequence of a PR-motivated and target-mongering approach to testing, rather than one that was seeking to rationally assess the testing programme to support a data-led policy. Such was driven by the need to make up in haste what was neglected at leisure. Ministerial public declarations of ambitious testing targets staked the credibility of government on meeting these arbitrary big numbers. This generated systematic pressures for creative accounting, data gaps and obfuscations. Moreover, if Dominic Cummings' testimony before the Parliamentary Select Committee (in May 2021) is to be believed, Hancock's obsession with testing targets ensured a massive misallocation of resources that could otherwise have been invested in getting off the ground a functional test-and-trace system that would have perhaps allowed avoidance of the second and third lockdowns.

> We had half the government, with me in number 10, calling round frantically saying, "do not do what Hancock says, build the thing properly for the medium term". And we had Hancock calling them all, saying, "down tools on this, do this, hold tests back so that I can hit my target". In my opinion he should have been fired for that alone. It was criminal, disgraceful behaviour that caused serious harm.[37]

Cummings' account certainly has basic intelligibility, if not plausibility, at least with regard to the alleged scuppering of test-and-trace by the Government's mass population testing targets. But he almost certainly exaggerated the degree of dissensus in ministerial circles over the target-mongering approach. This, after all, was a public relations exercise to demonstrate symbolically with high visibility "big numbers" that the Government was, after a wretched start to managing the pandemic, now assuming world leadership in the battle against the virus.

Contact tracing

From similarly inauspicious beginnings, progress on contact tracing, in contrast with that of community testing, remained painfully slow over the same period. This was during the summer of 2020, in the period between the first and second waves, when rapid progress ought to have been an absolute priority. It was not until 23 April that Matt Hancock declared that 18,000 people would be recruited to deliver the new test-and-trace system, which would roll out at some unspecified later date. Almost a month later, on 18 May, the Government announced that it had recruited 21,000 people to staff the system. This would not be rolled out until the end of the month,[38] however, and nor would it be fully operational "at the local level" until the end of June.[39] Later, on 17 June, the new NHSX contact-tracing downloadable application was declared by the minister for innovation at the DHSC not to be a government priority. This, he said, was not expected to be up-and-running before the winter. Indeed, a winter roll-out was said to be aspirational rather than certain.[40] Yet NHSX, trialled on the Isle of Wight in May,[41] was supposed to be an integral part of the new system, and was originally scheduled for national release in mid-May.

So, having been presented as an indispensable tool to contain the spread of COVID-19, now the ill-fated application was reclassified as being an inessential extra, more of a "cherry on the cake" for the new contact test-and-trace system that was on the way.[42] The application had in fact been ditched owing to technical failings and data protection and privacy concerns (which would deter people from downloading it), the latter of which had been known to ministers since March. The Government then declared that the NHS would work with Apple and Google to incorporate the latter's new track-and-trace software into a new application. (Apple and Google launched a version of the technology – which other governments' health authorities were building into their own track-and-trace apps – on 20 May).[43] This new application was trialled, again on the Isle of Wight in mid-August, and was eventually rolled out nationally on 24 September. This was more than four months behind schedule.[44] This was far too late to have any impact whatsoever in managing or mitigating the virus's second wave.

The Government's centralized contact test-and-trace system (NHS Test and Trace, or NHST&T) was eventually released nationally on 28 April 2020. But the system has since (up until the time of writing this chapter) majorly underperformed, "with ongoing challenges around test capacity and contacting both cases and their contacts".[45] Between May and October, the number of tests processed daily was running at only 68 percent of capacity.[46] GPs and frontline healthcare staff reported four-day delays in getting a test and five-day delays in getting the results as well as being instructed to travel hundreds of miles to get tested. This was mostly owing to the failure of planners to anticipate increasing demand for tests in the autumn as the schools, colleges and universities reopened.[47] As the National Audit Office (NAO) concluded:

> NHST&T did not plan for the sharp rise in testing demand in September . . . Laboratories processing community swab tests were unable to keep pace with the volume of tests and experienced large backlogs, which meant NHST&T had to limit the number of tests available and commission extra help from other laboratories. Rationing of tests meant some people were told to visit test sites hundreds of miles away.[48]

The Health Foundation reported in September 2020 that "only between 50% and 60% of contacts of known cases are being advised to isolate. Yet SAGE estimated that, for a contact test-and-trace system to be effective, it needed to trace around 80% of contacts of an index case".[49] According to analysis carried out by Reuters, between 28 May and 4 November 2020, the system had reached only half of the contacts of people who were infected by the virus – two-thirds of infected people and two-thirds of their contacts. Most of these were "household contacts" (i.e. members of the same household) who ought to have been self-quarantining anyway.[50]

In December, the NAO reported that the system was "contacting two out of every three people who have been close to someone who has tested positive, with about 40% of test results delivered within 24 hours, well below the Government's targets". Delivery of in-person test results within the appropriate 24-hour time-frame was fluctuating widely month by month. In June, 93 percent of test results were turned around in 24 hours, but in November it was 38 percent, and in October just 14 percent.[51] The Reuters study found that it was taking "on average at least a week" for contacts of infected persons to be traced and asked to self-isolate.[52] This was simply insufficient to break transmission chains. Many people traced on that timescale would no longer be infectious, having previously been free to transmit the virus.

Anecdotal evidence suggests as well a fundamental failure to trace people who were contacts of persons who were contact traced and possibly asymptomatically infected Interest declared, my ex-partner, who is a key worker in the residential care sector, tested COVID-19 positive in September 2020. I was then contact traced, asked by text message to self-isolate for 14 days, and directed to the NHS website in order to fill out an online form that enquired if I had relevant symptoms. Since I did not, I reported this as such. I was then surprised to find that I was offered no option to identify any persons that I may have been in contact with on the relevant timescale. It was as if recognition of asymptomatic transmission was not even programmed into the system.

Despite reforms, NHST&T has not sufficiently upped its level of performance in 2021, despite declarations to the contrary. According to research by the NAO: "In the six months from November last year [2020] to April this year [2021], it failed to reach nearly 100,000 people who had tested positive for Covid and as result failed to identify their contacts who could potentially infect others". The NAO's analysis also found that the system had managed to misplace 550 million COVID-19 tests between the start of March and 26 May 2021. This was in the sense that these had not been logged or registered as used. Of 655 million that were distributed over this period, just 96 million (or 14 percent) were logged, and the system's administrators reported that they had no idea if the unregistered tests had been used.[53]

Since its start in 2020 up until the time of penning this chapter (5 August 2021), the system has also been dogged by an atrocious utilization rate. By utilization rate is meant the proportion of time spent by staff in a working day or working week actually dispensing relevant functions or tasks. This is indicative, as the NAO report put it, that "substantial public resources have been spent on staff who provided minimal services in return". In June 2020, this was a meagre 1 percent for call handler staff and 4 percent for healthcare professionals. This rate was improved thereafter but was still substantially below the 50 percent target that was set for it. The utilization rate "remained well below a target of 50% throughout September and for much of October" 2020.[54] In February 2021, it plummeted to 11 percent, down from what has turned out to be its (anomalous) peak of 49 percent in November of the year before.[55]

The cost of this failed system has been astronomical. Tens of billions of taxpayers' money have been spent on it. Its budget for 2020/2021 was £22 billion.[56] This rose to £37 billion in 2021 in an attempt to dissolve its problems by throwing more cash at them.[57] This failed because under-resourcing was not the issue. Rather, the problem has been outsourcing, which is necessitated by the systematic scaling down of funding for healthcare services under neoliberal austerity, which left these under-resourced for the pandemic. Outsourcing is misallocation and waste on a grand scale for the simple reason that it presents a bonanza of riches for those whose *raison d'etre* is profit-making rather than public service.

Consequently, a considerable chunk of the budget of NHST&T has been swallowed up by the inflated salaries of the executives (who of course had to be remunerated at CEO rates) and thousands of private corporate-sector consultants who were brought in to advise or oversee or discuss the organization and administration of the system. The Public Accounts Committee (PAC) reported in March 2021,

> at the beginning of November 2020, there were 2,300 consultants and contractors working for 73 different suppliers in NHST&T, with a total consultancy cost of approximately £375 million up to that point. However, when giving evidence to the Science and Technology Committee on 3 February, NHST&T said that it was still employing around 2,500 consultants. When we took evidence in mid-January, the Department estimated around 900 contractors from Deloitte alone were still on NHST&T's books. The Department reported to us that the average cost per consultant was about £1,100 a day, up to a maximum of £6,624 for some consultancy staff.[58]

According to the chair of the committee, Meg Hillier, NHST&T was employing "more consultants in April 2021 than it did in November 2020. Despite being nearly a year old, nearly half the central staff are consultants".[59] Given the crucial importance of a properly functioning test-and-trace system to combating the pandemic for the foreseeable future, it would seem that such roles ought to be recognized as requiring filling by staff on permanent or fixed-term contracts rather than those who have no commitment to the programme or the public healthcare system onto which it is grafted. As Hillier rightly observed: "The danger is that institutional memory will disappear as consultants walk off with their fat pay cheques".[60]

Outsourcing is also a recipe for scaling down investment in the frontline service providers since the Government's motive for outsourcing is to reduce costs whereas the motive of the outsourced company is a healthy rate of profit. This means that the wages of the outsourced service workers must be significantly less than those employed by the state in order to court the business of the corporate sector so that recruitment or retention of those with the right skills to deliver a quality service is problematized.

> Handing over a central tracing service to 25,000 people with no experience and very little training in a skilled area . . . demands that processes are standardised and computerised to the point of ineffectiveness, with all discretion removed. The results have been all too painful to see. Success in tracing the contacts of those testing positive is far lower in the central service outsourced to Serco et al (around 64%, at the latest count) than in the smaller number of more complex cases handled by local public health teams (over 97%). Better performance can be found in countries where a substantial public health service has remained at the core of the process. Germany's well-established public health network was able to manage the efforts of thousands of extra tracers expertly.[61]

Huge amounts of public money were also hoovered up by a rafter of private-sector companies that would outfit or supply the programme. By the end of 2020, the DHSC had awarded "over 600 contracts for NHST&T-related services", according to testimony given by officials to the PAC.[62] The NAO reported in December: "Contracts worth £7 billion have been signed with 217 public and private organisations to provide supplies, services and infrastructure, including test laboratories and call handlers for tracing. NHST&T has plans to sign a further 154 contracts, worth £16.2 billion, by March 2021".[63] The programme was "principally run by 22 private companies, including Serco, Deloitte, Boots, DHL and Amazon",[64] which would rake in the bulk of the £37 billion that was allocated to the programme before March's end.

Much money was also squandered in the emergency fast-track tendering process, which was a green light to cronyism. Contracts were awarded at high cost to the public purse, often without competitive bidding to demonstrate value-for-money or efficiencies,[65] doubtless to assorted entrepreneurial friends and allies of ministers. By October 2020's end, NHST&T had signed contracts with 207 organizations, of which 121 "were assigned as direct awards without competition under emergency measures".[66] In November and December of 2020, the DHSC reported to the PAC that NHST&T had "awarded a further 207 contracts worth £1.3 billion, of which around 30 were direct awards under emergency regulations".[67] Dido Harding, business executive and Conservative peer (also the wife of a Conservative MP), who would bring to the table zero experience of public health administration, was seen as the ideal person to lead the test-and-trace programme.

All of this was inevitable given the political instincts and ideological biases of ministers of the "party of business" in the age of neoliberal governance. Neoliberalism has virtually synthesized the power of authorization (politics) and the power of allocation (economics) in the apparatuses of the modern state. According to neoliberalism, only the market and the profit motive can deliver rational outcomes, so these must govern state enterprises and the running of public services. So it is that the neoliberal "business state" in Britain has actively sought to subordinate the ethics of public service to the norms of entrepreneurialism, or rather to redefine the latter as indispensable to the former. Thus, it was no surprise that ministerial decision-making when it came to setting up the nationwide test-and-trace programme would default by way of reflex to neoliberal common sense and its fetish for public–private "partnerships".

For sure, under-resourcing of the NHS, generated by austerity politics, spurred outsourcing as a practical solution to setting up a test-and-trace system quickly. But this was driven also by the deeply ingrained distrust of public enterprise and worship of private enterprise in the neoliberal and Tory imagination. Naturally, this meant that local authorities and public sector healthcare professionals and administrators – who would reasonably be expected to know a thing or two about how to organize and deliver an effective public health programme (since they had experience in doing so) – were either bypassed or sidelined or placed in the thrall of those whose expertise lay mostly in self-enrichment and optimizing shareholder value.

But, remarkably, ministers have insisted that the "teething troubles" of the test-and-trace system were ironed out by the start of 2021. Even if true, this was too late for the programme to fulfil its goals. The main purpose of test-and-trace was to sufficiently disrupt the transmission of COVID-19 so that caseloads were held in check, the NHS was protected from mass hospitalizations, so that a second national lockdown (indeed even local lockdowns under the tier system) would be avoided. The tardiness and inefficiency of the system ensured that none of these objectives were achievable. Rather, as caseloads escalated, the system could not cope with the demands placed on it. This was inevitable given that it was failing to deliver on targets during a lengthy period (June and July 2020) when the pressures placed on it were relatively low as the virus ebbed from its April first-wave peak. The evidence of this resides simply in the events. As a matter of fact, the November/ December (2020) circuit-breaker lockdown, having failed to quell the virus, was followed by protracted lockdown at the start of 2021. As the chair of PAC put it, "despite the unimaginable resources thrown at this project Test and Trace cannot point to a measurable difference to the progress of the pandemic, and the promise on which this huge expense was justified – avoiding another lockdown – has been broken, twice".[68]

If a fourth lockdown is averted this autumn or winter, nor will NHST&T play any role in preventing it. At the time of writing (5 August 2021), with "Freedom Day" just two weeks in the past, the Government is seemingly intent on undermining the system that it promised would be a world-beater when it was launched in April 2020, which it has defended ever since as delivering on its objectives, and which is has lavished tens of billions of taxpayers' money on. Hence, motivated by the expectation that the "Great Unlocking" of 19 July, coinciding as it is with a period where COVID-19 infections are resurging driven by Delta, will unleash a deluge of contact alerts requiring people to self-isolate and take a test, ministers now declare that the system is overly sensitive and will be reigned-in. This is in order to avert or diminish a "pingdemic" (a plethora of unnecessary and superfluous alerts that may lead people to think that there is still a pandemic going on). Such (the full restoration of economic "business as usual") would threaten to undermine the whole purpose of "Freedom Day" as the fourth wave of the virus rages. If the system is recalibrated, at least this may allow it to cope with the demands placed on it. However, this would also further diminish the effectiveness of the programme (as will also the rhetoric of pingdemic) as people are incentivized to simply ignore contact alerts.

5 August 2021

Notes

1   Perraudin, F. (2020). 'UK government's coronavirus response beset by mixed messages and U-turns'. *Guardian*. (19 April).
2   Baynes, M. (2020). 'UK schools could reopen on May 11 – Boris handed option to save GCSE and A-level exams'. *Express*. (19 April); Stewart, H., Proctor, K. and Adams, R. (2020). 'Picnics and sunbathing on cards as PM expected to allow more time outside'. *Guardian*. (6 May); Mason, R. and Sample, I. (2020). '"Mixed messages": UK government's strategy fuels fears of rule-breaking'. *Guardian*. (7 May).
3   Mason and Sample (2020). See also: Blackall, M. and Orbordo, R. (2020). '"I cry every day": anxiety over plans to cut furlough scheme'. *Guardian*. (6 May); Partington, R. (2020). 'Rishi Sunak preparing to wind down coronavirus furlough scheme from July'. *Guardian*. (6 May); Proctor, K. (2020). 'Longer lockdown for over-70s "could create sense of victimisation"'. *Guardian* (online). (29 April).
4   *BBC News* (2020). 'Coronavirus: minister defends "stay alert" advice amid backlash'. (10 May).
5   *BBC News* (10 May, 2020).
6   *BBC News* (2020). 'Coronavirus: further 2,988 cases confirmed in UK'. (6 September); *BBC News* (2020). 'Coronavirus: Hancock concern over "sharp rise" in cases'. (8 September); Rosney, D. (2020). 'Coronavirus: young people breaking rules risk "second wave"'. Interview with Matt Hancock. (7 September).
7   *BBC News* (8 September, 2020).
8   *BBC News* (7 September, 2020).
9   *BBC News* (2020). 'Coronavirus: lockdown to be relaxed in England as 2m rule eased'. (23 June). See also: Cabinet Office (2020). *Review of Two Metre Social Distancing Guidance*. GOV.UK (online). (revised 26 June). Available at: www.gov.uk/government/publications/review-of-two-metre-social-distancing-guidance/review-of-two-metre-social-distancing-guidance.
10   Schraer, R. (2020). 'Coronavirus: what tests are being done in the UK'? *BBC News*. (14 May).
11   Davis, N. (2020). 'Is the spread of coronavirus in the UK really slowing down'? *Guardian*. (30 March).
12   Kitt, H. (2020). 'Contact tracers could deal with five people a week before scheme ended'. *Evening Standard*. (31 March); Tapper, J. '"Recruit volunteer army to trace Covid-19 contacts now"', urge top scientists'. *Guardian*. (4 April).
13   *BBC News* (2020). 'Coronavirus: essential workers in England to get tests'. (23 April).
14   *BBC News* (2020). Coronavirus: test website closes after "significant demand"'. (24 April).

15 Ford, M. (2020). 'Care UK reveals five-week delay on staff coronavirus testing'. *Nursing Times* (online). (31 July). Available at: www.nursingtimes.net/news/coronavirus/care-uk-reveals-five-week-delay-on-staff-coronavirus-testing-31-07-2020/#:~:text=The%20government%20has%20failed%20to,social%20care%20and%20care%20homes.

16 Ford, M. (2020). 'Covid-19 test results for care home nurses "consistently delayed and lost"'. *Nursing Times* (online). (15 September). Available at: www.nursingtimes.net/news/coronavirus/covid-19-test-results-for-care-home-nurses-consistently-delayed-and-lost-15-09-2020/

17 Campbell, L. and Walker, A. (2020). 'UK coronavirus live: rate of infection doubling every three to four days, says Gove'. *Guardian.* (27 March).

18 Mason, R. (2020). 'Coronavirus: just 2,000 NHS frontline workers tested so far'. *Guardian.* (1 April).

19 Ford, M. (2020). 'Compelling case' for weekly Covid-19 testing of NHS staff, say MPs'. *Nursing Times* (online). (1 October). Available at: www.nursingtimes.net/news/coronavirus/compelling-case-for-weekly-covid-19-testing-of-nhs-staff-say-mps-01-10-2020/

20 Lintern, S. (2020). 'Coronavirus: deaths of hundreds of frontline NHS and care workers to be investigated'. *Independent.* (11 August).

21 Parliamentary Select Committee (2020). *Delivering Core NHS and Care Services During the Pandemic and Beyond.* (1 October). Available at: https://publications.parliament.uk/pa/cm5801/cmselect/cmhealth/320/32002.htm

22 Schraer, R. (2020). 'Coronavirus: NHS staff need tests "twice a week"'. *BBC News.* (17 June).

23 Parliamentary Select Committee (1 October, 2020).

24 Ford (2020).

25 Perraudin, F. and Duncan, D. (2020). 'Britain's coronavirus testing scandal: a timeline of mixed messages'. *Guardian.* (3 April).

26 Perraudin and Duncan (2020).

27 Perraudin and Duncan (2020).

28 Woodcock, A. (2020). 'Government 'absolutely' stands by 100,000 coronavirus testing target by end of April – a day after only 19,000 carried out'. *Independent.* (21 April).

29 BBC News (23 April, 2020).(

30 Stewart, H. and Campbell, D. (2020). 'Hancock says UK hit 100,000 tests amid claims tally is artificially boosted'. *Guardian.* (1 May).

31 Schraer, R. (2020). 'Coronavirus: how to get a Covid test'. *BBC News.* (17 September).

32 Statista (2020). *Rate of Coronavirus (COVID-19) Tests Performed in the Most Impacted Countries Worldwide as of October 16, 2020 (Per Million Population).* (16 October). Available at: www.statista.com/statistics/1104645/covid19-testing-rate-select-countries-worldwide/

33 BBC News (2020). 'Coronavirus: government criticised over use of testing data'. (2 June).

34 *FullFact* (2020). 'Lots of people are getting confused over testing figures'. (18 September). Available at: https://fullfact.org/health/question-time-testing-figures/

35 BBC News (2 June, 2020).

36 *Fullfact* (18 September, 2020).

37 Lacobucci, G. (2021). 'Covid-19: PM's former chief aide accuses health secretary of lying over PPE and access to treatment'. *British Medical Journal* (online), 373 (1369). (26 May). Available at: www.bmj.com/content/373/bmj.n1369.

38 *PoliticsHome* (2020). 'Matt Hancock says 21,000 coronavirus contact tracers now hired as tests expanded to all symptomatic people over five'. (18 May). Available at: www.politicshome.com/news/article/matt-hancock-says-21000-coronavirus-contact-tracers-now-hired-as-tests-expanded-to-all-symptomatic-people-over-five.

39 Neville, S., Warrell, H. and Hughes, L. (2020). 'Technical glitches overshadow English track and trace launch'. *Financial Times.* (3 June).

40 BBC News (2020). 'Coronavirus: health minister says app should roll out by winter'. (17 June); Cellan-Jones, R. (2020). 'Germany has its Covid-19 app, so where's the UK's'? *BBC News.* (16 June).

41 *BBC News* (2020). 'Coronavirus: key workers to trial NHS tracing app'. (5 May).
42 Downey, A. (2020). 'Where are we with the NHS contact tracing app'? *Digital Health* (online). (28 September). Available at: www.digitalhealth.net/2020/09/timeline-what-happened-to-the-nhs-contact-tracing-app/.
43 Crouch, H. (2020). 'Apple and Google release their contact-tracing software'. *Digital Health* (online). (22 May). Available at: www.digitalhealth.net/2020/05/google-apple-contact-tracing-software-release/.
44 Downey (2020).
45 Brigg, A., Jenkins, D. and Fraser, C. (2020). *NHS Test and Trace: The Journey So Far.* The Health Foundation (online). (23 September). Available at: www.health.org.uk/publications/long-reads/nhs-test-and-trace-the-journey-so-far
46 National Audit Office (2020). *The Government's Approach to Test and Trace in England – Interim Report.* Press release. (11 December). Available at: www.nao.org.uk/press-release/the-governments-approach-to-test-and-trace-in-england-interim-report/.
47 Campbell, D. (2020). '"Utter shambles": GPs and medics decry NHS test-and-trace system'. *Guardian.* (14 September).
48 National Audit Office (2020).
49 Brigg et al. (2020).
50 McNeill, R. and Grey, S. (2020). 'Britain's COVID-19 track and trace failures, in numbers'. *Reuters.* (24 November).
51 As reported in the *Guardian.* See: Syal, R. (2020).'England's test and trace repeatedly failed to hit goals despite £22bn cost'. *Guardian.* (11 December).
52 McNeill and Grey (2020).
53 NAO data as reported in the *Huffington Post.* See: Waugh, P. (2021). 'Test and trace has lost track of nearly 600 million Covid tests'. *Huffington Post.* (25 June).
54 National Audit Office (2020).
55 NAO data cited by Waugh (2021).
56 National Audit Office (2020).
57 NAO data cited by Waugh (2021).
58 Parliamentary Accounts Committee (2021). *COVID-19: Test, Track and Trace (Part 1).* Parliament.uk (online). (10 March). Available at: https://publications.parliament.uk/pa/cm5801/cmselect/cmpubacc/932/93202.htm.
59 Cited in Waugh (2021).
60 Cited in Waugh (2021).
61 Brooks, R. (2020). 'The failure of test and trace shows the folly of handing huge contracts to private giants'. *Guardian.* (13 October).
62 PAC (2021).
63 National Audit Office (2020).
64 Woods, R. (2021). 'Multi-billion-pound UK track and trace system failed to reduce COVID-19 spread'. *World Socialist Web Site.* (29 March). Available at: www.wsws.org/en/articles/2021/03/30/trtr-m30.html.
65 National Audit Office (2020).
66 PAC (2021).
67 PAC (2021).
68 UK Parliament (2021). *Unimaginable" Cost of Test & Trace Failed to Deliver Central Promise of Averting Another Lockdown.* Public Accounts Committee. (10 March). Available at: https://committees.parliament.uk/committee/127/public-accounts-committee/news/150988/unimaginable-cost-of-test-trace-failed-to-deliver-central-promise-of-averting-another-lockdown/.

7

MASK SCEPTICISM

What may be termed as "mask scepticism" was another striking feature of British exceptionalism. This refers obviously to official attitudes towards donning face coverings as an aspect of anti-Covid non-pharmaceutical interventions (NPIs). This, like certain other aspects of the exceptionalism spectrum, was not merely an attitude of government, but was also seemingly hard-wired into the mindset of its scientific advisers (the chief medical and scientific officers, Whitty and Vallance, their deputies, the members of the SAGE group and its subgroups). Only "scepticism" is not really the best term to describe this phenomenon. This was much more than scepticism and altogether far less healthy and excusable than mere scepticism ever could be. A descriptively better term would be mask cynicism for reasons that I will discuss. This chapter will offer a short history of mask-scepticism in official circles from the start of the British pandemic up until and including the summer of 2020. The phenomenon was to dramatically resurface in the run-up to "Freedom Day" on 19 July 2021. But this aspect of it will be addressed in Chapter 8.

Most western governments (or governments in the Global North) were doubtful of the public health benefits of mask-wearing at the outset of the pandemic. However, for the most part, they set these doubts aside, either recommending or mandating the practice under specific circumstances and in particular places – mostly in indoor settings where two-metre distancing was not possible and on public transport. They did this, presumably, for two main reasons. First, because scientific evidence available at the time (of which there was not much) did not *disprove* the potential efficacy of mask-wearing for reducing person-to-person transmission. Indeed, this appeared to provide *some* evidence (albeit indecisive) that the practice would be beneficial. Second, because recommending or mandating public mask-wearing was simply an easy step for any government to take. There were no logistical issues. There were no practical difficulties. The costs of mass-producing or mass-procuring masks were relatively low. A fearful public would perhaps be

DOI: 10.4324/9781003275039-8

easily incentivized to tolerate the inconvenience of wearing them. So, there were in potential real public health wins and no losses.

The peculiarity of British mask scepticism

British scepticism at the level of government and government-approved science, by contrast, was indeed exceptional. This was more mask-cynicism than mask-scepticism. This was outright mask resistance and opposition. Throughout the lock-down and much of the runup to it, the Government insisted (contrary to evolving WTO guidance on the matter, and in sharp difference to pandemic control policy in most other countries)[1] that there were negligible health-protection advantages in people donning face coverings in any public places where physical distancing was challenging.[2] For the British, unlike virtually everyone else, there was no point, according to the Government and its scientific appointees, in wearing a face cover-ing. As Chris Whitty put it (on 4 March 2020): "Wearing a mask if you don't have an infection reduces the risk almost to nothing at all".[3] Now, this was not exactly the position of the WTO – not even at the early stages of the pandemic, when the organization was seemingly also sceptical about the general benefits of mask-wearing.

At the start of March (2020), the WTO's position on public face-masking, as stated by Dr N. Paranietharan, the organization's representative in Indonesia, was indeed that the practice "can give a false sense of protection for healthy people". This was because if "you do not wear the mask properly, touch the mask with unwashed hands, or remove it incorrectly, you can actually place yourself at greater risk of inadvertently transmitting germs and making yourself or others sick".[4] But the WTO soon revised its guidance. The WHO's subsequent position (not itself without ambiguities and equivocations) was that mask-wearing may be considered a practice that would act "as a preventive measure" for those in mass gatherings or congested spaces or if in contact with an infected person. In particular, face-covering may "reduce the risk of exposure of people before they display symptoms".[5]

But, even before then, Paranietharan was not saying that wearing face coverings would not offer the public protection from the virus or be ineffective in reducing transmission. Mask-wearing would be efficacious, he said, for those healthy mem-bers of the public caring for or in close proximity with infected persons. "If you are healthy, you do not need to wear a mask, unless you are taking care of a person with suspected Covid-19 infection". People should also, he said, wear a mask if they were "coughing or sneezing". This was actually logically supportive of general mask-wearing in crowded indoor spaces, though the WTO did not recommend this at that stage. Rather, Paranietharan's point was that, if mask-wearing was to be beneficial, people needed to do it properly, dispose of their masks safely, and not use these as substitute for other protective measures "Masks are *effective* [my emphasis] only when used in combination with frequent hand-cleaning with soap and water or alcohol-based hand rub".[6]

By contrast, the stance of the UK government and its scientific advisers towards face coverings was simply and straightforwardly negative. Far from mask-wearing being encouraged, this was to be deterred. On 12 March, Chris Whitty's deputy, Dr Jenny Harries, in an interview for the BBC, cautioned members of the general public to *avoid* wearing face masks. This was justified on the grounds (borrowed selectively from the WHO) that if these were used incorrectly this would generate greater rather than lesser health risks. Fiddling with the mask, for example, could lead to people self-infecting themselves, as they transmit the virus from surfaces they have touched to their own airways. The wearer would also be placed at risk if the mask was loose or ill-fitting. The WHO's caution on public mask-wearing and stress on the need to educate the user if the practice was to be efficacious was thus "translated" locally as being straightforwardly inefficacious because people were bound to get it wrong. Moreover, even if people did wear the masks correctly, the health benefits were bound to be negligible. On 4 April, Professor Jonathan Van Tam, another of the Government's medical advisers, stated unequivocally during a press briefing that

> there was no evidence that general wearing of face masks by the public who are well affects the spread of the disease in our society. . . . In terms of the hard evidence and what the UK Government recommends, we do not recommend face masks for general wearing by the public.[7]

There was no dalliance here with Paranietharan's position that mask-wearing under certain circumstances and scenarios may or would yield such benefits.

On 17 April, the Minister for Transport, Grant Shapps, reiterated the official line – there were no plans to encourage people to wear masks. This was in response to the US Centers for Disease Control and Prevention's (USDCPs) recommendation that people wear masks in crowded public spaces. Not only, claimed Shapps, was there no steer from SAGE that anyone other than healthcare professionals caring for the sick should wear masks (since scientific evidence showing safety benefits was, as Chris Whitty put it, "weak"), but there was "also evidence out there that wearing it [a mask] could be counterproductive". This was because, according to "the science" and "experts", mask-wearing may provoke in the wearers a false sense of security, leading them to disregard two-metre distancing and regular handwashing.[8] On 23 April, Jenny Harries dismissed the efficacy of mask-wearing even in densely packed indoor spaces without ventilation (the London tube being the example she was presented with). The benefits were, she said, at best (i.e. in "potential"), "very, very small". This was just as SAGE's deliberations of that same day repeated Whitty's judgement that evidence in favour of masks was "weak".[9]

Of course, none of these perspectives on either the supposedly miniscule (if that) advantages of mask-wearing or the supposedly much bigger disadvantages of doing so were in fact science-led or data-led, since there was insufficient scientific evidence to support them. Rather, these were the speculations of mask-sceptics in government and amongst its scientific and medical appointees. The requirement that mask-wearing could only be legitimized by Van Tam's "hard" evidence meant that "soft" evidence could be disregarded. At the same time, mask-scepticism was not even supported by "soft" evidence. For there was no evidence that mask-wearing could not yield benefits, only that it was not absolutely clear that there were substantial benefits. To put the matter more diplomatically, indeed remarkably so, as Emily So and Hannah Baker do, "the scientific advisors . . . [were] . . . demanding much too high of a standard of evidence than . . . [was] . . . warranted by the current situation".

> The Precautionary Principle seems to argue that masks should be recommended even if the case for adopting them is not 100% watertight. Their cautious approach is also inconsistent since other highly uncertain strategies have been adopted, yet masks remain contentious.[10]

Not only were these judgements speculative, but they were also threadbare rationales rooted in confirmation bias. Those countries that were destined to do better at containing the virus and limiting its damage were those that embraced public mask-wearing as well as all those other practices that Harries and Shapps chose to believe would be hampered or offset by mask-wearing. This was the case for most of the countries in Southeast Asia, for example, where physical distancing (along with border controls, travel restrictions, and robust quarantining) co-existed with mask-wearing, with these practices likely reinforcing rather than obstructing each other.

Assuming the contrary would be the case in the UK was also simply counter-intuitive. In Southeast Asia, the public would be incentivized to take the threat of the pandemic seriously by virtue of the fact that this was seen to merit a rafter of measures being put in place (including compulsory mask-wearing) to control it. Here masking-up was a visually symbolic confirmation of the need to respect physical distancing, not its disincentive. Even if the *literal* impact of public mask-wearing on transmission rates was small, as the Government and government scientists thought, the *symbolic* impact of the practice may generate far greater benefits in reducing the spread of the virus. This is because widespread mask-donning in busy public areas (shops, supermarkets, malls, leisure or sports centres, etc.) may reinforce the message that there is a major life-threatening disease on the loose and thereby encourage more vigilant physical distancing. This possibility was seemingly not considered at all.

Why would it be any different in the UK to elsewhere? Could it be because British exceptionalism holds that the British people are "exceptional" in that they are impervious to good sense? But, even if it was different in the UK, inasmuch as mask-wearing would encourage disregard of physical distancing, why would it be beyond the power of government messaging to educate the public that physical distancing, even more so than mask-wearing, was indispensable to preventing the spread of the virus? Again, as Emily So and Hannah Baker rightly (and politely) put the matter:

> The reticence of UK scientists seems to be driven by their sense of how we as a nation would behave with masks, and they will only consider their health effects after some assurance of compliance. But we have all had to change our behaviours for Covid-19, so why would this be one step too far?[11]

To assume otherwise (i.e. that people in the UK could not be persuaded that mask-wearing would not be an alternative to handwashing or two-metre physical distancing), as ministers and the Government's scientists evidently did, was also to infantilize the public. To deem mask-wearing potentially injurious to public health, on the grounds that ordinary people could not be trusted to wear the correct masks or to wear them correctly, was more of the same. Putting on a face covering, learning how it ought to be worn, as well as the behaviours to avoid when wearing it, how to dispose of it, and so on, was hardly intellectually challenging.

In sharp contrast to the UK government's attitude to face coverings, confronted with the pandemic's first wave, most European governments shifted from embracing mask scepticism to either recommending or legally mandating mask-use in certain settings or under specific circumstances since before the spring of 2020. Mandatory mask-wearing was introduced in the Czech Republic on 19 March, in Slovakia on 25 March, in Austria on 6 April, in Germany on 22 April, in Greece on 29 April, in France on 11 May, and in Spain on 21 May.[12] Face masks were officially recommended for use in Italy early in April and were made mandatory in the Lombardy region on the same timescale.[13] The Portuguese government announced that it was recommending public mask-wearing on 13 April.[14] In Germany, people were given an official steer to voluntarily wear face masks also from mid-April.[15] And, of course, in many countries in Southeast Asia – with a rich history of coping with outbreaks of infectious diseases that could potentially become epidemics – face-masking was an established public practice, backed by health professionals and by government, long before the novel coronavirus.

Public health experts and scientists in these countries were exactly those that officials in Hancock's DHSC and the UK government's chief scientific advisers ought to have been consulting with in order to inform judgement on public mask-wearing. However, British exceptionalism ruled this out. The attachment of Southeast Asian countries and peoples to mask-wearing was dismissed, in Van Tam's words, as something "wired" into their cultures,[16] an aspect of custom, rather than as something informed by practical judgement, by experiences of coping with viruses such as SARS, and a "better safe than sorry" attitude to public health.[17] Westerners did not understand and still needed to learn that the long history of popular mask-wearing in East Asia in particular was not motivated by individualistic judgements of the efficacy of mask-wearing for one's own health and safety, but by commitment to protecting the health and safety of others by simply minimizing or disrupting the transmission of germs.[18]

The Government eventually made mask-wearing mandatory on 15 June 2020 – up to a point.[19] Now mask-wearing became law on public transport. This was more than a month after it had settled for advising or recommending that people should mask up on public transport or in certain shops under Phase 1 of its unlocking of lockdown roadmap. In all other public settings, this remained a matter for individual decision-making, however. It was not until 14 July that the Government announced that compulsory mask-wearing would be extended also to members of the general public when entering shops, department stores and supermarkets – but this would not come into force until 24 July.[20] Mandatory face-masking was later extended to include cinemas and houses of worship on 8 August.[21] Finally, in the autumn of 2020 (on 22 September), under the impress of the COVID-19 second wave, ministers announced that mandatory face coverings would be required for staff in all retail settings in England starting on 24 September.[22]

There was no explanation for the further delay (i.e. from the 14 July mandate to its 24 July implementation), which defied rational explanation, since the case for it was conceded, and implementing the new policy posed no practical difficulties that would require advance preparations. This caused exasperation and consternation in the medical profession whose members overwhelmingly supported compulsory mask-wearing especially in the context of the unlocking of other restrictions. As the BMA council chair Chaand Nagpaul put it:

> Up until now . . . Westminster . . . has refused to put in place this logical policy to prevent spread of the virus, and which has been the norm in around 120 countries globally including most of Europe – so this step is long overdue.[23]

Boris Johnson himself was photographed donning a face mask in public for the first time on 15 July (hence taking more than two months to heed the public safety advice of his own government).[24]

These developments were not only trailing those elsewhere across the world, but they were lagging behind the evolving guidance furnished by the WTO and the Government's own scientific advisers on the efficacy of public mask-wearing. On 6 April 2020, the WTO updated its advice, now recommending mask-wearing in those countries where other preventative measures were impracticable.[25] The next day the European Centre for Disease Prevention and Control published new recommendations for combating the spread of the virus that included public mask-wearing.[26] On 5 May, the Government's Chief Scientific Officer, Patrick Vallance, reported to the Parliamentary Health and Social Care Committee that SAGE now considered that recent scientific studies provided "some evidence" that mask-wearing made a "marginal but positive" contribution to preventing person-to-person infection. For, even though "the major root of infection is probably droplet spread, rather than through aerosol . . . there may be some aerosol components as well".[27]

This was rather understating the matter. A range of scientific studies had by the summer of 2020 evidenced that face coverings significantly if not majorly reduced viral transmission. For example, a study published in *Nature Medicine* on 3 April concluded:

> Our findings indicate that surgical masks can efficaciously reduce the emission of influenza virus particles into the environment in respiratory droplets, but not in aerosols . . . We also demonstrated the efficacy of surgical masks to reduce coronavirus detection and viral copies in large respiratory droplets and in aerosols. . . . Face masks significantly reduced detection of influenza virus RNA in respiratory droplets and coronavirus RNA in aerosols, with a trend toward reduced detection of coronavirus RNA in respiratory droplets. This has important implications for control of COVID-19, suggesting that surgical face masks could be used by ill people to reduce onward transmission.[28]

Another April study reported "the results of a laser light-scattering experiment in which speech-generated droplets and their trajectories were visualized". This study tracked the movement of droplets exhaled by speech through a light sheet using high-speed filming techniques. Such was relevant to assessing the efficacy of face masks in preventing onward transmission of viruses because "studies have shown that the number of droplets produced by speaking is similar to the number produced by coughing". The findings were indicative that specialized face coverings would be very effective in blocking the expulsion of droplets beyond the barrier provided by the mask. This was demonstrated indirectly by showing that merely placing a damp dishcloth over the mouth and nose when making certain speech sounds was effective in blocking onward transmission.

> We found that when the person said, "stay healthy," numerous droplets ranging from 20 to 500 μm were generated. These droplets produced flashes as they passed through the light sheet. . . . When the same phrase was uttered three times through a slightly damp washcloth over the speaker's mouth, the flash count remained close to the background level (mean, 0.1 flashes); this showed a decrease in the number of forward-moving droplets.

At the start of June, *The Lancet* published a meta-review of all studies investigating the efficacy of mask-wearing which found that this *majorly* reduced the risk of infection. This was so much so that mask-wearers (so long as they wore the masks correctly) would reduce their risk of catching COVID-19 to just 3 percent in those settings where the masks were worn. Such was the case with the highest-grade medical masks, but other masks (disposable surgical and reusable cotton ones) also substantially reduced infection risk. These findings were based on the analysis of data drawn from 172 studies in 16 countries.[29]

Substantial benefits were also reported from studies carried out by researchers at Cambridge University, Edinburgh University and Oxford University in June and July. The Cambridge study was indicative that wearing even simple homemade masks would be effective in reducing transmission, whether or not the wearers were symptomatic. As Dr Richard Stutt summarized the findings:

> Our analyses support the immediate and universal adoption of face masks by the public. If widespread face mask use by the public is combined with physical distancing and some lockdown, it may offer an acceptable way of managing the pandemic and reopening economic activity long before there is a working vaccine.[30]

The Edinburgh study "assessed different face coverings using a technique – called Background Oriented Schlieren imaging". This is a method that allows researchers "to measure the distance and direction travelled by air expelled when a person breathes or coughs". Subjects wore face masks of different types, in lying or standing positions, and measurements were made of how far forward their breaths travelled. The study found that wearing "all face coverings without an outlet valve . . . reduce[d] . . . the forward distance travelled by a deep breath out by at least 90 per cent".[31]

The Oxford study found that

> face masks and coverings for the general public are effective in improving: i) source protection, i.e., reduced virus transmission from the wearer when they are of optimal material and construction and fitted correctly; and ii) wearer protection, i.e., reduced rate of infection of those who wear them.[32]

> The use of cotton masks is associated with a 54% lower relative odds of infection in comparison to the no mask groups (RR=0.46; 95% CI: 0.22–0.97; N=746) with a coefficient heterogeneity I2 of 66.6% (Q-test P=0.05). For paper masks, the relative odds of infection were 39% lower than in the no mask group (RR=0.61; 95% CI: 0.41–0.90; N=166; I2 = 0.0%).[33]

Summarizing the results, lead researcher Professor Melinda Mills, concluded:

> Next to hand washing and social distancing, face masks and coverings are one of the most of widely adopted non-pharmaceutical interventions for reducing the transmission of respiratory infections. . . . The evidence is clear that people should wear masks to reduce virus transmission and protect themselves, with most countries recommending the public to wear them.

Mills expressed bafflement over why "policy resistance" to public face-masking by certain governments (especially by the UK government and its scientific advisers) "has been so high". Such policy resistance was a threat to public health because it also encouraged mask scepticism and disregard for masking-up in the general public. The Oxford researchers noted that mask-wearing was much lower in the

UK than in other countries with no prior history of the practice. By the end of April 2020, there was a take-up rate of just 26 percent in England compared to 83 percent in Italy, 66 percent in the US, 64 percent in Spain, 45 percent in France, 35 percent in Belgium, and 32 percent in Germany.[34] Despite much evidence in favour of mask-wearing, and despite most governments worldwide supporting and mandating it, "clear policy recommendations that the public should . . . has been unclear and inconsistent in some countries such as England".[35]

This resistance was warranted by "the science" only on a specific and overly restrictive concept of scientific evidence. There was, said the Oxford research-ers, "over-reliance on an evidence-based approach and assertion that evidence was weak due to few conclusive RCT (randomized control trial) results in community settings, discounting high quality non-RCT evidence".[36] But, as Mills pointed out, "RCTs don't fit well when looking at behaviour and it was clear that high quality observational and behavioural research had been largely discarded".[37] The paradox (or double standards) here was that standards of evidence based on clinical trials were not regarded as being necessary to support the adoption of physical distancing and quarantining policies, yet these were deemed as essential to enlist government support for public mask-wearing.[38]

Explaining mask scepticism

The rationales presented by ministers and government scientists (from the start of the pandemic right up to May) for why mask-wearing should not be officially encouraged or mandated were so weak it is hard to believe they were regarded as credible, even by those who promulgated them. These appear more as legitima-tions for mask refusal that was endorsed for other unacknowledged reasons. The impression is reinforced by the fact that, even after SAGE came round to the idea that mask-wearing was not irrelevant or worse, it took the Cabinet a further two months to legally mandate the practice. If so, what were these unacknowledged reasons for refusing to countenance donning face coverings?

Part of it was perhaps the impact on thinking (on "establishment" scientists and ministers) of the old colonial outlook that "Britain knows best" and that there is little to be learned from the public health practices of other countries. Such an outlook was hardly likely to be dented in the post-Brexit political context that was seeing ministers lauding a newly resurgent Britain going it alone on the global stage and repositioning itself as a world leader – on the promotion of free trade, on sci-entific and technological innovation, in reducing carbon emissions, in combatting international terrorism, and so on. The UK was, after all, at the forefront of pan-demic preparedness, according to these same scientists and ministers, whereas mask-wearing was merely an arbitrary cultural tradition of East Asian countries rather than one based on discernible objective benefits. Since that was the assumption – because mask-wearing originated outside the "rational" cultures of the West – then it was no surprise that dismissal was the default position.

But, as far as explaining the specifically *scientific* scepticism, other factors may be germane. Government-appointed experts have a tendency towards conservativism or circumspection in the advice they offer to ministers inasmuch as this, if it went "too far", could upset the status quo. This would be especially the case where the Government of the day is committed to conserving rather than reforming the status quo. These "official" experts are also specifically appointees and sometimes employees of a particular kind of political authority – a neoliberal capitalist state and governance that is simply not well-disposed to any form of public policy that places restrictions on the exercise of individual rights, whatever the social or community benefits of doing so. Since these "political" or "state" scientists know what is expected of them, or how far they can go (if their advice it so be heeded), they will tailor it so that the ears of ministers may be receptive. The reluctance of the official scientific and public health advisers to steer the Government towards a mask-wearing policy may reflect a lack of confidence that such advice would be taken seriously unless the evidence in favour of it was "hard" or incontrovertible.

But there is perhaps something else to be said about the possible motives behind the mask-denial of the Government's scientific and medical advisors. Elite "establishment" or "managerial" or "corporate" scientists or clinicians (as Whitty and Vallance undoubtedly are) are not members of a classless tribe committed to "pure" science or maximal public health to the exclusion of all else. Rather, they are – by virtue of birth, education, command over authoritative and allocative resources, and the social circles they inhabit – members of the higher professional-managerial and propertied classes whose members run the executive and legislative apparatuses of state and the corporate economy. As such they will have a strong tendency to share the property-friendly and market-friendly beliefs and values and attitudes of those who share their class situation and who occupy as they do authoritative roles in the state and in corporations. Not least this is because these cultural sensibilities are consistent with their material interests as these are given by their positions in society *vis-à-vis* various resources and other people differently placed in society.

In short, those health and scientific experts that the Government considered as a "safe pair of hands", inasmuch as they could be trusted to grasp the necessity of reconciling public health and safety matters with the preservation of the economic and political status quo (indeed the avoidance of even its disruption), are exactly those who would be appointed into authoritative positions in the state. Reconciliation of public health needs with the political and economic imperatives of profit-fuelled capitalist expansion must always dilute and compromise the former. Indeed, since the capitalist imperative of accumulation for accumulation's sake, of growth for survival's sake, is incompatible with public health, the danger under neoliberal governance is that dilution or compromise of the latter in the service of the former is turned into its capitulation or outright subordination.

Such is demanded by "realism" – and this is the burden not only of power-holders but of those experts integrated into the state whose job is to advise them. These experts would be those who were inclined to self-filter the advice and guidance they offered to government, so that this did not stray outside the neoliberal capitalism-serving ideological framework that governs state policy action in the UK. This is precisely because they would themselves identify with that framework.

In that case, their mask-scepticism may be rooted not in scientific caution but in political predispositions that are shared with ministers and politicians.

If this is the case, to understand the mask-denial of the Government's experts, we need to understand the mask-denial of government. Of all of the many and different elements of British exceptionalism, dogged ministerial resistance to public mask-wearing appears by far as the most puzzling. There were, after all, no economic deficits in embracing the practice and incentivizing the public to get on board with it – as there were with physical distancing and self-isolation restrictions. Now, it would be tempting to view this protracted mask-denial as simply the disingenuous behaviour of politicians who having insisted at the beginning that the benefits were non-existent sought to avoid losing face by sticking to their guns. However, for a government forced into so many policy U-turns by its own inadequacies of policy response, one other about-face would not seem to pose significant risk of causing further damage to public perceptions of its competence.

Rather, mask-refusal as government policy was likely simply motivated by the "libertarian" element of neoliberal politics and ideology that is ingrained in the sensibilities of ministers and substantial numbers of MPs – especially though not exclusively on one side of the commons. Mask-wearing, especially for right-wing neoliberals, is emblematic of illiberalism: the suspension of certain individual liberties (especially the freedom to trade and to shop and to work) owing to physical distancing and lockdown restrictions. Mask-wearing, in other words, for many MPs, became visually symbolic of the general loss of freedom under the wheels of a "nanny state" emboldened by the pandemic. (Nanny-state aversion is of course a long-standing preoccupation of the New Right whose state-actors basically pioneered neoliberalism in 1980s Britain). Since physical distancing rules could not be avoided if a public health catastrophe was to be averted – or, rather, if a far bigger one was to be averted – at least there could be for them resistance to this particular image, or more literally façade, of illiberalism.

Such explains why the issue of mask-wearing so excites or agitates (and indeed irks and enrages) especially Conservative passions. A matter of minor personal inconvenience compared to all of the other COVID-19 restrictions was amplified in the Tory (and neoliberal) imagination into an assault on the foundations of citizenship itself. This accounts for the long resistance of ministers to either supporting or mandating face-masking. This also explains why its legal support was ditched at the first opportunity (i.e. on 19 July 2021's "Freedom Day") alongside attempts to legitimize non-mask-wearing behaviour when the logical case for continuing to mandate and incentivize the practice was overwhelming. If "Freedom Day" should lead to hospitalizations spiralling out of control, the ditching of mandatory face coverings could even help sustain another round of lockdown avoidance. This is inasmuch as restoring mandatory mask coverings may then function as the fillip that would allow the Government to resist re-introducing more substantive restrictions.

3 August 2020 (updated 14 July 2021)

Notes

1 As Professor Melinda Mills observed, following on from the WHO's declaration of a global pandemic in mid-March, 70 national governments immediately recommended mask wearing. By early July 2020, in more than 120 countries, mask-wearing was mandatory in all or most public settings. See University of Oxford (2020). 'Oxford COVID-19 study: face masks and coverings work – act now'. *Oxford University* (online). News Release. (8 July). Available at: www.ox.ac.uk/news/2020-07-08-oxford-covid-19-study-face-masks-and-coverings-work-act-now.

2 Gehrke, L. and Furlong, A. (2020). 'Timeline: how Europe embraced the coronavirus face mask'. *Politico*. (16 July).

3 Cited in: Gehrke and Furlong (2020). The most remarkable thing about this statement was that it was not science- or data-led at all. Rather, the matter of the efficacy of mask-wearing was yet to be determined by scientific study. There were good logical reasons for thinking that mask-wearing would offer some protection from transmitting the virus. These are so obvious they need not be stated. Indeed, there was "weak" evidence in favour, as Whitty himself said.

4 WHO (2020). *Media Statement: The Role and Need of Masks During COVID-19 Outbreak*. WHO (online). (6 March). Available at: www.who.int/indonesia/news/detail/06-03-2020-media-statement-the-role-and-need-of-masks-during-covid-19-outbreak.

5 Stubley, P. (2020). 'Coronavirus: WHO updates face mask advice but does not recommend wider use among public'. *Independent*. (7 April). Available at: www.independent.co.uk/news/health/coronavirus-face-mask-guidance-official-evidence-who-trump-a9453001.html.

6 WHO (2020).

7 So, E. and Baker, H. (2020). *Mask or No Mask? A Look at UK's Policy Over Time*. Centre for Research in the Arts, Social Sciences and Humanities (online). (9 June). Available at: www.crassh.cam.ac.uk/blog/post/mask-or-no-mask-a-look-at-uks-policy-over-time.

8 *BBC News* (2020). 'Coronavirus: UK to be "guided by scientists" on face masks'. (17 April).

9 So and Baker (2020).

10 So and Baker (2020).

11 So and Baker (2020).

12 *BBC News* (2020). 'Coronavirus: Germany's states make face masks compulsory'. (22 April); Gehrke and Furlong (2020).

13 Giuffrida, A. and Beaumont, P. (2020). 'Lombardy insists on face masks outside homes to stop Covid-19'. *Guardian*. (5 April).

14 Gehrke and Furlong (2020).

15 *BBC News* (17 April, 2020).

16 So and Baker (2020).

17 As So and Baker (2020) describe it.

18 Sand, J. (2020). 'We share what we exhale: a short cultural history of mask-wearing'. *Times Literary Supplement*, 6109 (1 May).

19 Department for Transport (2020). *Face Coverings to Become Mandatory on Public Transport*. GOV.UK (online). (4 June). Available at: www.gov.uk/government/news/face-coverings-to-become-mandatory-on-public-transport.

20 *BBC News* (2020). 'Coronavirus: face masks and coverings to be compulsory in England's shops'. (14 July). Typically, there were illogical exemptions. Children under 11 years of age, for example, were not required to wear them. This was presumably based on the myth that children were less likely to either catch or transmit the virus than adults.

21 *BBC News* (2020). 'Coronavirus: Boris Johnson postpones lockdown easing in England'. (31 July).

22 *BBC News* (2020). 'Coronavirus: new Covid restrictions could last six months, says Boris Johnson'. (22 September).

23 Blackburn, P. (2020). 'Government makes wearing face masks mandatory'. *British Medical Association* (online). (14 July). Available at: www.bma.org.uk/news-and-opinion/government-makes-wearing-face-masks-mandatory.

24 Gehrke and Furlong (2020).

25 Martuscelli, C. (2020). 'WHO softens its stance on masks, with caveats'. *Politico*. (6 April).

26 Gehrke and Furlong (2020).

27 *BBC News* (2020). 'Coronavirus: mass testing earlier "would have been beneficial"'. (5 May).

28 Leung, N. et al. (2020). 'Respiratory virus shedding in exhaled breath and efficacy of face masks'. *Nature Medicine*, 26 (3 April), pp. 676–80 (p. 679).

29 Chu, D.K., Aki, E.A., Duda, S., Solo, K., Yaacoub, S. and Shunemann, J. (2020). 'Physical distancing, face masks, and eye protection to prevent person-to-person transmission of SARS-CoV-2 and COVID-19: a systematic review and meta-analysis'. *The Lancet*, 395 (10242) (1 June), pp. 1973–87.

30 Brackley, P. (2020). *Coronavirus: Face Masks are Key to Preventing Second Wave of Covid-19 – and We Should All Wear Them, Say University of Cambridge Researchers*. University of Cambridge (online). (11 June). Available at: www.cambridgeindependent.co.uk/news/face-masks-are-key-to-preventing-second-wave-of-covid-19-and-we-should-all-wear-them-say-cambridge-researchers-9112778/.

31 Sridhar, D. and King, L. (2020). *Why Wearing a Face Covering Can Make a Difference*. University of Edinburgh (online). (2 July). Available at: www.ed.ac.uk/covid-19-response/expert-insights/why-wearing-face-covering-can-make-difference.

32 The Royal Society and The British Academy (2020). *Face Masks and Coverings for the General Public: Behavioural Knowledge, Effectiveness of Cloth Coverings and Public Messaging*. Royal Society and British Academy (online). (26 June), p. 2. Available at: https://royalsociety.org/-/media/policy/projects/set-c/set-c-facemasks.pdf?la=en-GB&hash=A22A87CB28F7D6AD9BD93BBCBFC2BB24.

33 RS and BA (2020), p. 7.

34 RS and BA (2020), p. 20.

35 University of Oxford. (8 July, 2020).

36 RS and BA (2020), p. 2.

37 University of Oxford (8 July, 2020).

38 RS and BA (2020), p. 2.

8
FREEDOM DAY

"Freedom Day" (19 July 2021) promises to be the most recent case of British exceptionalism, which this time is carried forth by vaccine triumphalism, if not fetishism. This is whereby the Government insists that the only necessary protection against the virus is mass inoculation. This is clear enough from contemporary events in the run-up to 19 July. Events leading up to 19 July will be addressed here in this chapter. So too will what is proposed for "Freedom Day". I will also offer a forecast of likely developments owing to 19 July. This is ventured on the assumption that at the time of writing these words (15 July 2021) the Great Unlocking that is mooted will proceed as seems inevitable.

The resurgence of the virus on the cusp of the summer of 2021, after a hiatus extending around eight weeks from early March until the start of May, paralleled the Government's step-by-step scaling down of lockdown restrictions. Boris Johnson released his most recent roadmap to what he dubbed as "Freedom Day" on 22 February, according to which the bulk of remaining physical distancing would be dispensed with more than a week before June's end.[1] This was three-and-a-half months after the unlocking started with school and college returns. This roadmap plan, like its predecessor, was to unfold in stages, each tied to a specific date, yet supposedly subject to passing tests (on vaccine targets and efficacy – including against new variants – plus infection rates).

Stage 1 was the reopening of schools and colleges on 8 March. Stage 2, starting on 29 March, would resume outdoor gatherings of up to six persons as well as sports activities. Stage 3, starting on 12 April, would see the restoration of all non-essential shops, plus the reopening of a rafter of lifestyle and fitness venues (outdoor hospitality, gyms, hairdressers, etc.). Stage 4 extended the "rule of six" of permitted social gatherings to pub and bar venues and permitted members of two households to mix socially in indoor settings. The final stage would basically terminate all

DOI: 10.4324/9781003275039-9

remaining physical distancing rules outside hospitals, care homes and national exit and entry ports. This was proposed for 21 June.[2]

Johnson's 22 February statement in the House of Commons commended the plan as "cautious but irreversible", as "led by data rather than dates".[3] Yet the peak of the calamitous second (or third) wave was barely a month in the past and the seven-day average of daily new cases had barely dipped beneath 10,000, and this with an accompanying seven-day average of 330 deaths. This was pretty much at the same stage of the pandemic's downswing as was the case on the cusp of the first (premature) unlocking. At the start of the previous unlocking process, the seven-day average of daily deaths was running at 360. However, at least this time the first moves to wind down restrictions were still a couple of weeks away.[4] Of course, Johnson's statement was self-contradictory. If the unlocking was to be led by data, there was no sense in setting definite dates to each of its stages. And, if the unlocking was irreversible, then it could neither be "cautious" nor data-led, since the "wrong" data would not be permitted to delay or suspend it.[5] Thus, the suspicion was that the roadmap would be cautious only rhetorically by virtue of what was claimed for it.

There is some evidence supportive of that interpretation. The third lockdown, like the second, was less comprehensive and more equivocal than the first, despite the greater negative impact of the virus's second and third waves – as measured in terms of infections, hospitalizations and mortalities. This partly explained why the transmission rate during the third lockdown was not suppressed by anywhere as much as it was on the first shutdown before the current period of unlocking got started, despite its longer duration. In the week prior to the 22 February roadmap plans being set in motion (with the 8 March school and college re-openings), 41,594 new cases of infection were recorded. This compared to 28,460 in the week before the 13 May start of the first roadmap out of lockdown restrictions.[6] During the period where the ebbing of the first wave bottomed-out at its lower scales (i.e. from 22 June to 28 July 2020), there were 24,466 new cases. This was an average of 661 per day. During the equivalent longer period of the bottoming-out at the lower scales of the second or, on my representation, third wave (i.e. from 4 April to 16 July 2021) there were 95,055 new cases. This was an average of 2,211 per day.[7]

However, the unlocking was more drawn out than it was the first time round – by more than a month. This (along with frequent government pronouncements over the spring and summer months affirming that their approach was indeed cautious and based on scientific judgement) helped sustain what may be termed as an ideology of evidence-based caution that disguised an underlying reality that was much less clear-cut.[8] Noisy recursive affirmations of policy led by "data not dates" deflects the public mind from recognizing that roadmaps are based on politics rather than science and are doubtless intended to protect political leaders from accusations of taking risks with public health.

This has been exposed by the most recent developments. In the current times, even the rhetoric of data-led caution has been pushed into the background. Rather, the removal of Health Secretary Matt Hancock from his post on 27 June and his replacement by former chancellor Sajid Javid heralded the Government's default to its earlier risk-taking (with public safety) *modus operandi* by means of a headlong rush to restoring full economic normalcy. Such has been facilitated by the success of the vaccination programme in extending maximal double-dose protection to the high-priority groups and lesser single-dose protection to most other adult cohorts. This has afforded Johnson renewed confidence to re-embark on his "hope for the best" and "suck it and see" approach in the context of full unlocking. The government insists that further delay of "Freedom Day" beyond 19 July (owing to a Delta-fuelled rise in caseloads) would not be countenanced no matter what.

Matt Hancock, who had positioned himself as a force for caution and moderation in the Government, and under pressure from scientists and the BMA,[9] had joined with cabinet big-hitters Rishi Sunak and Michael Gove to browbeat Boris Johnson into delaying by a month the final ditching of virtually all remaining lockdown measures – which had been planned for 21 June. This was owing to a resurgence of the virus conveyed especially by the Delta variant.[10] Johnson was obviously reluctant, claiming (wrongly) that the data did not warrant postponement beyond 21 June, since this he said showed "stability" of infection rates at the lower scales, whereas in fact caseloads were increasing as Delta became dominant.[11] But, in the end, Johnson deferred to the trio, even though support for Hancock in the Cabinet and on the backbenches had virtually evaporated owing to the delay.[12] Hancock's removal, by contrast, radically strengthened the influence of the long-standing lockdown sceptics on the PM's thinking.[13]

Johnson's own distaste for physical distancing rules and his desire to justify getting rid of them at the first opportunity was also emboldened by Chris Whitty's (contentious – even on scientific grounds) assessment delivered to the Cabinet on 28 June that if physical distancing restrictions were to be lifted all in one go it would be better to do that in the summer rather than in the autumn with winter approaching. As Whitty put it in a subsequent press briefing: "At a certain point, you move to the situation where instead of actually averting hospitalisations and deaths, you move over to just delaying them".[14] Whitty's assessments were hardly unequivocal support for simply ditching all community-facing restrictions, but it was inevitable that the PM and Tory lockdown sceptics would exploit their ambivalence as such, as Whitty ought to have known.[15]

Whitty's views were remarkable not simply for their defeatism but for the fact that they were strikingly reminiscent of his (and Patrick Vallance's) legitimizations of Johnson's disastrous approach to the unfolding crisis in the weeks leading up to the first lockdown in March the year before. This response, as we have seen, was notable for its tardiness and reactiveness, leading to thousands of unnecessary deaths. Back then, on the eve of the crisis, Whitty and Vallance had advised the Government that the virus could not be blocked, nor its ill effects radically reduced. Rather, all that could be accomplished was to delay its spread, steer (i.e. "flatten" or "soften") the rise and fall of its trajectory, and thereby mitigate the damage it would cause by cushioning the NHS from having to deal with too many cases in one go. Whitty's summer interventions, then, were a case of "back to the future", suggestive of a fairly radical failure of self-reflection on his part.

These allowed a veneer of scientific legitimation to be imparted to the agitations of the already powerful and influential anti-lockdown lobby among the MPs and wider party spearheaded by the Covid Recovery Group (whose views commanded the sympathy if not support of the majority of MPs and likely of members as well), imparting confidence to the gung-ho constituency who regarded lockdown as misguided from the start. This also marginalized further the few remaining voices for moderation. Such reportedly was decisive, post-Hancock, in securing the Cabinet's collective go-ahead to "Freedom Day".[16]

Hancock's replacement, Sajid Javid, in his first statement to the press (on 27 June) affirmed his intention to restore normality "as quickly as possible".[17] The next day he declared in parliament that from now on the Government would be replacing a policy informed by "data rather than dates" with one informed by "dates not data", since no "date we choose comes with zero risk".[18] This meant that the roadmap plan to dump the remaining physical distancing controls which had been deferred until 19 July would proceed "irreversibly" on that date, since "restrictions on our freedoms . . . must come to an end", and with "no going back". "Freedom Day" would not only be "the end of the line" but "the start of an exciting new journey for our country".[19]

Javid's "top priority", in his own words, was not so much protecting the public from COVID-19 as "restoring our freedoms".[20] This was clear enough even at the level of semantics. "My primary goal is to help return the economic and cultural life that makes this country so great, while, of course, protecting life and the NHS".[21] There was, he said, "no reason to go beyond" 19 July because, although infections were increasing, the number of deaths was "mercifully low". At the same time, "people and businesses need certainty, so we want every step to be irreversible".[22]

Prioritizing business "security" and freedom over norms intended to safeguard public health may be considered a rather unfortunate priority for a new *health* secretary to embrace from the very start of his tenure, yet Javid (Johnson's former chancellor) was undeterred. His claim that there was *no reason* for delay was obviously assertive rather than cautiously equivocal, despite his corresponding claim that caution was being exercised. This assertion was also simply false. There was, of course, evidence-based reason for delay. This was on the grounds of a number of targets that the Government had set for itself and which it had said would need to be met for full and complete unlocking under Phase 4 to go ahead. However, since not all the targets were likely to be met, and none unambiguously so,[23] this may explain why Javid did not refer to the test criteria in his press briefings or statement to the House of 28 June 2021.

Javid's declarations of intent thus crystallized the Government's resolve to risk major public health deficits (including significantly higher numbers of deaths) for the sake of full and immediate economic renewal. As Javid later made clear, his intention was indeed to make a bonfire of virtually all physical distancing norms:

> We will revoke all social distancing guidance, including the two-metre rule, except for in specific settings such as ports of entry and medical settings,

where of course it would continue to make sense. . . . It will no longer be necessary to work from home. There will be no limits on the number of people we can meet. There will no limits on the number of people who can attend life events such as weddings and funerals, and there will be no restrictions on communal worship or singing. . .. All businesses that were forced to close their doors will be able to open them once again. And we will lift the cap on named care home visitors so that families can come together in the ways they choose to do so.[24]

But this was just as infection rates were increasing rapidly to their highest levels since the tail end of January and as the number of daily deaths, though low in comparison with the earlier waves, increased majorly. Between 4 July and 15 July, there were another 408 deaths. This was a daily mortality rate three times higher (at 37.1 per day on average) than the preceding period from the start of the present wave, that is, from 30 May to 3 July.[25] With the daily death toll, as predicted by pandemic modellers, set to increase by anywhere from between 100 and 400 deaths a day by mid-August, in the context of predicted daily caseloads of 100,000 plus, it was clear that the pandemic was resurging.

Javid and Johnson circulated further details of the 19 July plans over the next few days. Mass spectator (e.g. sporting and music) events would be permitted to resume. Organizers of such events would not be compelled to require participants to demonstrate they were either vaccinated or COVID-19 tested, though this was to be "encouraged". Nightclubs would reopen. There would be no restrictions on home social entertainment or leisure events such as house parties, though of course people should exercise restraint. Customers in pubs or clubs would be able to present their custom at the bar rather than place their orders using an app, though businesses may retain the practice if they preferred. Businesses would not be required to gather information from customers for contact tracking/tracing purposes, though they were free to do so if they wished. There would no longer be any requirement for clients or customers to scan a QR code when frequenting any venue (e.g. restaurants, bars, gyms), though businesses venues may request this of customers. Not only was the requirement that people should go to work only if homeworking was not feasible scrapped, but there would be no legal entitlement for workers to homework if they preferred to on health and safety grounds.[26]

Aspects of this were bizarrely ambivalent. This was especially with regard to the rhetoric of "freedom" or even "encouragement" of people or businesses to retain certain precautions that were to be legally abolished. If these practices were necessary, why undercut their normative supports? Why would anyone be motivated to exercise their freedom to voluntarily impose such controls on themselves or others when the Government did not consider these important enough to warrant legal backing? Why would any retail or hospitality business retain non-mandatory physical distancing controls under circumstances in which doing was likely to place it at competitive disadvantage with those rival businesses that ditched them? The ambivalence of the messaging accompanying the upcoming ditching of restrictions likely reflected the "bad conscience" of ministers. This was in the sense that, since they were fully aware of the public health gamble that "Freedom Day" posed, it was necessary for them to get their alibi on record in advance of Operation Unlocking, in case the experiment went awry. This alibi would be simply that people had abused their freedoms by not continuing with self-limiting practices which they were at liberty to retain and which they were "encouraged" to retain.

Yet, even before "Freedom Day," the Government had resumed large-scale spectator events, despite the rising caseload. These were presented as "controlled experiments" in unlockings that would measure case-by-case the public health impact of reopening such stadia events. The biggest "test-case" was the UEFA European Football Championship from 11 June to 11 July, which featured games with large crowds, especially in the later stages. There were 60,000 spectators for the England versus Denmark semi-final and for the England versus Italy match in the tournament final, for example. These vast numbers were due to Johnson's relaxing of restrictions (set up before the start of the competition) on the number of attendees in the knock-out phase. This was as it sought to hitch a ride on the wave of euphoric national chauvinism that competitive team sports tends to provoke, especially in the former colonizer countries, and especially when a national team is doing well. Here, in these packed stadia, there was little opportunity for physical distancing, and as TV cameras showed, scarcely anyone paid the slightest attention to one-metre plus distancing or mask-wearing, which then remained legal mandates. Moreover, supporters congregated outside stadiums and in the streets, again with very few respecting physical distancing or mask-wearing rules.

Business Secretary Kwasi Kwarteng commented in the press, on the eve of the Denmark match, that the Government could not "guarantee" that this would not trigger a super-spreader spike of cases. After all, "there's always risk in life", he philosophized, so this would be a case of "see what happens". Nonetheless, ministers were, Kwarteng said, "confident" there would be no "big outbreak".[27] This confidence was not shared by health experts. As Antoine Flahault, Professor of Public Health at the University of Geneva, cautioned: "It is possible, probable even, that regions very little affected in the UK will find themselves infected by supporters returning from London".[28] Kwarteng's confidence was also unshaken by the fact that public health authorities in a number of other countries with supporters at the Euros (including Denmark and Finland) detected outbreaks of the virus among returning fans. Some 1,300 Scottish fans who travelled to London for the England versus Scotland fixture (400 of whom were inside Wembley for the game) tested positive on their return to Scotland.[29] This was even though the Government was then still committed, in rhetoric at least, to a data-led COVID-19 policy.

Even though "Freedom Day" was to mark the end of physical distancing restrictions, nonetheless self-isolation or quarantine rules were to remain in place, Javid said. But, from 16 August, there was to be a marked scaling-down of the latter as well. Twice-vaccinated people, and those under 18 years of age, would no longer be required to self-isolate if they had been in close contact with an infected person. This was even though transmission among the young was driving the latest wave of infections and the effectiveness of vaccination in preventing infection by the Delta variant was hardly clear-cut. The school bubble system would also be terminated, whereupon children identified by test-and-trace would no longer be required to quarantine. Nor would fully vaccinated UK residents returning home from amber-flagged countries (for COVID-19 risk) any longer be required to self-isolate.[30]

Moreover, although the test-and-trace system would be retained, the NHS app that carried it would be reset to make it more "sensitive" or "proportionate" to the post-vaccination climate. In other words, the app would be recalibrated, if this was possible, so that the volume of people who were contacted and asked to self-isolate because of their close contact with an infected person would be dramatically reduced. This was considered necessary to avoid a "pingdemic" of stay-home alerts generated by mushrooming caseloads in the months following unlocking.[31] Such would disrupt full capitalist restoration, after all, by forcing millions to take time off work. Since this would be the inevitable consequence of allowing the virus to run amok, doctoring the alert system was the Government's technical fix to a problem of public health risk that it was itself generating. Doubtless, too, this was seen as a fix that would have the advantage of reducing public alarm as caseloads, hospitalizations, and deaths built up. The hubris of "pingdemic" would also inevitably provide tacit encouragement for people to take the pandemic much less seriously than before, thereby incentivizing larger numbers from not engaging with the test-and-trace system.

From 19 July onwards, Javid said, people would have to "learn to live with the virus", accepting its consequences whatever these may be in the post-vaccination context.[32] This was even though the consequences may include, as Javid opined, a hundred thousand plus new infections a day within a short space of time after all restrictions were lifted.[33] These were the facts that would need to be faced, according to his "broad and balanced" view. Javid even compared these post-vaccination consequences with those that would typically result from an outbreak of seasonal influenza – much to the dismay of scientists.[34] "We are going to have to learn to accept the existence of Covid and find ways to cope with it – just as we already do with flu".[35]

This was a remarkable back-to-the-future moment, a rewind to the complacent attitude of government in the run-up to the start of the UK crisis only 15 months earlier. Back then, in advance of COVID-19 reaching these shores, right through to the start of the pandemic in Britain, ministers had dismissed the virus as little more than a flu.[36] Johnson himself dubbed it back then as the "new swine flu" and (presumably jokingly) invited Chris Whitty to inject him with it on national TV to reassure the public that the pandemic was a storm in a teacup.[37] As Stephen Reicher, Professor of Behavioural Psychology, and one of the Government's own scientific advisers, responded to Javid's statement:

> It is frightening to have a health secretary who still thinks Covid is flu. Who is unconcerned at levels of infection. . .. Who wants to ditch all protections while only half of us are vaccinated. . .. Above all, it is frightening to have a health secretary who wants to make all protections a matter of personal choice when the key message of the pandemic is this isn't an "I" thing, it's a "we" thing.[38]

During the week following Javid's "bullish" or "ebullient" (as it was described in the press) parliamentary declaration of intent of 28 June to imminently and irreversibly normalize economic life, the prime minister repeatedly reiterated the new party line. Following Javid's example, he too presented COVID-19 as a fact of life that had to be lived with (rather than as he did before an "enemy to be vanquished"),[39] just as he minimized the virus as a problem on a par with flu.[40] He too shrugged his shoulders at the inevitability of rising caseloads as he urged the public to "reconcile" itself, albeit "sadly", to "more deaths".[41]

Johnson explicitly presented 19 July as a return to "pretty much life before Covid".[42] "Freedom Day", he promised, would mark the end of government "diktats" on physical distancing in favour of individuals being freed to make "responsible" choices about their own safety and the safety of others.[43] State management of the virus would be replaced by its personal management by citizens, since the "move away from legal restrictions" would free people "to make their own informed decisions" about physical distancing.[44] The Government thus envisaged 19 July not so much as the moment it restored the public's freedom from the burden of social restrictions but rather more as the point at which it claimed its own freedom from the most basic job of government – protecting the health of its own citizens. By its own decree, all future hospitalizations and deaths, and any disruption caused to social life by escalating caseloads, would post-19 July cease to be the Government's responsibility. Instead, these would be the fault of those people who did not take upon themselves responsibility for the protection of self and others.[45]

Johnson released his press briefings on "Freedom Day" just as assorted ministers and MPs were dispatched to media outlets to hard sell it as the restoration civil liberties as a matter of moral imperative and civic duty. Remarkably, included among the freedoms to be recovered once-and-for-all was the right of people even to dispense with more-than-one-metre distancing or donning a face mask, whether in crowded outdoor places, confined indoor spaces (with the possible exception of health and care establishments), or on public transport. To mask or not to mask, or to keep one's distance or not, this was voluntary, a matter for the individual conscience.[46] Bang on cue, Tory politicians represented even these undoubtedly minor or trivial impositions on daily conduct (inasmuch as these were imposed by legal norms and backed up by judicial sanctions) as an intolerable moral affront to individual rights that could no longer be a matter of compulsion in a post-vaccine Britain.

Environment Minister George Eustice provided an earlier indication of things to come. As he put it: "I have to be honest, once I'm told that it's safe not to, I want to get back to normal. I think a lot of people will want to shed those masks".[47] Subsequently, Chancellor Rishi Sunak and Minister for Local Government Robert Jenrick announced that they would no longer wear face masks starting on "Freedom Day". We should respect that other "people will come to different conclusions" over mask-wearing, but everyone must be trusted to "exercise good judgement", opined Jenrick. Care Minister Helen Whately ventured that mask-wearing in whatever setting was legitimate for some, but equally not so for others, though she would consider doing so as a personal choice under certain circumstances, or in response to guidance. However, mask-shedding would be for her liberating. "I can't wait not to have to", she declared.[48] Whately even considered face-masking to be a source of social disadvantage for some. "I think face masks have a real downside", she declared, citing the predicament of the aurally impaired.[49] Simultaneously, assorted Conservative MPs brought to the airwaves threadbare justifications of why mask-wearing was rightfully and justly a matter of individual discretion, since this was, as they insisted, very much more than mere personal inconvenience for the sake of the safety of others.[50]

Naturally, emboldened by the dearth of political dissent to 19 July on the opposition benches, the unlockings this promised did not go far enough to satisfy the bulk of Tory MPs or their corporate backers. Despite projected caseloads of 100,000 plus a day (and of two million new infections in total) by mid-August,[51] this was for them no good reason why it was necessary to wait until 16 August to end self-isolation or quarantine rules for those people flagged as being in close contact with an infected person. This was, in their view, simply indecision and over-caution.[52] True to form, government spokespersons responded by hinting in the media that, for NHS workers at least, there may be a case for exemption from home quarantine for twice-vaccinated persons.[53]

By contrast, 19 July provoked considerable disquiet among public health experts, for very good reasons.[54] This was not simply because ditching face masks and physical distancing created public health risks for the sake of conceding only the most trivial of "freedoms". This was also because this was the latest in a long series of "confused messages" from ministers. Now, the problem with ambivalent government messaging is that it undermines public vigilance and dissipates public support for sensible interpersonal protection measures by denying these any kind of official steer or support.[55] But the bigger issue in this case was less the ambivalence of messaging and more the content of policy.

In this case, policy was freeing people to retreat from responsibility for the protection of others on the grounds that this was exactly what the Government was proposing to do. Such could hardly deter people from asking themselves the question: if "they" (the elected political authority) are withdrawing from a commitment to physical distancing, why should "we" (the citizenry) take over the burden of responsibility for it? Moreover, because the face mask symbolizes in the most visible way the daily risk of infection and the need for respect of the wellbeing of others, the Government's undermining of the practice could only give people cause to imagine that *all* self-controls or self-discipline (from hand sanitizing to the basic respect of personal space) were no longer necessary.[56] After all, ministerial justification of "Freedom Day" was that vaccination had "severed" (in Johnson's words) the link between viral transmission and significant levels of major illness.[57] By contrast, for Chris Whitty, this link had only been "weakened" (albeit substantially).[58]

The triviality of the freedom offered by legalizing non-wearing for many would confirm the new triviality of the disease post-vaccination that it was supposed to help protect against. But the symbolic power of this particular aspect of the final unlocking of lockdown protections was also bound to provoke a vast groundswell of public alarm – as it did.[59] As such, this was also bound to polarize opinion between pro-maskers and anti-maskers – as it did.[60] This indeed raised the spectre of potential conflict among practitioners of each in public settings. Since the decisions of people to unmask in crowded or poorly ventilated environments would impose themselves on the security and wellbeing of those who continue to mask themselves, this promised a moral incentivization of interpersonal conflict. Such is the inevitable consequence of the new doctrine of personal choice as this filled the space left by the withdrawal of state authority. This is because mask-wearing confers protections not on the wearer but on those the mask-wearer comes into contact with, so that one's own safety is reliant on the mask-wearing of others, not one's own.

"Freedom Day" thus not only removes state controls over the spread of the virus but also simultaneously manages the feat of weakening controls at the community and interpersonal levels. But there is a further problem with the way that the 19 July unlocking has been marketed by government. Dubbing this "Freedom Day" was manifestly inappropriate because it was crassly insensitive to all of those who had lost their lives or been bereaved or suffered long-term debilitating illnesses from COVID-19. Where was their freedom? It was crassly insensitive as well to all of those clinically vulnerable people whose lives and wellbeing were threatened by the abolition of restrictions and by the commitment never to bring them back no matter what. For them, the freedoms of others (including the most mundane libidinal and consumerist of these freedoms) would mean their own lives would have to become even less free and even more controlled to minimize the risk posed to them by those who would voluntarily disregard distancing and other precautions.[61]

From the perspective of wider public health safety, the semantics of 19 July would even provide tacit *encouragement* to people to dispense with physical distancing and face-masking. This is not simply a matter of this behaviour being made permissible by the lifting of legal restrictions. Rather, this is a matter of people being presented with the idea that what is permissible is also morally defensible, even morally desirable. This is because, on this representation of the meaning of 19 July, "freedom" (however that is exercised) is, as far as COVID-19 is concerned, simply virtue, just as virtue is "anything goes".

Whichever choice is made (to distance or not, to mask or unmask) is of the same status (as an exercise of choice) in this enchanted realm of abstract decontextualized libertarianism. If this was not the case, the lifting of all legal controls on social conduct relevant to the pandemic could not be represented (as it was) as simply the restoration of liberty.[62] At a more mundane level, the hubris of "Freedom Day" sanctions instrumental conduct that is de-civilizing or corrosive of the communal bond. Since eschewing physical distancing or mask-donning for one's "own good reasons" is simply freedom (and since freedom is an unqualified good because that is, after all, the purpose of 19 July), people are thereby licensed to morally legitimize anti-social behaviours that in reality are motivated by the mundane egoism of personal preference or convenience.

This pattern of government "guidance" by which the public were almost encouraged to ditch physical distancing and related precautionary behaviours was also a case of back to the future, for something similar was in evidence as the Government began the process of easing the first lockdown in the spring of 2020. As I discussed earlier, as caseloads and hospitalizations began to recede in the earlier period, ministers were not content to simply embark on the roadmap to normality by means of the step-by-step lifting of restrictions. Rather, they also acted to mobilize people to embrace the opportunities that were afforded by the piecemeal unlockings. The public were urged to return to sports and leisure centres, pubs and restaurants. Indeed, in some cases, they were provided with financial incentives to do so (namely, under the "Eat Out to Help Out" scheme).[63] This was on the grounds that this kind of behaviour would be civic virtue, or patriotic duty, in the service of rescuing the economy, or at the very least saving the hospitality and leisure industries.[64] As Chancellor, Rishi Sunak, put it, when launching Eat Out to Help Out:

> Our Eat Out to Help Out scheme's number one aim is to help protect the jobs of 1.8 million chefs, waiters and restaurateurs by boosting demand and getting customers through the door. More than 72,000 establishments will be serving discounted meals across the country, with the government paying half the bill. The industry is a vital ingredient to our economy and it's been hit hard by coronavirus, so enjoy summer safely by showing your favourite places your support – we'll pay half.[65]

This public incentivization by government for fast-tracked normalization of social leisure was doubtless part of the explanation of why infection rates were not depressed sufficiently over the spring and summer months to prevent the virus resurging rapidly in the autumn of 2020 as conditions more favourable for its transmission were restored. Eat Out to Help Out is estimated as having been "responsible for eight to 17 per cent of newly detected Covid-19 clusters in August and early September",[66] according to researchers at Warwick University. As Stephen Reicher explains, "we never got infections low enough to be able to deal with the disease and so when conditions changed in the autumn, when schools went back and people went back to work and universities went back and the weather got worse and we went inside, so infections spiked". Reicher's concern that "we're on line to repeat the mistakes of last summer" seems prescient.

> I think this time round, we should learn from that [premature unlockings and incitements to relax social distancing] . . . and we should get infections low to a point where we we're in a much better place in the autumn, where we don't have to reimpose restrictions. . . . It seems to me that if we got right the basic public health moves to suppress infection, we wouldn't be talking about a high reservoir of infection which can then spike very quickly when conditions change.[67]

Quite so. I would add to Reicher's concern that, given that COVID-19 caseloads were on an upward curve much in advance of "Freedom Day", these mistakes of government are, if anything, set to be repeated on an even bigger and bolder scale than before.

Remarkably, if not unsurprisingly, the Government itself was caught off-guard by the negative public response to their own promised impending "liberty", this reflecting its characteristically narcissistic lack of basic self-reflection and understanding of the public mind. Within two weeks of Javid's declaration of the Government's irreversible commitment to "Freedom Day", ministers were changing their tune on physical distancing, including on the unmasking issue. Apparently prompted by a rethink at No. 10,[68] they started de-emphasizing the "libertarian" aspects of abandoning all physical distancing and setting aside mask-wearing and eschewing description of mask-shedding as simply a matter of choice. Johnson, having declared (on 28 June) that "Freedom Day" would mark a return "pretty much to life before Covid", was (by 12 July) urging people "*not* [my emphasis] to return to life as normal after July 19" or else they would "risk restrictions being reimposed".[69]

Almost overnight, the rhetoric of mask-doffing as a necessary freedom from illiberal restriction disappeared. The new steer became that members of the public should continue to wear face-masks under exactly the same circumstances as before on and after 19 July, because that would be "responsible citizenship" (as Javid put it),[70] once the legal requirement to do so ended. Johnson himself advised or recommended that people should continue to wear masks in crowded indoor places beyond "Freedom Day".[71] Indeed, this was (according to vaccinations minister Nadhim Zahawi) *expected* behaviour.[72] That this was a case of disingenuous gesture politics, however, was exposed by the Government's decision to abolish mandatory face coverings in parliament from 19 July, with MPs thereafter only "advised" or "encouraged" (by whom exactly?) to wear these in the chambers or in the wider parliamentary estate. By contrast, parliamentary staff would still be required to wear masks, since they unlike MPs were government employees.[73]

This sea change may be read as a partial victory for those scientific and public health experts who had raised objections. They had possibly raised the jitters of ministers, in the context of fast-rising increases in the rate of virus infection.[74] Or perhaps simply the sharply increasing caseload was by itself sufficient to provoke this response from a government mindful of the need to avoid the appearance of recklessness. This conceivably encouraged ministers to at least offer a gesture towards re-responsibilization of the public for anti-COVID-19 precautions having washed their own hands of this responsibility.[75]

The more likely reason for the about-turn, however, was the Government's recognition that it had misjudged the public mood on physical distancing issues, in that it imagined that most people shared above and all else its impatience for ditching them altogether. Anxiety and disapproval over mask-ditching reflected deeper popular unhappiness with the Great Unlocking of which masks were symbolic.[76] (The solipsist simply presumes that his or her own beliefs and values are those of everyone else – until these are contested.) This is because ministers were of course fully aware that there was already a return to mass infection and they would reasonably conclude that post-19 July these could escalate to levels not yet experienced. They would know as well that this would soon lead to far higher rates of hospitalization and mortality than had been seen in the spring.

Javid's own statements to the House had emphasized that releasing all physical distancing controls was not risk free. This was far from ideal, but was rather better than the alternative, he asserted. Javid even acknowledged that this would place the country in "unchartered territory".[77] This was tacit admission that unlocking as caseloads skyrocketed was in fact a laboratory experiment or "great gamble" (as sympathetic and unsympathetic press commentators alike put it) with public safety.[78] So, ministers were committed to full unlocking because they had decided that the price of expendable lives, whatever that price would be, was worth paying. They had even conceded implicitly that they had no way of judging how high that price (of lost lives) would be. Rather, whatever the public health deficit would be, this was quietly accepted, since that is the consequence of plunging headlong into *uncharted* territory. What is unchartered is unknown and can only be guessed at, so rational risk assessments are undermined.

But the problem that the Government encountered with its unwavering commitment to "Freedom Day" was simply that the public (or major constituencies of it) did not share its high tolerance for difficult-to-measure (yet potentially astronomical) public health risk. Rather, they still wanted that risk to be managed responsibly.[79] Many as well were unimpressed by the Government's association of liberty with mere individual preferences of convenience at the expense of social care for others – especially care for the clinically vulnerable for whom the vaccines offer lesser protection than is typical or none at all.[80] Consequently, ministers may have recognized potential injury to self-interest (electoral hazard) from appearing to have overdone the gung-ho embrace of 19 July as the libertarian casting off of all restrictions. Not for the first time the citizenry (or substantial numbers of citizens) manifested a stronger sense of collective responsibility for and commitment to the cause of public safety than their own government could muster.

Nonetheless, irrespective of the vicissitudes of the Government's attitude to face masks and physical distancing, "Freedom Day" itself is unlikely to be postponed again. This is despite the weakness of the case for it. Johnson's own rubber-stamping of 19 July was perfunctory by way of justification. This simply presented the public with Whitty's dilemma: either unlock fully now during summertime or else later as winter approaches and the NHS is placed under greater strain by the virus.

> If we can't reopen our society in the next few weeks, when we'll be helped by the arrival of summer and the school holidays, we must ask ourselves – when will we return to normal? And to those who say we should delay again – the alternative to that is to open up in winter when the virus will have an advantage, or not at all this year.[81]

This was false dilemma because there was no reason (other than the fact that Javid had ruled one out under any circumstances) for supposing a summer unlocking would preclude the need for a winter lockdown later on. The UK had already experienced three lockdowns in response to three waves of infection and was, despite vaccination, in the middle of yet another surge of infections that threatened to dwarf the previous ones. How, then, would a total summer unlocking that gave the virus free reign rule out also a major winter crisis? The only sensible answer to this question would be that such a later winter crisis may be averted by the further progress of the vaccination programme.[82] But the logical problem with this answer for ministers is that it actually provides no support for the summer unlocking. This beggars the obvious question: why not delay the release of the remaining controls until after double-dose protection of the adult population is accomplished? Indeed, why not tighten these controls up, given that the virus has yet again slipped its leash?

The illogic of Johnson's rationale for "Freedom Day" may be summarized as follows. First, since he had himself claimed that the virus would be reinvigorated by winter *irrespective of the summer unlocking*, this undermined his own case for going ahead with it. As Dr Nathalie McDermott, an expert in infectious diseases at King's College London pointed out, unlocking restrictions with infection rates headed up rather than down would simply generate the high likelihood of a "bigger problem in the autumn". This would be when winter was just a few weeks away, that is, at exactly the worst time to be creating such a problem. "The last thing that we want to do now is to allow a virus to gain a foothold and circulate significantly within our population as we come into the winter months".[83]

Second, if the virus would be conferred major advantage by virtue of a later (autumn or winter) unlocking of the last vestiges of lockdown, then this showed that it was not yet close to being defeated. The link between infection and public health risk was not, after all, as Johnson claimed, "severed". Yet the defeat of COVID-19 in terms of its capacity to endanger public health as this was bestowed by mass vaccination was exactly the Government's reason for accepting no further delays to its 19 July bonfire of restrictions.

Third, Johnson's concept of "complete normality" was in any case deeply flawed and aiming for it was misguided. This is because this "final step fetishism" simply assumes that this is feasible or even desirable. For that is the Promised Land set for 19 July. But this is not the view of much medical, public health or scientific opinion. According to this, the "new normal" must include a measure of physical distancing (such as mask-wearing and respecting the at-least-one-metre rule), precisely because the protections offered by the vaccines (whether in terms of reducing transmissions or illness) are neither perfect nor fixed once-and-for-all.[84] Indeed, scientists and public health experts had urged ministers not to go for an all-eggs-in-one-basket approach to solving the pandemic (i.e. complete reliance on mass vaccination), stressing the continued wisdom of sticking with the additional safeguards of personal hygiene practices and physical distancing regulations.

This was on the grounds that not enough yet was known for certain about the degree of protection that the vaccines provided (since research is relatively new and constantly developing), or if the estimated protections would alone suffice to suppress the virus,[85] or how much protection they would offer in a situation where virus transmission rates spiralled (as they are currently in the UK). In particular, not enough was known about if the vaccines would be as effective against the doubly-mutated Delta variant as they were apparently against earlier strains, given that early results suggested these were perhaps less effective.[86] The latter concern seems especially pertinent in that Delta is regarded as the "fittest" variant so far, responsible for 99 percent of current cases in the UK, and is thought to be 60 percent more infectious than the Alpha (Kent) variant. Delta "may . . . be linked to a greater risk of hospitalisation and is somewhat more resistant to vaccines, particularly after one dose".[87] As Professor of Virology at Leeds University Stephen Griffin explains:

> This is the problem with hanging everything on vaccines until you've got something near a population immunity threshold . . . you need a much higher coverage to protect against a variant that's more transmissible. . . . It just speaks to the fact that we really, really must keep cases down at the same time as rolling the vaccines out. . . . The ideal scenario is that you build your vaccine wall before you get exposed to variants because that means that even if you do get an outbreak, you've got sufficiently few people that are susceptible that the R never gets above 1, you don't see an increase in that outbreak. . . . The problem is that we haven't reached that protective level, and so if you do get infections and cases growing there's plenty of susceptible people to pass that infection on to.[88]

Finally, it is clear that a later unlocking (rather than the present one) would benefit from further progress in the vaccination programme, so that whatever "advantage" the virus enjoyed in winter would be diminished. As of 10 July 2021, around 87 percent of the adult population (45.7 million people) were once-jabbed, whereas approximately 65 percent (34 million people) were double-jabbed.[89] This meant there were still considerable gaps in public protection. Taking the population as a whole, only 67 percent were once-jabbed, and only 51 percent were double-jabbed. Vaccination of young adults was only recently started and rollout to 18-year olds began only on 17 June.[90] Yet it was these who were the main sources of virus transmission in the current upsurge and who were to be exposed to high risk of infection by the 19 July unlocking.[91]

Research indicates that young adults and children are much less vulnerable than older people to becoming seriously ill from immediate or initial COVID-19 infection. This is the Government's justification for unlocking before the vaccination programme is anywhere close to running its course. But this research provides little guidance on whether or not young adults or subadults are at lesser or greater risk than older adults of becoming ill later on from Post-COVID-19 Syndrome (or

Long Covid, as it is commonly known). "As of 6 June 2021, an estimated 962,000 people in the UK were experiencing self-reported Long Covid symptoms, according to ONS figures. This amounts to 1.5 per cent of the population".[92]

Long Covid may affect people who were asymptomatic or who had minor symptoms when they first contracted the virus, and many sufferers are still unwell a year after being infected. Moreover, people who experienced minor or no symptoms on the initial infection often experience far more radical ill effects later on. According to a study of 800 Long Covid sufferers across 15 NHS trusts by a team of researchers at UCL, people with the condition experience a poorer quality of life than those suffering from advanced lung cancer.

> Long Covid patients reported, on average, a quality of life score around 50 on a 0 to 100 scale, where 0 is "the worst imaginable state of health" and 100 is the "best imaginable state of health". By comparison, patients with advanced – metastatic – lung cancer typically report values above 60 on the same quality of life measure.[93]

Sufferers were found to be "severely impaired" in the key domains of their everyday lives – working, shopping, childcare, paying household bills, maintaining intimate relationships, and pursuing social and leisure activities. Their mean scores on this "work and social adjustment scale" were 21, whereas any score above 20 is indicative of severe disability. Their mean scores on the "fatigue scale" (or FACIT-F) were 21, whereas scores over 30 are classed as normal, and those of 40 are indicative of average good health. Their mean scores on the "anxiety scale" (or GAD-7) were 8.7, whereas on the "depression scale" (PQH-8) these were 11.2. On the former, a score of more than eight is indicative of clinical anxiety, whereas, on the latter, a score of more than ten is indicative of clinical depression.[94]

Thus, as academic clinician David Strain points out, unwillingness of government to take measures to prevent the mass infection of young people amounts to conducting a

> dangerous experiment with the next generation . . . It is a fact that the more Covid . . . [there is] . . . the more Long Covid . . . [there is]. And the big worry is this is affecting the younger generation that the entire country is dependent on to get the country moving again.[95]

Not only would 18-year-olds be without double-dose vaccine protection by 19 July, but nor were children vaccinated, not even once. Indeed, all the signs were that the Government had no plans to inoculate children (i.e. persons under 18) at all in the vaccine programme.[96] Yet the notion embraced by Government that children were not only scarcely ever made ill from the virus but also highly unlikely to catch it or pass it on (and *considerably* less so than adults) has not been supported by research. This, along with a political discourse that children's psychological wellbeing and educational needs (especially of those from economically disadvantaged families and neighbourhoods) were being severely if not fatally damaged by having to be schooled online from home rather than on-site, has over the course of the pandemic ideologized delayed school shutdowns and fast-tracked re-openings.

Microbiologist Professor Ravi Gupta has summarized the overall picture as follows: "You have lots of vaccinated people, those who are semi-immune because they've already been infected, unvaccinated people, and a lot of young people". This complexity and unevenness of vaccine coverage and the real unknowns about vaccine protection, Gupta points out, makes modelling the course and impact of the current wave prohibitively difficult.[97] Ten percent of people who are double-jabbed will still become ill from the virus, even if most of these mildly, for the simple reason that vaccination does not provide full and complete immunity.[98]

Unevenness of vaccine coverage does not merely generate gaps among the less clinically vulnerable, but also persisting ones among clinically vulnerable groups. Included among those in the vaccine gaps are the 10 percent of people who did not respond to invitations to receive their jabs, among them significant numbers of the elderly. "Either they didn't want it, didn't turn up, or they couldn't have it for some sort of medical reason", Michael Landray, Professor of Epidemiology at Oxford University, explains. Landray reminds us that there are also significant numbers of old people whose immune systems would not be sufficiently boosted by the vaccines to give them enough protection from major illnesses. He also cautions us that, since the oldest of the 65-plus group would be those who received their jabs at the earlier stages of the programme, they may have diminished protection from the virus, just as "Freedom Day" beckons.[99] This creates significant, if not major, risk that under conditions of relaxed physical distancing the virus will find them and kill them. Such is a real possibility because the duration of protection from the virus provided by the vaccines is unknown.

Modelling of the third (or fourth) wave is also problematized by uncertainty over the impact of the Delta variant. This is owing to Delta's accelerated infectiousness compared to previous strains of the virus (this has an estimated R number of between five and seven if unchecked by restrictions),[100] and some evidence that the existing vaccines have less efficacy than previously thought in lowering transmission rates.[101] These factors combined have radicalized the objections of scientists, health managers and medics to "Freedom Day". As Stephen Griffin of Leeds University puts it: "Whilst there is need to further validate the . . . [data], it adds to the concerns over the dropping of mitigation . . .".[102]

The same conclusions were drawn by the COVID-19 Response Team at Imperial College London's School of Hygiene and Tropical Medicine. Their research highlights the radical uncertainty of accurately projecting how the current (third or fourth) wave will unfold and the magnitude of its impact.[103] This is in part owing to incomplete and uneven vaccine coverage and insufficient data to make secure judgements over the efficacy of the vaccines against Delta (especially over time), but also owing to other unknowns that complexify the outlook. The team projected that outcomes arising from "Freedom Day" during the present wave may vary from a range of between 9,400 deaths (with an estimated range of 4,600–19,800 deaths) on the best-case scenario to one of 115,800 deaths (with an estimated range of 81,700–143,600 deaths) on the worst-case scenario.[104]

Which of these scenarios would play out would depend not only on how the vaccines cope under the pressures of massively accelerated caseloads, but on how the public respond to the Government's abolition of legal controls binding them to physical distancing and other precautionary behaviours (hand sanitization, mask-wearing, self-isolation, etc.). On the one hand, if the public responds (or substantial numbers of the public respond) to "Freedom Day" by immediately abandoning the protections afforded by physical distancing and related practices, the worst-case scenarios were feasible. If, on the other hand, the public's response (or the response of most of the public) to the lifting of restrictions was to continue with precautionary behaviours or to scale these down gradually, exercising caution, the best-case scenarios were feasible.[105]

As Neil Ferguson (one of the co-authors) summarized the conclusions of the study:

> The lifting of mandatory restrictions on 19th July is a calculated risk. If individuals remain cautious in the face of rising levels of infection, our analysis suggests that the third wave will be substantially smaller than if contacts immediately revert to pre-pandemic levels. However, a large third wave of infections is inevitable if mandatory restrictions are lifted. It is much harder to predict what this will translate into in terms of hospitalisations and deaths. The link between cases and hospitalisations has been weakened but not severed.[106]

This radical uncertainty was the consequence of the Government's legal mandate for people to disregard physical distancing, indeed its tacit encouragement for people to disregard it, by representing this as the restoration of liberty, and owing to their mixed messaging.

As always, with Boris Johnson's government, it was hard to judge whether ambivalent or outrightly inconsistent public messaging on how people should respond to the abolition of legal restrictions on physical distancing was simply incompetence or was an exercise of Machiavellian intent. Did they want to undermine public responsibilization for COVID-19 having abandoned their own, in order to fast-track herd immunity by means of rapid mass infection, irrespective of the costs? This would be a push for herd immunity in the population before autumn saw millions headed for schools, colleges and universities and as colder climes drove everyone indoors.

Or were ministers so carried away by vaccination success (owing to small hospital caseloads alongside higher rates of infection) that they simply misled themselves that the public mind was as one with their own for complete unlocking, so that they were thrown into disunity as reality dawned? If it was the former, ministers could hardly be upfront about it. It would be electorally unwise to simply urge people to relax physical distancing, for that would certainly appear reckless and indifferent. Much better, instead, to affirm the liberatory nature of disbanding physical distancing norms alongside appeals for people to be "responsible" with their liberty. Then, if things go badly, the irresponsible public can always be blamed.

Either way, 19 July was another massive gamble with public health, a default to "wait and see" and "hope for the best", which had characterized the Government's response since the beginning of the pandemic. This would be where "the best" that was hoped for by ministers was a scenario where economic normalcy and all its benefits would coincide with a fatality rate that the public would regard as acceptable, posing low electoral risk for the ruling party. Alas, with substantial numbers of people desensitized to mass death, and weary of lockdowns, the Government's gamble was perhaps that the bulk of the public would be tolerant of anything up to a peak of 400 deaths a day as the price to pay for recovery of all of their freedoms. Johnson's own scientific modellers anticipated that the unlocking would generate 100–200 deaths a day at the peak of the present wave of infections later in the summer. This was on the basis of a predicted peak of 100,000 cases a day and on a particular estimate of vaccine efficacy that saw the jabs reducing hospitalization rates by fourfold and the mortality rate by tenfold compared to the previous wave.[107]

As for Ferguson's own conclusions derived from the work of his team at Imperial College, these were misplaced in one important respect. *Calculated* risk? How could this be when the potential scenarios rested on unknowable judgements of public response to the Government's great unlocking of restrictions that gave rise to widely differing estimates of the potential impact? Earlier, before the publication of the study, in response to the Government's reiteration of its intention to liberate itself from responsibility for protecting the public from the virus, Ferguson declared that the risk involved was "justifiable", hence providing (as did Whitty) a stamp of pseudo-scientific legitimation to Johnson's "great gamble".[108] In doing so he placed himself on the outermost fringe of independent scientific opinion,[109] the vast bulk of which quite rightly regarded 19 July as reckless unethical subordination of science to politics.[110]

As Richard Horton, Editor-in-Chief of *The Lancet*, commented: "The government plan is not, as some have characterised it, a reasonable gamble – it is an entirely unnecessary and self-inflicted hazard that will cause real harm to health". The grounds for that virtual scientific consensus which Horton expresses were made clear by the content of an open letter to the Government bearing the signatures of 122 international scientists:

> The UK government must reconsider its current strategy and take urgent steps to protect the public, including children. We believe the government is embarking on a dangerous and unethical experiment, and we call on it to pause plans to abandon mitigations on 19 July, 2021 . . . Implicit in this decision is the acceptance that infections will surge, but that this does not matter because "vaccines have broken the link between infections and mortality". On July 19 2021 – branded Freedom Day – almost all restrictions are set to end. We believe this decision is dangerous and premature . . . In light of these grave risks, and given that vaccination offers the prospect of quickly reaching the same goal of population immunity without incurring them, we consider any strategy that tolerates high level of infection to be both unethical and illogical.[111]

The majority view was certainly data-led. As noted previously, the Government's own scientific modellers had plotted a likely scenario in which the post-19 July upsurge could at its peak generate thousands of hospitalizations and 100–200-plus deaths per day, whereas the independent Scientific Pandemic Influenza Group on Modelling (SPI-M) considered that a more likely outcome of 19 July was a death toll that could rise up to 400 a day by the time of its expected mid-August 2021 peak.[112]

Science and healthcare expertise certainly did not speak with one voice on the question of what appropriate policy in coping with the pandemic would be looking ahead to autumn. Dr Chaand Nagpaul, chairperson of the BMA, for example, was not set against further unlocking of restrictions on 19 July, so long as these did not include ditching mandatory one-metre-plus distancing and mask-wearing.[113] As he put it: "We know that masks are effective in stopping the spread, so it is nonsensical and dangerous for the government to abandon compulsory mask wearing in indoor public settings, such as public transport, on July 19th".[114]

Contrary to Ferguson (and Whitty), however, for most, the most prudent course was to step back from "Freedom Day", by either postponing further de-escalation of compulsory physical distancing, or indeed by restoring some earlier controls.[115] This would provide time for the vaccination programme to offer at least a single jab to all adults (and better still two and perhaps single jabs to children as well). Such would have been a policy that offered perhaps the best (if not only) chance of preventing the present wave spiralling out of control and protecting the public from the risks of mass infection.[116] Such would be a policy led by scientific facts and ethical judgement. But, as Maria Van Kerkhove, the WHO's technical COVID-19 lead put it (in a thinly veiled reference to Johnson's 19 July plans), any government that chose not to implement "consistently proven actions that prevent infections, reduce spread, prevent disease and save lives", would be acting in a way that was "immoral, unethical and non-scientific".[117]

The biggest risk factor associated with abandoning legally prescribed physical distancing is actually beyond the reach of the scientific modellers to predict. This is incalculable and hence uninsurable risk. This is the risk posed by mass community infection and transmission of the acceleration of the virus's capacity to adapt, to mutate, to diversify, i.e. to manufacture new variants.[118] As Paul Hunter, Professor of Medicine at East Anglia University, pointed out, when discussing India's pandemic, it is "not surprising" that India produced the most dangerous variant to date (Delta), nor that the other dangerous variants were incubated in South Africa, Brazil, and the UK.

> If you think about where the main variants have arisen . . . all of these are countries that have really struggled to keep case numbers down. . . . India has got a huge pandemic, and therefore that's where you're going to be getting the variant.[119]

"Freedom Day", then, is not a recipe for keeping case numbers low. Quite the opposite. Astronomical infection caseloads (such as those that are likely to be generated by the abolition of legal controls that would bind people to physical distancing behaviours) will radically increase the sheer number of opportunities that the virus has to attack the host population. From accelerated opportunity to infect people comes also accelerated opportunity for the virus to find new ways to challenge or attack or offset the immune systems of hosts. A fundamental part of that process of challenge is mutation: random adaptations, which if these have greater reproductive fitness than existing ones, will become dominant. In Professor Susan Michie's words: "Allowing community transmission to surge is like building new 'variant factories' at a very fast rate".[120] High case volumes "challenge the virus", as Dr Mike Tildesley puts it.[121] This is presumably in the sense that where infection rates are spiralling competition for access to hosts is dramatically increased, which provides a spur for the breeding of mutants strains, which will obtain an advantage in the race to infect (reproduce).

Since increased infectiousness would confer reproductive advantage on the virus, new variants are selected because they spread and transmit with greater efficiency, outcompeting less infectious ones. If the infected population is diverse, owing to a high degree of demographic or ethnic heterogeneity (as most national populations in the cosmopolitan age are), the challenge this will present to the virus will also create selection pressures for adaptive flexibility, so that there may develop multiple avenues of attack, and which may impact differentially on different groups. Occasionally, with the acceleration of the selection dynamic, variants which are successful because they are more transmittable will also have other random mutations that render them more dangerous or injurious to their hosts in terms of the diseases or illnesses they cause. Occasionally too, this process will select variants that are better adapted to evading or diminishing vaccine protections. Put simply, with higher rates of community transmission, there is higher risk of the mutation of new variants, and of certain of these becoming more successful and deadly, whereas such risks are much reduced under conditions where the rate of community transmission is kept in check.

Of course, the unvaccinated are always, as Dr William Schaffner of Vanderbilt University's Medical Center puts it,

> potential vaccine factories. . . . The more unvaccinated people there are, the more opportunities for the virus to multiply. . . .. When it does, it mutates, and it could throw off a variant mutation that is even more serious down the road.[122]

This is especially where infection rates are accelerating. But the danger of factory-producing mutant strains of the virus under circumstances of mass infection is also acute in a partially or largely vaccinated population where there nonetheless remain significant (if not major) gaps in overall coverage, such as is the case in the UK.

As Professor of Virology Christina Pagel explains:

> When you have incredibly high levels of Covid, which we have now in England – and it's not going to go away any time soon – and a partially vaccinated population, any mutation that can infect vaccinated people better has a big selection advantage and can spread.[123]

This is because vaccination itself exerts selection pressures on the virus to adapt in ways that will allow it to infect inoculated people, just as the protection gaps or shortfalls in the population provide it with an opportunity to evolve exactly those adaptative solutions. The unvaccinated population become enclaves for the random production of new variants that are better equipped to infect the vaccinated and which by virtue of that become dominant. In effect, the enclaves become potentially bridgeheads for the transmission of vaccine-resistant strains into the vaccinated population, whereas thereafter natural selection will tend to reinforce that tendency owing to the reproductive advantages this confers.

This confirms the utter irrationality from the scientific perspective of Johnson's "Freedom Day", since this threatens to undo his government's only success story in dealing with the pandemic, i.e. the vaccine programme, as virologist Dr Jemma Geoghegan explains:

> If you are going to train a virus to escape vaccine-induced immunity, you would do exactly what they're [the UK government is] doing. You're basically providing a training ground for the virus to overcome those selection pressures. You're allowing the virus to continue to spread. With this moderately immune population and with the Delta variant that has an R . . . that's estimated to be probably five or six, you need a threshold [of vaccine coverage] to be much, much, much higher than they (the UK population) currently have.[124]

Of course, sometimes a gambler's risks do not end badly. The nature of gambling is that sometimes you win, sometimes you lose. Johnson's latest gamble with the public health of those he is charged with responsibility for protecting may not generate another massive crisis of hospitalizations and deaths or a vast overhang of Long-Covid cases. The potential threat of large numbers of younger people (and even children) finding their life chances damaged by COVID-19 infection in the longer term may not come to pass. It may even be the case that the current wave will not lead to the deaths or affliction with life-threatening illness of those with compromised immune systems or of the most frail or elderly whose vaccination protections have become a little long in the tooth or which were less effective in the first place. Mass infection in a semi-immunized population may not generate a variant that can evade or diminish the vaccines or radicalize the symptoms of infection.

But simply to point out these potential positive scenarios is to draw attention to their negative contraries. These are a *lot of risks* – and the likelihood of some or all of them coming to pass evades rational risk assessment upon which the scientific modelling of scenarios depends. Risking public health on the spin of the roulette wheel (in the service of the liberalization of commerce) can never be the policy approach of responsible, ethical government. But there is another danger looking beyond 19 July that has not been acknowledged. This is that scientific pandemic modelling has not considered at all (with its estimates of 100,000-plus daily infections at the peak of the current wave) the potential of "Freedom Day" and its aftermath to seriously undermine the accuracy of transmission data records – or at least not as far as I can tell.

July 19 is predicated on the illusion or myth, for all practical intents and purposes, that the pandemic is over, superseded by the "endemic". The threat posed by the virus is no longer to public health, according to this discourse, but to economic renewal, as millions of people are kept away from work and other more pleasurable pursuits (such as summer holidays) by a "pingdemic" of self-isolation texts. This basically incentivizes people to avoid getting tested, if they should receive a prompt, because if they should get the wrong result from the test, this would interrupt their newly restored "liberties". In any case, since the virus's capacity to inflict serious harm is, as Johnson has decreed it, "severed" by vaccination, why is the inconvenience of getting tested even if one is feeling unwell from self-suspected COVID-19 infection any longer necessary? The hubris of "Freedom" Day" would hardly deter people from drawing that conclusion. This means that rational accounting will be imperilled and with it the potential for data-led responses.

Consequently, "Freedom Day" may not, in fact, lead to anywhere close to the 100,000 cases per day predicted by the modellers for late summer, not on the official count. Rather, the officially acknowledged caseload could be considerably less, even if large volumes of people disregarded altogether physical distancing and face-mask wearing. This would be simply because the hubris of 19 July has seriously undermined the process of mass population testing, hence the accuracy of data production, so that official counts may be rendered even greater under-estimates of the real situation on the ground than they were during the first wave where population testing-and-tracing did not exist.

In that case, a scenario could emerge where the ratio of deaths to recorded infection rates is considerably higher than is predicted by scientific modelling. Instead of 100–200 deaths on an "official" caseload of 100,000 a day, for example, the same number or more on an "official" caseload of between 25,000 and 50,000, this seems feasible. But, even if so, we can count on the fact that the Government will exploit the apparently lower-than-expected caseloads after 19 July to trumpet the foresight and wisdom of the judgement call that drove "Freedom Day", declaring that this has indeed been confirmed by events as scarcely risky at all, contrary to the fears of over-cautious scientists. Alas, such is also likely to be ideologically weaponized by ministers to resist calls for restoration of some controls as the body bags mount up.

19 July 2021 (updated 15 August 2021)

Notes

1 *BBC News* (2021). 'Lockdown: Boris Johnson unveils plan to end England restrictions by 21 June'. (22 February).

2 *BBC News* (22 February).

3 Johnson, B. (2021). *PM Statement to the House of Commons on Roadmap for Easing Lockdown Restrictions in England: 22 February 2021*. Coronavirus (COVID-19): rules, guidance and support. GOV.UK (online). Available at: www.gov.uk/government/speeches/pm-statement-to-the-house-of-commons-on-roadmap-for-easing-lockdown-restrictions-in-england-22-february-2021.

4 PHE (2021). *Coronavirus (COVID-19) in the UK*. GOV.UK (online). Available at: https://coronavirus.data.gov.uk/. See data under "Cases" and "Deaths". Accessed: 09/06/2021.

5 Skopeliti, C. (2021). 'Don't drop "data, not dates" approach, UK adviser warns as Covid cases surge'. *Guardian*. (29 May).

6 Worldometer (2021). *Covid-19 Coronavirus Pandemic: Countries: United Kingdom – Daily New Cases*. Available at: www.worldometers.info/coronavirus/country/uk/. Accessed: 15/07/2021; GOV.UK (2021). *Coronavirus (COVID-19) in the UK: Cases by Specimen Date*. Available at: https://coronavirus.data.gov.uk/details/cases. Accessed: 15/07/2021.

7 PHE (2021). *Coronavirus (COVID-19) in the UK: Cases by Specimen Date*. GOV.UK (online). Available at: https://coronavirus.data.gov.uk/details/cases. Accessed: 15/07/2021.

8 The slogan "cautious but irreversible" with reference to removal of social distancing restrictions culminating in the "Freedom Day" of 21 June became the Government's stock-in-trade from 22 February onwards.

9 Mason, R. (2021). 'Scientists urge Matt Hancock to delay England's June 21 re-opening'. *National*. (7 June); O'Connor, M. (2021). 'Government "open" to delaying 21 June England lockdown end date'. *BBC News*. (6 June); Pickover, E. (2021). 'Delay reopening by "a few weeks"' say scientists'. *Evening Standard*. (7 June); Somerville, E. and McTaggart, I. (2021). 'June 21 reopening to be delayed by up to four weeks'. *Telegraph*. (12 June); Wright, K. (2021). 'UK in early stages of third wave – scientist'. *BBC News*. (31 May).

10 Morton, B. (2021). 'Lockdown easing in England delayed to 19 July'. *BBC News*. (14 June); McTaggart, I. and Neilan, C. (2021). *"Now Is the Time to Ease off the Accelerator", Boris Johnson Says as He Announces Four-Week Delay to End of Lockdown'*. (14 June). Available at: www.telegraph.co.uk/politics/2021/06/14/politics-latest-news-boris-johnson-announcement-news-lockdown/.

11 Elgot, J. and Davies, C. (2021). 'Boris Johnson says no evidence to delay England reopening'. *Guardian*. (1 June).

12 In the run-up to the events that triggered Hancock's sacking/resignation, there was evidence of a campaign at work within the Government to undermine him. See Ahmed, N. (2021). 'Matt Hancock "suppressing" Covid data from government departments, says whistleblower'. *Byline Times*. (10 June).

13 Gye, H. (2021). 'Sajid Javid's arrival shifts the balance of opinion on lockdowns'. *I-News*. (28 June).

14 Parker, G. (2021). 'Whitty assessment provided Johnson with cover to lift Covid restrictions'. *Financial Times*. (10 July).

15 Even when conceding delay, Johnson had affirmed his "determination" to avoid further deferrals, describing 19 July as a "terminus date" for social restrictions. See: Shearing, H. (2021). 'PM insists July unlocking will go ahead in England'. *BBC News*. (15 June).

16 Parker (2021).

17 Therrien, A. (2021). 'Sajid Javid wants return to normal "as soon as possible"'. *BBC News*. (27 June).

18 Skopeliti (2021).

19 Allegretti, A. (2021). 'Sajid Javid: Covid restrictions in England must end on 19 July'. *Guardian*. (28 June); *ITN News* (2021). 'New at Ten'. (28 June); Gye (2021); Merrick, R. (2021). 'Sajid Javid rules out further lockdowns: "there's no going back"'.

Independent. (28 June); Shearing, H. (2021). 'Covid-19: end of England's Covid rules still set for 19 July'. *BBC News*. (28 June).

20 Davis, A. (2021). 'U.K.'s Javid says his priority is to get country back to normal'. *Bloomberg*. (27 June); Gye (2021); Therrien, A. (2021). 'Sajid Javid wants return to normal "as soon as possible"'. *BBC News*. (27 June).

21 Allegretti (28 June, 2021).

22 Shearing (2021).

23 Merrick, J. (2021). 'The four tests for 19 July might not pass – but that is unlikely to stop Boris Johnson lifting restrictions'. *I-News*. (10 July). The four tests to be met were as follows. (1) Continued progress with the vaccine roll-out so that the population is sufficiently protected by 19 July. (There was continued progress but there would still be substantial coverage gaps). (2) If data shows that the vaccines are successful in breaking or radically undermining the link between infections, hospitalizations, and deaths. (Data at that point indicated a major weakening (not breaking or undermining) of the link between infections and hospitalizations but not of the link between vaccines and infections. The data was also uncertain owing to the newness of Delta). (3) Infection and transmission rates are unlikely to spiral to such a degree that intense pressures are placed on healthcare services that could endanger their capacity to cope. (The likelihood was simply unknown at that point because the new Covid wave was at an early stage. But given the rate of its growth there was high possibility of intense pressures on the NHS). (5) Risk assessment of the Covid threat currently posed is not potentially in "fundamental" need of rebalancing by the emergence of new variants. (Delta was a relatively new variant that was under study).

24 Javid, S. (2021). 'Covid-19 Update'. *Statement to the House of Commons*. Hansard: UK Parliament. (5 July). Available at: https://hansard.parliament.uk/commons/2021-07-05/debates/803398B1-F845-43BA-A159-22E4CC6B9ECD/Covid-19Update.

25 GOV.UK (2021). *Coronavirus (COVID-19) in the UK: Deaths Within 28 Days of Positive Test by Date of Death: Daily*. Available at: https://coronavirus.data.gov.uk/details/deaths. Accessed: 15/07/2021; GOV.UK (2021). *Coronavirus (COVID-19) in the UK: Cases in United Kingdom: Cases by Specimen Date*. Available at: https://coronavirus.data.gov.uk/details/cases. Accessed: 15/07/2021.

26 Morton (2021); Dinnen (2021). 'Boris Johnson confirms nearly all Covid restrictions to be lifted on July 19 in England'. ITV News. (12 July); McGuinness, A. (2021). 'What is "freedom day" in England likely to look like – and will it go ahead on 19 July'? Sky News. (5 July).

27 Forrest, A. (2021). 'Euro 2020: risk of big Covid outbreak from England-Denmark game, government admits'. *Independent*. (7 July).

28 *France 24* (2021). 'Euro 2021: England vs Italy final fuels Covid-19 outbreak fears'. (11 July).

29 Forrest (2021).

30 Ross, T. and Donaldson, K. (2021). 'Self-isolation rules ease as U.K. faces 100,000 cases a day'. *Bloomberg*. (6 July).

31 Merrick, R. and Woodcock, A. (2021). 'Sensitivity of covid app could be reduced to save millions from being "pinged"'. *Independent*. (8 July).

32 *ITN News* (28 June, 2021); Cameron-Chileshe, J. and Parker, G. (2021). 'UK must "learn to live" with Covid, says new health secretary'. *Financial Times*. (28 June); Devlin, K. (2021). 'Javid warns UK has to learn to live with Covid but 19 July will be start of "exciting new journey"'. *Independent*. (29 June).

33 Parker, G. (2021). 'UK Covid cases may soar to 100,000 a day, Sajid Javid warns'. *Financial Times*. (6 July).

34 Butterworth, B. (2021). 'Scientists warn against "frightening" comparisons between Covid and flu'. *I-News*. (5 July).

35 Clark, S. (2021). 'Sajid Javid says 19 July will go ahead but "we have to be honest about the fact" cases will rise significantly'. *I-News*. (4 July).

36 Of course, this underselling of COVID-19 was also underselling of flu, since flu is hardly inconsequential. Tens of thousands are killed by it in a bad year in the UK, the vast majority of them over 75 years of age. See: Krelle, H. and Tallack, C. (2021). *One*

Year on: Three Myths About COVID-19 That the Data Proved Wrong. The Health Foundation (online). (23 March). Available at: www.health.org.uk/publications/long-reads/one-year-on-three-myths-about-COVID-19-that-the-data-proved-wrong.

37 Wearmouth, R. (2021). 'Boris Johnson "Dismissed Covid as Swine Flu and Joked He Would be Injected Live on TV"'. *Huffington Post*. (26 May).

38 Allegretti, A. and Geddes, L. (2021). 'PM to confirm 19 July end to Covid rules despite scientists' warnings'. *Guardian*. (4 July); Merrick, R. (2021). 'Boris Johnson set to announce easing of social distancing rules despite backlash from scientists'. *Independent*. (5 July).

39 *ITV News* (2021). 'Boris Johnson to restore freedoms as he tells public to "learn to live" with Covid-19'. (5 July); Bloom, D. (2020). 'Boris Johnson claims Britain can "defeat" coronavirus "by the Spring"'. *Mirror*. (2 November); Woodcock, A. (2020). 'Battle with disease could be over as early as the spring, Boris Johnson claims'. *Independent*. (2 November); O'Grady, S. (2021). 'Boris Johnson has surrendered to Covid – he should never be forgiven'. *Independent*. (5 July).

40 Butterworth (2021).

41 Lawless, J. (2021). 'Johnson says restrictions to ease, UK must live with virus'. *Associated Press News*. (5 July).

42 Wright, K. and Snowdon, K. (2021). 'Covid: easing measures on 19 July very likely, says Boris Johnson'. *BBC News*. (28 June).

43 Morton, B. (2021). '**Boris Johnson upbeat about easing lockdown in England on 19 July**'. *BBC News*. (1 July); Smith, M. and Bloom, D. (2021). 'Boris Johnson confirms freedom day plans from July 19 tearing up almost all Covid laws'. *Mirror*. (5 July); Bowden, G. (2021). 'Covid: most rules set to end in England, says PM'. *BBC News*. (5 July).

44 Johnson cited in *The Week* (2021). '"Britain's great gamble": who is saying what about freedom day unlocking'. (6 July).

45 A point well made by columnist Sean O'Grady. See: O'Grady, S. (2021). 'There could be 15,000 unnecessary Covid deaths by January – and Boris Johnson will blame you'. *Independent*. (6 July).

46 Javid (5 July, 2021); Morris, S. (2021). 'PM confirms face masks to become "personal choice" – but calls mount to keep legal requirement on public transport'. *Sky News*. (5 July); Woodcock, A. (2021). 'Boris Johnson says rules on masks and social distancing set to be torn up on 19 July'. *Independent*. (5 July).

47 Merrick, J. (2021). 'Face masks to be optional after 19 July, George Eustice says'. *I-News*. (24 June); *Reuters* (2021). 'Face masks to become a personal choice in England, minister says'. (4 July).

48 Allegretti, A. (2021). 'Ministers accused of causing confusion over face masks in England'. *Guardian*. (5 July); Whitehead, J. (2021). '"Not taking precautions is enormously selfish"': meet the people who will keep wearing face masks after 19 July'. *Independent*. (5 July).

49 Stone, J. (2021). 'Health minister refuses to say virus is under control ahead of lockdown rules lifting announcement'. *Guardian*. (5 July).

50 For example, Tory MP Laura Farris's faithful recital of the script on BBC's *Newsnight* current affairs programme (5 July 2021). Politicians were not the only ones who allowed perspective to party with the fairies over the crucial importance of getting rid of compulsory face-mask wearing in select settings to the cause of civil liberties. *Times* columnist Janice Turner, for example, described masking-up as "the most visible, divisive and loathed . . . remaining restrictions on our freedoms". Ditching them, she said, would restore "full-face normality". See: Turner, J. (2021). 'This time I'm ready to throw away my mask'. *Sunday Times* (online). (3 July).

51 *ITV News* (6 July, 2021).

52 Craig, J. (2021). 'PM heading for showdown with MPs amid predictions millions of Britons could get coronavirus this summer'. *Sky News*. (7 July).

53 Yorke, H., Donnelly, L. and Roberts, L. (2021). 'Vaccinated NHS staff could be freed from self-isolation rules before August 16'. *Telegraph*. (9 July); *Sky News* (2021). 'NHS staff could be made exempt from self-isolation rules when restrictions lift on 19 July'. (10 July).

54 Allegretti (2021). As reported by *Newsnight* (5 July 2021), Whitty (along with the Government's Chief Scientific Officer Patrick Vallance) was at the very least placing a very different "emphasis" on social distancing than government ministers.

55 A point made by Stephen Reicher (Professor of Behaviour Science at the University of St Andrews), cited in Allegretti (2021).

56 Shaw, N. (2021). 'People will stop thinking Covid is serious after July 19, say experts'. *Wales Online*. (7 July). Available at: www.walesonline.co.uk/news/uk-news/people-stop-thinking-covid-serious-20987871.

57 Hughes, D. (2021). 'Johnson claims link between coronavirus cases and deaths has been "severed"'. *Evening Standard*. (7 July).

58 Wright, O. and Smythe, C. (2021). 'We won't return to some sort of normality until spring, says Chris Whitty'. *Times*. (7 July).

59 Glaze, B. (2021). 'Plan to axe face masks sparks alarm – as most want them to stay on public transport'. *Mirror*. (5 July); Helm, T. and Savage, M. (2021). 'Public alarm grows at Boris Johnson's plan for Covid "freedom day"'. *Guardian*. (10 July).

60 Gye, H. (2021). 'Face masks set to become next culture war as wearers call those who plan to ditch them from 19 July "reckless"'. *I-News*. (9 July). Gye cites a survey by Redfield and Wilton Strategies which reveals that public opinion is evenly divided for and against the abolition of social distancing protections post-19 July. But the survey found that a large majority were in favour of public mask-wearing. Forty-seven percent of respondents said they would continue wearing face masks "all or most of the time" in public settings whereas 29 percent said they would wear them "some of the time". Only 21 percent said they would not wear them at all or wear them rarely. Sixty-nine percent of respondents who said they would continue with marks reported that they would view non-wearers as "reckless".

61 This issue escaped the notice of the right-wing corporate media in Britain whose own crassness of insensitivity to the vulnerable echoed that of the Government. See *The Week* (6 July, 2021).

62 Such a formula can hardly stand up in the broader societal context, of course. "It's like having a government that thinks road safety should be completely up to 'individual responsibility': no traffic lights, no highway code, no law about driving on the left, no crash barriers", as Professor of Public Health at UCL Robert West rightly observed (cited in Merrick, 5 July, 2021). Indeed.

63 HM Treasury (2020). *Eat Out to Help Out Launches Today – With Government Paying Half on Restaurant Bills*. Press Release. GOV.UK (online). (3 August). Available at: www.gov.uk/government/news/eat-out-to-help-out-launches-today-with-government-paying-half-on-restaurant-bills.

64 Dole, N. (2020). 'UK government urges people to "eat out for England"'. *ABC News*. (4 August); Stubley, P. (2020). 'Lockdown: Rishi Sunak urges public to head back to pubs and restaurants to save economy'. *Independent*. (4 July); *Reuters* (2020). 'Keep on dining out, UK minister urges as popular cut-price offer ends'. (31 August).

65 HM Treasury (2020).

66 Chief researcher, Professor Thiemo Fetzer, cited in: Skopeliti, C. (2020). '"Eat out to help out" scheme accelerated coronavirus second wave across UK, study says'. *Independent*. (30 October).

67 Reicher cited in: Middleton, J. (2021). 'UK on course to repeat Covid mistakes of last summer, Sage expert warns'. *Independent*. (30 June).

68 Stewart, H., Allegretti, Grower, N. and Brooks, L. (2021). 'Boris Johnson may tone down "freedom" rhetoric amid reopening jitters'. *Guardian*. (10 July).

69 Smyth, C. (2021). 'July 19: Boris Johnson offers freedom day with health warning'. *Times*. (16 July); Wright and Snowden (2021).

70 The same Javid who just a few days earlier in his statement to the House declared that only "entry ports" and "healthcare settings" were places where there was a "case" for continued face-masking after 19 July.

71 Stevens, J. and Haywood, E. (2021). 'The great masks muddle: Boris Johnson says law on face coverings will be axed . . . then sparks confusion by urging us to put them back on again!' *Mail* (online). (5 July).

72 MacKay, S. (2021). 'Covid-19: masks still expected to be worn indoors after 19 July – Zahawi'. *BBC News*. (12 July); Merrick, J. (2021). 'Fears over 19 July have triggered a marked shift in tone from ministers on face masks'. *I-News*. (11 July); Walker, P. (2021). 'Nadhim Zahawi says mask wearing will be "expected" after 19 July'. *Guardian*. (11 July).

73 *BBC News* (2021). 'Ban MPs from the Commons if they refuse to wear a mask, say unions'. (14 July); Heffer, G. (2021). 'COVID-19: parliament staff "incredulous and angry" at MPs not having to wear masks from Monday'. *Sky News*. (15 July).

74 Nick Triggle, BBC health correspondent, cited in Morton (2021).

75 Peck, T. (2021). 'The only ones who'll get any sort of freedom on "freedom day" are the government – the freedom to stop worrying about the pandemic'. *Independent*. (24 June); Flinders, M. (2021). 'July 19 "Freedom Day": Boris Johnson's biggest gamble is trusting the public'. *Conversation*. (7 July).

76 The Redfield and Wilton Strategies survey (conducted by Politico in July) revealed an even divide of respondents in favour of or opposed to the 19 July lifting of restrictions. See: McDonald, A. (2021). 'Almost half of Brits think Boris Johnson eased coronavirus rules too soon: Poll'. Politico. (30 July). But a poll of 2,001 adults conducted by Opinium for the Observer on 8 and 9 June found that half of respondents wanted "Freedom Day" to be put on ice compared to 31 percent who wanted it to go ahead. See: Helm and Savage (2021). A YouGov poll cited by The Week. (6 July 2021) found that 70 percent of respondents wanted mask-wearing to be compulsory on public transport post-19 July and 66 percent of them wanted this to be mandatory in shops and enclosed spaces.

77 Parker (2021).

78 For example: *The Week* (6 July, 2021); Whipple (2021). 'Freedom Day: Britain's great gamble with Covid unlocking begins'. *Times*. (6 July); Flinders (2021); Balls, K. (2021). 'If Boris Johnson's gamble over lockdown goes awry, he will struggle to find anyone else to blame'. *I-News*. (7 July).

79 This is also evidenced by the public attitudes survey cited by Gys (2021) and by the *Observer* poll (cited in Helm and Savage, 2021).

80 The most clinically vulnerable who have the most to lose from the end of restrictions are the 3.7 million people in the UK with conditions that render them immuno-deficient. One of those clinically vulnerable persons, 74-year-old Rosie Duffin, retired NHS worker, doubtless spoke for millions when, interviewed by the BBC, she opined: "I don't see the problem with wearing face masks. . . . It doesn't make sense does it? . . . When it comes to my own protection, and the protection of others, surely it's a small thing to do". See Lee, J. and Gillet, F. (2021). 'Covid-19: "For us it's not freedom day, is it?" *BBC News*. (6 July).

81 Johnson, B. (2021). *PM Statement at Coronavirus Press Conference: 5 July 2021*. Coronavirus (COVID-19): rules, guidance and support. GOV.UK (online). Available at: www.gov. uk/government/speeches/pm-statement-at-coronavirus-press-conference-5-july-2021.

82 This is because the virus has the capacity to re-infect the same person (and on the repeat dose cause greater illness) over the course of the same outbreak.

83 Dr. Nathalie McDermott interviewed on BBC's *Newsnight* current affairs programme (9pm, 6 July, 2021).

84 *BBC News* (2021). 'Covid: "society might not return to normal until 2022"'. (4 February); Binding, L. (2021). 'COVID-19: tougher rules around face masks and social distancing needed as lockdown lifts, scientists say'. *Sky News*. (31 March); Hayworth, E. (2021). 'Freedom may only last for weeks: experts raise fears of another autumn lockdown and warn some changes to our lifestyles could be permanent because allowing Covid cases to rise is a "significant risk"'. *Mail*. (5 July).

85 See Gorvett, Z. (2021). 'How effective is a single vaccine dose against Covid-19'? *BBC Global News*. (15 January); Dolgin, E. (2021). 'Is one vaccine dose enough if you've had COVID? What the science says'. *Nature* (online). (25 June). Available at: www.nature.com/articles/d41586-021-01609-4; Schuster-Bruce, C. (2021). 'How much protection you get from one shot of the Pfizer, AstraZeneca, and Moderna vaccines, according to the best available data'. *Business Insider*. (9 July).

86 See Sakay, Y.N. (2021). 'Here's how well COVID-19 vaccines work against the Delta variant'. *Healthline* (online). (16 July). Available at: www.healthline.com/health-news/heres-how-well-covid-19-vaccines-work-against-the-delta-variant.

87 Grover, N. (2021). 'Delta Covid variant may be edging race against vaccines'. *Guardian*. (27 June).

88 Cited in Grover (2021).

89 Visual Data and Journalism Team (2021). 'Covid vaccine: how many people in the UK have been vaccinated so far'? *BBC News*. (10 July).

90 NHS (2021). *NHS Invites All Adults to Get a COVID Jab in Final Push*. (17 June). Available at: www.england.nhs.uk/2021/06/nhs-invites-all-adults-to-get-a-covid-jab-in-final-push/; Marris, J. (2021). 'COVID-19: young people step forward for coronavirus vaccine in record numbers'. *Sky News*. (9 June).

91 Bryant, M. (2021). 'Third wave of Covid "definitely under way" in UK, says expert'. *Guardian*. (19 June).

92 Blackall, M. (2021). 'Long Covid: NHS taskforce scientist says letting coronavirus circulate among young is a "dangerous experiment"'. *I-News*. (9 July).

93 Manuel Gomes, one of the UCL researchers, cited in: Bawden (2021). 'Long Covid feels worse than advanced lung cancer for many patients, study finds'. *I-News*. (28 June).

94 Bawden (2021).

95 David Strain cited in Blackall (2021).

96 Forrest, A. (2021). 'No decision yet on whether UK children will get Covid vaccine, says government adviser'. *Independent*. (24 March); Roxby, P. and Triggle, N. (2021). 'Covid: children aged 12–17 unlikely to be offered vaccine in UK'. *BBC News*. (16 June).

97 Gupta quoted in: Cox, D. (2021). 'The third wave of Covid is here . . . and it's weird'. *Wired*. (28 June).

98 Wood, P. (2021). 'Easing lockdown rules on 19 July will make unvaccinated people Covid "variant factories", scientists warn'. *I-News*. (5 July).

99 Landray cited in Cox (2021).

100 According to Professor Martin McKee of the London School of Hygiene and Tropical Diseases (cited in Cox, 2021).

101 Bawden, T. (2021). 'Covid vaccines may be less effective at cutting infections, but remain effective against serious illness'. *I-News*. (12 July). The evidence for this, as Professor Karl Friston of Imperial College London, explains, is that the current acceleration of Covid cases is much higher than would be expected based on the infectiousness of Delta and the state of progress of the vaccination programme.

102 Griffin cited in Bawden (2021).

103 Sonabend, R. et al. (2021). *Evaluating the Roadmap Out of Lockdown for England: Modelling the Delayed Step 4 of the Roadmap in the Context of the Delta Variant*. Imperial College London, MRC Centre for Global Infectious Disease Analysis. (7 July). Available at: https://assets.publishing.service.gov.uk/government/uploads/system/uploads/attachment_data/file/1001177/S1303_Imperial_College_London_Evaluating_the_Roadmap_out_of_Lockdown_for_England_modelling_the_delayed_step_4.2_of_the_roadmap_in_the_context_of_the_Delta_variant__7_July_2021__1_.pdf.

104 Sonabend et al. (2021), pp. 8–9.

105 Sonabend et al. (2021), pp. 3–8.

106 O'Hare, R. and Mehta, R. (2021). 'Magnitude of Third Wave Highly Uncertain, Suggests New Analysis'. *Imperial College London: News* (online). (12 July). Available at: www.imperial.ac.uk/news/226213/magnitude-third-wave-highly-uncertain-suggests/.

107 Vaughan, A. (2021). 'Covid-19 deaths in England could peak at 100 per day in August'. *New Scientist*. (12 July). Available at: www.newscientist.com/article/2283813-covid-19-deaths-in-england-could-peak-at-100-per-day-in-august/.

108 How many deaths or hospitalizations Ferguson considered as acceptable on his empirical cost-benefit analysis of tolerable risk is not clear. At least 4,600 fatalities, obviously. Thankfully, the bulk of scientific and public health expert opinion resisted the imperative of the empirical-instrumental imagination (exemplified by Ferguson) to eschew ethical judgements in favour of purely quantitative ones.

109 Ferguson was not alone. Paul Hunter, Professor of Medicine at East Anglia University, and Alyson Pollock, Professor of public health at Newcastle University, also found the policy of complete unlocking a "sensible" one. See: Geddes, L. (2021). 'UK scientists caution that lifting of Covid rules is like building "variant factories"'. *Guardian*. (4 July).

110 Forrest, A. and Stone, J. (2021). 'Boris Johnson pursuing Covid policy of mass infection that poses "danger to the world", scientists warn: international experts convene emergency summit ahead of England's unlocking'. *Independent*. (17 July); Quinn, B. (2021). 'England's Covid unlocking is threat to world, say 1,200 scientists'. *Guardian*. (16 July).

111 Cited in Cowburn, A. (2021). 'Boris Johnson urged to abandon "dangerous and unethical" plan to lift Covid restrictions on 19 July'. *Independent*. (8 July).

112 Elgot, J. (2021). 'Doctors warn of "devastating consequences" of lifting Covid rules in England'. *Guardian*. (13 July).

113 *Sky News* (2021). 'Doctors call for "targeted coronavirus prevention measures" to stay after 19 July'. (3 July); Snowdon, K. (2021). 'Doctors want to keep some measures after 19 July'. *BBC News*. (3 July).

114 Cited in Cowburn (2021).

115 Editor-in-Chief of *The Lancet*, Richard Horton, expressed bafflement at the minority view of the handful of scientists to offer support to Johnson's plans for total unlocking. Speaking, for example, of Whitty's tepid "now is better than later" rationale for the plan, Horton pointed out that this commanded little support among experts. Whitty's claim to the contrary was, he said, "wilfully misrepresenting scientific opinion". (Horton cited in Forrest and Stone, 2021).

116 This was exactly the critique mobilized by a chorus of public health professionals and scientists of various hues (in the UK and overseas, and including those of current and former members of the SAGE group advising the Government). See Allegretti and Geddes (4 July, 2021); Blackall (9 July, 2021); Blackall, M. (2021). 'Lockdown easing: doctors warn full lifting of Covid rules on 19 July could have "devastating consequences"'. *I-News*. (13 July); Forrest, A. and Stone, J. (2021). 'Boris Johnson pursuing Covid policy of mass infection that poses "danger to the world", scientists warn'. *Independent*. (16 July); Giordano, C. (2021). '"Irresponsible and perilous" to press ahead with lockdown lifting in England, doctors warn'. *Independent*. (13 July); Gurdasani, D. et al. (2021). 'Mass infection is not an option: we must do more to protect our young'. *The Lancet*, 398 (10297), pp. 297–98; Mahase, E. (2021) 'Covid-19: experts condemn UK "freedom day" as dangerous and unethical'. *British Medical Journal*, 374 (1829) (19 July). Available at: www.bmj.com/content/374/bmj.n1829; Middleton, J. (2021). 'New Zealand scientists say UK's "awful experiment" on Covid will threaten the country'. *Independent*. (14 July); *Sky News*. (3 July, 2021); *ITV News* (2021). '"Dangerous" to return to life as normal on July 19, expert warns'. (10 July); Wise, J. (2021). 'Covid-19: ending all restrictions in England on 19 July "dangerous and premature," say experts'. *British Medical Journal*, 374 (8300) (9 July). Available at: www.bmj.com/content/374/bmj.n1751; *TWN World News* (2021). ' Doctors "profoundly concerned" about 19 July amid "dramatic" rise in cases'. (7 July); *TWN World News* (2021). 'Government adviser warns of mutation risk as doctors voice concern over rising cases'. (4 July).

117 Helm and Savage (10 July, 2021).
118 As the SAGE group warned (Hayworth, 2021).
119 *ITV News* (2021). 'Covid: cases of India coronavirus variant found in UK features two mutations that could be "of concern"' (16 April).
120 Cited in Geddes (2021).
121 *World News* (2021). ' Government adviser warns of mutation risk as doctors voice concern over rising cases'. (10 July).
122 Cited in Wood (2021).
123 Cited in Forrest and Stone (2021).
124 Cited in Middleton (2021).

CONCLUSIONS

Beyond freedom?

The pandemic situation since mid-July 2021 has of course continued to evolve, both domestically and internationally. The number of officially recorded infections worldwide stood at 544,390,605 by 20 June 2022. The number of officially recorded fatalities by then had reached 6,341,027. The peak number of daily deaths worldwide from the first worldwide surge of the pandemic was 120,642. This was on 28 May 2020. This number increased more than sevenfold to 851,980 on 7 January 2021 at the peak of the second international wave. A third bigger international peak of fatalities was reached on 23 April 2021. This saw 901,627 deaths officially registered. This was followed by a fourth wave that peaked on 19 August with 756,141 officially recognized deaths. But towards the end of 2021 a fifth international wave of infections began to build that dwarfed all of the predecessors. This peaked at 3,840,220 on 21 January 2022 before beginning its slow descent. Global deaths from this wave did not dip below one million until early April this year (2022).[1]

Yet there has also been a degree of pandemic continuity amid the global ups and downs. This is with regard to the status of the UK within the bigger international context. At the time of writing this chapter (20 June 2022), the UK has held on to its unenviable position as the European leader for COVID-19 deaths, excepting only Europe's great outlier state, Russia. By then, the death tally stood at 179,537 on the UK government's official count, which as we will see is a radical undercount. This was much in excess of the number in Germany (140,292), in France (149,039), and in the early COVID-19 frontrunner European countries of Italy (167,721) and Spain (107,482). The UK is also still a European leader in the number of deaths per million of the population (with 2,618), ahead of Russia (with 2,605), and second only to Italy (with 2,782). Not only that, the UK remains still in second place among the G7 and the countries of the Global North in terms of mortalities, just as it has been throughout the pandemic, second only to the other great bastion of neoliberal governance, the US.[2]

DOI: 10.4324/9781003275039-10

The explanation for this persisting state of affairs, I contend, is British exceptionalism. For this reason, there is utility in examining the unfolding of government policy with regard to COVID-19 since July 19 (2021's) "Freedom Day". Moreover, a few words that would distil from the foregoing how British exceptionalism may be explained is warranted. These tasks ought to suffice by way of conclusion.

British exceptionalism since "Freedom Day"

This book has argued that British exceptionalism has drastically radicalized the negative impact of the pandemic on public health. The unreformed pattern of government policy in relation to COVID-19, which has not only stripped away the residual physical distancing but also substantially undermined even effective monitoring of the virus, has continued to perpetrate these harms ever since, as I will briefly illustrate. Since this is the case, when the next pandemic arrives, which will be sooner rather than later, there are few prospects that British exceptionalism will not simply repeat.

What was promised for "Freedom Day" by its artificers was, as we have seen, the virtual disbandment of legally mandated NPIs as a line of defence against the pandemic. What was not promised to commence exactly on 19 July 2021 was to be rolled out in short order afterwards. The rationale was explicitly that COVID-19 would hitherto be regarded as posing a threat to public health that was not significantly greater than that of a nasty case of flu. This was owing to the success of the vaccination programme in "substantially breaking" the connection between anyone contracting the virus and becoming seriously ill from the mischance of doing so. Before the summer of 2021 was over, the policies that would make regard or disregard for physical distancing behaviours simply a matter of personal choice were implemented on exactly the timescales that were proposed for them. As the Government's own retrospective account of its actions spins the matter:

> Although other countries now exceed the UK's proportion of the total population vaccinated, the speed and highly targeted nature of the vaccination programme had a direct impact on the Government's ability to open up the economy and ease social restrictions sooner than other comparator countries, without placing the NHS under unsustainable pressure. . . . On 19 July 2021, the Government removed most restrictions in England at step 4 of the Roadmap and, in doing so, opened up earlier than many other comparable countries. The Government made a deliberate choice to do so at this point as it coincided with the end of the school term and meant that restrictions were removed over the summer period when more activities take place outdoors and there is less pressure on the NHS.[3]

This is British exceptionalism unrepentant. It is for its architects a matter of pride and a marker of success that the economy is reopened faster than anywhere else, indeed starting from much in advance of "Freedom Day". So too for them is it a matter of pride and prestige that 19 July, in scrapping virtually all controls (including those – such as mask-wearing – which carried no economic penalties whatsoever), acted as a trailblazer among the high-income countries in casting off public health precautions. As for the "highly-targeted" vaccination programme, this was mythology, inasmuch as the original plan to double-dose the old and vulnerable as a first priority was replaced by a dash for mass population coverage, age cohort by age cohort, so that workers could be returned to the workplace and children to the schools as quickly as possible.

By contrast, by and large, EU governments scaled back on physical distancing and other NPIs much more cautiously than did Johnson's gang. Entering the current year most were committed to them still (public mask-wearing, Covid passes, restrictions on certain venues, limited closures, etc.). It was not until February 2022 that Denmark led the way in following the UK example, with others then taking the same path, at varying speeds.[4] This is certainly not to idealize the EU. Incaution and imprudence is relative, not absolute. The competitive nature of international capitalism is such that the pressures to simply ditch physical distancing (indeed even COVID-19 testing and tracing) while the pandemic still rages, as it definitely still is, are universally experienced. And where certain of the leading economic players of world capitalism fast-track the casting off of social restrictions, the others are placed under greater pressure to follow suit.

This is exactly what is happening as, for example, the leading EU states perceive commercial rivals, such as the UK, as potentially grabbing a competitive advantage by re-opening their economies faster. Unsurprisingly, then, across the channel, politicians increasingly spout the same kinds of ideologically loaded rationalizations for total freedoms from pandemic precautions that have been common currency in the UK for far longer – such as that COVID-19 is no longer a threat to society or especially injurious to public health. This is much to the chagrin of the WHO, which at least understands that Omicron (the most recent Covid-variant) is no flu. The organization has long cautioned governments not to adopt an "all eggs in one basket" of mass vaccination as public health policy.[5] This was oft repeated on the run-up to the UK's "Freedom Day".[6] Alarmed by pandemic denialism on the continent, the WHO has since the start of the new year urged the EU not to dismantle all physical distancing protections, to no avail.[7]

Despite itself, the Government's self-account of its action up to mid-February 2022 makes it clear enough what its priorities for 19 July were. This was not a matter of saving vulnerable lives or avoiding potentially high risk of unknowable levels of long-term health damage to unknown numbers of people (i.e. due to "Long Covid"). Rather, this was about fast-tracking full capitalist restoration all-in-one-go in the summer of 2021 where the risk of over-stressing the healthcare system would, in theory, be significantly less than if the unlocking gamble proceeded later in the year. In other words, since the dismantling of physical distancing controls before the autumn of 2021 *no matter what* was a given, a red line that could not be crossed, it was better that this was done sooner rather than later. This was not least because that would hopefully evade the media spectacle (and negative press for the Government) of an overloaded NHS. Where was the concern with actual *lives* in all of this?

As for policy developments since the summer of 2021, these obviously fit the pattern that was set by 19 July. Nonetheless, the incaution these have demonstrated, even by the standards set by "Freedom Day" itself, have been remarkable. In September 2021, the PM proposed his "Plan A" for managing the pandemic over the rest of the autumn and for the winter months to follow. This self-styled "comprehensive" plan basically reduced to booster vaccinations, the continuation of established practices of testing and self-isolation, and border control measures.[8] That is, it contained hardly anything at all, and nothing that committed the Government itself to "comprehensive planning". There was also a "Plan B" to be deployed if circumstances made it necessary. This plan too was fairly minimalist. This was a steer for workers and employers to reintroduce work-at-home practices wherever possible and the reintroduction of the recently unnecessarily ditched mandatory mask-donning in certain indoor settings but excluding hospitalities.[9]

In the event, owing to the importation of the highly infectious Omicron variant, and its rapid community spread, driving a fresh wave of infections, Johnson was compelled to announce a switch to Plan B on 8 December 2021.[10] True to precedent, the decision to make the change was a tardy one, following a period of intense lobbying by medical professionals.[11] Independent SAGE lobbied for a precautionary 10-day lockdown on the grounds that there was insufficient data on the infectiousness and pathogenic potential of Omicron to assess its impact on hospitalization rates. It was better, the scientists pointed out, to avert a potential crisis rather than wait for one to materialize and then try to deal with it. For exactly the same reason (paucity of data on Omicron impacts), however, Chris Whitty, representing government science, rejected a circuit-breaker lockdown. After all, that would not be data-led.[12] The "data" in question, Whitty neglected to say, would be people in MVUs and dead bodies in mortuaries

SAGE, clinicians and other healthcare experts nonetheless were fruitlessly urging the Government to at least shift to Plan B. This was since October 2021, before Omicron, owing to fast-rising Delta caseloads and hospitalizations.[13] Given the threadbare protections offered by Plan B, it was fortunate indeed that although Omicron was the most transmissible variant yet, it was not as virulent as Delta, and nor was it able to breach the vaccine wall which was buttressed by the booster roll-out. Despite transmission rates still running at unprecedented thresholds throughout January of the current year, the Government announced the switch back from Plan B to Plan A just six weeks later.[14] There were 111,748 verified infections and 18,732 new hospitalizations on the same day (19 January 2022) that Javid announced the change. The peak of the first Omicron wave was just five days in the past.[15]

As for the Government's commitment to practices of mass testing and self-isolation for positively-testing persons, there was none. I forecasted before 19 July last year that a consequence of "Freedom Day" would be that the even residual effectiveness of test-and-trace would be dissolved. This was as people were disincentivized to report symptoms or take a test or voluntarily self-isolate. There-fore, the capacity of science to measure accurately the volume of caseloads would also be seriously compromised. This has undeniably come to pass, and it was rec-ognized and lamented by independent scientists faced with the summer upsurge of 2021. Initially, the caseloads of 100,000–120,000 per day that were forewarned by Javid and expected by the epidemiological modellers before autumn seemingly did not materialize (though they did come later).[16] This was to some degree at least, it was surmised, because much of it was just not visible due to much higher levels of non-testing and non-reporting than before.[17] This undermining of testing and reporting has meant as well that the emergence of new variants that pose higher risk is likely to be detected less quickly than before, with all of the enhanced danger to public health that this presents.

Ministers delivered further hatchet blows to the residual public safety protec-tions provided by COVID-19 testing a couple of months into the current year (2022). This was when the PM confirmed on 22 February earlier reports of the imminent repeal of all remaining pandemic laws in England under his "Living with Covid" (in reality *ignoring* it) plan. The "roadmap" set out in September the year before was that these remaining laws should all go on March 24, but these plans were now brought forward by a month. The test-and-trace system was disbanded on 24 February. Starting on 24 February as well, people were no longer legally required to self-isolate if they positively tested for COVID-19. This applied to vac-cinated and unvaccinated persons alike. Also commencing on that day, vaccinated people were no longer required to test for seven days if they had been in close con-tact with an infected person. Simultaneously, unvaccinated persons who were still required to self-test for seven days if they had been in close contact with an infected person were not required to stay at home.[18]

These moves basically freed people to place self-interest before collective well-being. This was because they extended to them the "right" to cause harm to others in pursuit of their own wants or preferences. This was either unwittingly (as in the case of people who continued as normal having chosen not to test themselves after being in close contact with someone who was infected) or knowingly (as in the case of people who continued to associate with others outside the home having failed a test). Not only that, these rule changes also provided tacit encouragement for people to do exactly that. This was because repealing these laws was not simply the removal of a constraint on conduct but also conveyed the message that sticking to these practices was no longer necessary to save lives or protect the NHS.

If this was necessary, after all, the Government would not be repealing these laws, which were supposedly being got rid of because COVID-19, like flu, is sim-ply an inconvenience. Now, people did not need to be hoodwinked by ministerial pandemic denialism to abandon self-isolation and self-testing. For many, it was enough that this was mandated, especially since they could "play along" with the denialism of others. As for those who were hoodwinked, some would be unwit-tingly co-opted into denialism, whereas others would doubtless self-convince over the correctness of denialism because this fits with confirmation bias (most people do not, after all, *want* to be physically distancing or self-isolating). Whatever the motives, public safety was the loser.

The Government then scrapped free PCRs and LFTs for members of the general public starting from 1 April 2022. From that point, people could no longer obtain kits for home-testing from workplaces or pharmacies. Instead, they would have to order them online and pay themselves. Predictably, this dramatically lowered the number of people taking tests, especially among those who are asymptomatic or experiencing mild symptoms.[19] This obviously further undermined surveillance of the pandemic, so that the magnitude of caseloads would hitherto be even more understated, further supporting pandemic denialism. Yet, as self-quarantine, home-testing and free testing were got rid of, Johnson and his ministers were simultaneously urging people to be "safe" and "responsible". This was by wearing masks, staying home, taking tests and reporting the results.[20]

The disingenuity of this was and is staggering, of course. How is self-isolation commendable if it does not particularly advance the cause of public health? If taking tests and reporting results is indeed the right thing to be doing, how then does disincentivizing the practice by making it more expensive and inconvenient assist the cause of "responsibility"? If testing and reporting (hence tracing) serves the cause of public safety (and if not why would it be the responsible course of action?), is it not obvious that the Government would need to facilitate these practices by putting money where its mouth is rather than simply passing over the responsibility to individuals?

In an earlier chapter of this book I discussed an aspect of British exceptionalism that I described as "communicative ambivalence". It is clear that the phenomenon is very much alive and kicking post-19 July 2021, where it doubtless continues to sow confusion in the public mind about exactly how to behave in response to the pandemic. I suspect that this mixed messaging (to use a more straightforward term) will persist until the pandemic is over. I surmised earlier in the present work that, although communicative ambivalence may be interpreted as chaotic and inadvertent, as simply the nincompoopery of the clueless, the reality is likely rather different. This is because such mixed messaging has been relentlessly consistent throughout the course of the pandemic. Communicative ambivalence reflects the Government's ambivalence of outlook towards the whole project of placing restrictions on the freedoms of commerce in the service of public health and safety. Mixed messaging not only reflects ambivalence of outlook but also is likely a self-conscious attempt to resolve it on the side of economic freedoms.

Johnson was forced, reluctantly and belatedly, into nationwide lockdown, and all of the associated NPIs. He needed to be convinced that an unmitigated public health catastrophe would result from eschewing these restrictions before he acquiesced to them. So, as soon as room for any doubt whatsoever is opened up over whether or not such restrictions are strictly necessary to avoid a worse-case scenario (which for the Government would be a situation where the NHS cannot cope), an interest is generated in undermining them, even as these are set out and formally endorsed. Communicative ambivalence may serve to dilute and weaken public support for physical distancing and related NPIs (which cannot simply be ditched or rejected by government if it wishes to retain public support), so that these practices fizzle out of their own accord. This may explain the mixed messaging of government in the midst of the first lockdown of March–May 2020. Or it can be used (as it has been post-19 July 2021) to disincentivize people's voluntary physical distancing and related behaviours once these are no longer legally mandated. Either way, communicative ambivalence surreptitiously serves the goal of fast-tracked economic normalization.

With regard to the Government's border-control policy, I noted in an earlier chapter the inconsistency of its plans to continue with the traffic-lighted system that restricted or blocked entrees from many parts of the world (and forcibly detained returnees in exorbitantly priced quarantine hotels) with within-border 19 July freedoms. The persistence of such controls, I speculated, may provide a propaganda benefit for the Government. This was by maintaining the fiction that ministers were still invested in the task of protecting the public from new variants and by promulgating the myth that these were more likely to be "alien" (i.e. imports from overseas) rather than locally grown as was made more likely by the dismantling of within-border NPIs.

But such ideological benefits, I suggested, were likely to be trumped by those practical economic ones that would result from the dismantling of border controls altogether. For a government such as the UK's, which was committed to all forms of profitable cross-border flows, and which presided over an economy with one of the biggest tourism industries in the world, this was likely to be sooner rather than later. Consequently, despite its September (2021) commitment to "measures at the border",[21] the Government announced it would scrap its amber list of travel-restricted countries in mid-September, which would come into force at the start of October of that year.[22] Simultaneously, the red list of the most radically travel-restricted countries (which barred entry from overseas nationals and which mandated hotel quarantine for returning UK residents or citizens living abroad) was rapidly scaled down. This survived, albeit only nominally, until mid-December, along supposedly with an idle skeleton crew of quarantine hotels. But it was emptied of all countries by the start of November.[23] On the cusp of the winter of 2021, then, there were no long border protections in force.

The fast-track virtual abolition of border security measures was forecasted in my book, but this hardly required futurology skills. But I also warned of the dangers of importing new dangerous variants from virus hotspots that the policy risked. The Omicron variant was duly exported to the UK (probably from South Africa – removed relatively recently from the red list) shortly afterwards, in November 2021. The Government congratulated itself for speedily acting to ban flights from South Africa and for adding South Africa and several other Omicron-stricken countries to the hitherto depopulated red list. However, Javid was compelled to admit that passengers arriving from South Africa after the travel ban was announced but before it was implemented were not Covid-tested on entry and were not prevented from using public transport to get to their destinations.[24] This was suggestive that, despite the Government's claim to the contrary, the red list system and supporting quarantine hotels were not simply idle but were actually defunct, so that there was nowhere that the arrivals could be quarantined.[25]

The pandemic since "Freedom Day"

The negative consequences of 19 July 2021's "Freedom Day" and those policies that followed in terms of the undermining of public health protections have been clear enough right up to the present day, though these have hardly been acknowledged by a government painstakingly devoted to the ideological task of representing COVID-19, post-vaccination, as little more than a nasty flu.[26] In place of the pre-vaccination pattern of the pandemic of steep rises in deaths and hospitalizations followed by (under tightening social restrictions) their steep decline until they plateaued at almost negligible scales, a new post-vaccination pattern has been consolidated. This has been one in which the daily average of people killed by it from mid-August onwards up until the year's end fluctuated from between 109 and 196, never thereafter dipping below that threshold, just as the virus was allowed free reign to spread and circulate. By the end of 2021, a further 20,567 people had lost their lives to COVID-19 since 19 July.[27]

Moreover, the situation worsened in the first month of 2022. The daily average for daily deaths fluctuated between 171 and 303 throughout January according to *Worldometer*. Between 6 January and 4 February, there were never fewer than 200 deaths per day.[28] February was a better month, though the daily mortality rate remained high, ranging from 119.7 and 218.1 on a seven-day average throughout the month.[29] Another 12,021 COVID-19 deaths were officially registered during that period. Since the start of March, the rate of mortalities has fallen. Nonetheless, another 15,046 people have been killed by the virus up to and including 20 June.[30] This brings the price of "freedom" in lost lives since 19 July 2021 in the UK to 48,024, as the virus is basically allowed a free lunch. These victims will be those who are from the most vulnerable groups (those for whom vaccines are less protective, the immune-compromised, those who are not vaccinated – often for medical reasons, those who are elderly and with underlying health conditions). To put that in perspective, when the first wave reached its peak for daily deaths (1,094), on 9 April 2020, the total official death toll stood at 11,830.[31]

This is not exactly how I forecasted the pandemic would play out in a post-distancing UK. Back in mid-July last year, I thought that the casualty toll could be much higher than even these rather sobering statistics indicate. For reasons set out in this book, the potential for a worser-case scenario was a very real one. This has been avoided because the gambler's gambles do not always backfire, or not as much as they could. But nor did the gamble with public health simply succeed in the sense of vindicating itself by virtue of other (economic) benefits. Rather, even from the Government's perspective, the public health outlook has remained troubling, and with the potential to tip over quite suddenly into another major crisis. At no point since "Freedom Day" did the daily death count rise as high as 400, as was predicted by some modellers, true. Deaths from the Delta-powered summer and autumn of 2021 waves peaked at 132 (9 September) and 155 (31 October), according to ONS data, whereas deaths from the first and second Omicron waves peaked at 265 on 27 January and 268 on 8 April.[32]

But high scales of mortality have persisted for much of the period since then, with the low rates of daily deaths that were engineered by more stringent (or indeed any) physical distancing controls a thing of the past, just as the virus has been able to mutate without the constraints on this behaviour that such controls provide. Between 6 May and 12 June 2021, owing to the success of the third lockdown in disrupting transmission chains, the seven-day average of COVID-19 deaths was never higher than ten. Between 30 July and 6 September 2020, owing to the success of the first lockdown in squeezing the virus's infection opportunities, exactly the same situation prevailed By contrast, the result of Johnson's "living with Covid" strategy has been an acceleration of new pandemic waves (three so far) fuelled by Omicron. This is alongside daily death tolls that during the lowest ebbs of the virus's cycles have never been less than three times higher and which typically have been between seven times and 11 times higher than during the previous lows.[33] So far the Omicron subvariants have not evaded vaccine protections, and neither BA.1 nor BA.2 (the jury is out on BA.4 and BA.5) have been associated with increased pathogenic harm. But the danger is ever present (including of evolution of a strain beyond Omicron that is a game-changer).

The Government's cause in continuing to eschew pandemic controls and in chipping away at those which remain has been assisted by its success in reassuring the public that the new normal of prolonged periods of high COVID-19 mortality exists more at the level of appearances than at the level of reality. This is by sowing the notion that Omicron deaths in recent months are not really Covid deaths at all. Rather, these are deaths of people who, even though they have contracted the disease, are not hospitalized for that reason. Or, these are the deaths of people who though hospitalized owing to COVID-19, are not killed by it, but by other conditions or causes.[34] The perspective supposedly supporting this notion is uncontentious. This is that the vaccines are for most people succeeding in minimizing harmful symptoms and that the Omicron subvariants that have become dominant may have marginally reduced harmfulness alongside enhanced infectiousness – up to now. Empirical support for this proposition is to be found in the fact that, since 5 November 2021, despite two new waves of infections, the number of hospitalized patients requiring MVUs has declined overall. By contrast, in the run-up to "Freedom Day" (19 July 2021), and for several months afterwards, the number of COVID-19 patients in MVUs rose steadily alongside climbing caseloads and hospitalizations.[35]

The difference between the two periods is that in the former, unlike the latter, Delta, not Omicron, was dominant. This was just as there were also substantial gaps in vaccine coverage in the earlier period that would later be made up. Nonetheless, the notion that COVID-19 is no longer a killer is empirically unsupported. Such is also evidenced by the GOV.UK data. These reveal that as caseloads rose sharply during the two most recent Covid waves, so simultaneously did hospitalizations and deaths. Between 8 December 2021 and 4 January 2022, during Omicron's winter upsurge, the number of infections increased fourfold, just as hospitalizations rose by 275 percent and deaths by 250 percent. In the most recent wave before the present one (which is building as I write this conclusion), which got started in earnest on 22 February and which peaked on 28 March, the number of infections and hospitalizations both rose by 250 percent, whereas the number of people who died rose by 180 percent.[36]

The two-time coincidence of upwards trends in all three data sets on the same timescales is unlikely to be accidental. A case could be made that the December/January (2021/22) Omicron wave may have killed people for seasonable reasons unconnected to COVID-19. But what is not in doubt is that, despite the BA.1 and BA.2 mutations that seemingly have made the virus less pathogenic, Omicron is still much deadlier than seasonable illnesses such as flu. This is not "just a flu" as is now commonly said. Moreover, the spring wave of Omicron would not have coincided with any increase in non-Covid seasonably linked CDs, so that COVID-19 itself is the only plausible cause of the bulk of deaths of those who perished within 28 days of a positive test.

However, it is data derived from death certificates that is most instructive in illuminating the real level of Omicron's harm. By 1 January 2022, according to the ONS, 174,000 deaths, based on information on death certificates, were registered in the UK.[37] Now, since the start of the year, Omicron has become completely dominant in the UK, as this has been carried by a rapid succession of variants: initially BA.1 and BA.2, from January into March; latterly, by subvariants of BA.1 and BA.2, and most recently of all by BA.4 and BA.5 Less than two months after its emergence, by 21 February, 9,000 people had been killed by Omicron, based on ONS data on death certificates.[38] According to Professor Christina Pagel, writing in the *British Medical Journal*, the number of Omicron deaths had grown to 20,000 by mid-June this year. This is the same number of people who were killed by Delta. This, again, is based on the number of death certificates which identify the disease as main or contributory cause.[39]

The spin of government ministers and certain establishment-friendly epide-miologists who were more-or-less supportive of "Freedom Day" that Omicron is largely emptied of its capacity to pose significant public danger is not generally shared by a majority of non-aligned scientists of disease and disease control. Pagel doubtless speaks for many as she observes:

> While omicron might be somewhat less severe than delta, and people have higher immunity through vaccination and previous infection, it is not mild. At a population level, its sheer transmissibility more than compensates for any reduction in experienced disease severity or symptoms for the individual.[40]

As for the present (June 2022) resurgence of Omicron, carried by the new BA.4 and BA.5 offshoots, Professor Danny Altmann of Imperial College London, regards this as "very concerning".

> We're now firmly into our next wave, the BA4/5 wave. "I see no ships" will get us only so far when we're once again up to two per cent prevalence, as we were a few months back, and hospital admissions creeping up again. This isn't really "living with COVID" when you consider that the Omicron wave brought another 615,000 into the Long Covid clinics, with all that entails in terms of human misery, people off work, kids off school.[41]

Indeed, on the subject of Long Covid, the ONS estimates that by the start of May this year there were 1.8 million people self-reporting as suffering from the condition.[42]

There are also early signs that the newest offshoots of Omicron may generate more severe symptoms and be more injurious to health than the earlier ones. As Paul Burton, Moderna's Chief Medical Officer, reports:

> There is emerging data that BA.4 and BA.5 is actually more pathogenic than BA.1 and BA.2, so there's a higher hospitalisation risk – so it's an important and worrisome variant. . . . Omicron is devastating. It's infected millions of people a day even in the US and hundreds of thousands in the UK and across Europe. We're going to be dealing with the ramifications of Omicron for years to come – long Covid, depression, neurological features, diabetes, cardiovascular disease – and stuff that will begin to emerge. Omicron is not mild.[43]

According to Professor Kei Sato's team of clinical researchers based at Tokyo University's Institute of Medical Research, the new subvariants of Omicron are also being associated with a greater tendency to attack the lungs than the earlier ones. This too is an obvious source of concern. As Sato reports: "We have data suggesting that BA.4/5 spike is more fusogenic than BA.2 spike. In our previous studies on Delta, BA.1 and BA.2, higher fusogenicity is closely associated with lung preference".[44]

But what about the workers? What has rather been forgotten or ignored in all of this talk of "living with Covid" are those who are actually most having to cope with the consequences of policies which are about disregarding COVID-19. Healthcare frontliners are already living with "Long Covid" in ever-growing numbers. "It was reported this month [June] that over 10,000 NHS workers have been off work for more than three months" owing to the condition.[45]

In Chapter 2 I discussed the shortages of PPE and MVUs and other healthcare resources that healthcare workers had to cope with during the first pandemic wave. In Chapter 3 I contextualized these issues in the long-standing crisis of the welfare state under neoliberal "restructuring" and in more recent times austerity politics.

The problem of the chronic under-resourcing and under-valuing of healthcare (and indeed social care) must impact negatively on the capacity of the system to cope with the ongoing pandemic in its present rhythms, let alone with a qualitatively bigger crisis that would arise if a new variant came along which just happens to breach the vaccine wall or become more virulent. There simply is no slack in the NHS to cope with radically upscaled demands.

Insofar as the NHS has coped with the pandemic, this has been at the cost of the broader health needs of the population, as the waiting lists for treatments of other illnesses grow longer. In January 2016, there were 3.29 million people on NHS waiting lists for consultant-led elective care. By February 2020, on the eve of the pandemic, this had grown to 4.43 million. Today there are 6.48 million people waiting for consultant-led elective care. In February 2022, only 61.8 percent of those referred by their GPs to the NHS for urgent cancer treatment were treated within two months compared to 78.8 percent in March 2020. In April 2022, only 79.1 percent of those referred to the NHS for an appointment with a consultant were consulted within two months compared to 91.9 percent in March 2020.[46]

This has also been at the cost of the wellbeing of healthcare staff. A succession of pandemic waves since the first one have piled unrelenting pressures on NHS workers, with only shortish respites in between the upsurges that bring large volumes of people into the hospitals. The recent Omicron waves have certainly hospitalized fewer people than the earlier ones. But the numbers have not been small in any absolute or numerical sense, so that the (already seriously under-resourced – as we have seen) healthcare system remains a stressed one, a system in perpetual crisis, with frontliners placed under pressures that never go away, unlike as was the case earlier due to the longer respites provided by the lockdowns.[47] Again, Christina Pagel draws attention to the consequences of this situation:

> The NHS is already in crisis with long waiting times in A&E, high response times for ambulances, and record numbers of people waiting for routine treatment. The number of people being admitted to hospital with covid has now started to rise again too. So in the short term, expect further pressure to pile on both secondary and primary care, as more people get sick and need care and more staff are off sick, making it even harder to provide care.[48]

This situation is simply unsustainable. Yet it will continue for the foreseeable future. This is as new COVID-19 upsurges conveyed by new variants and subvariants occur every three months or so under circumstances where there are simply no firebreaks. This is just as the effects of these waves are basically rendered almost invisible by the Government's pandemic denialism and those who acquiesce with it.

Explaining British exceptionalism

An explanation of all the various manifestations of British exceptionalism is ventured throughout this enterprise. The explanation is not complex. British exceptionalism is a pattern of policy responses to the pandemic that compromised public health owing the overriding priority accorded by the Government to capitalist economics and free markets above all else. As such, British exceptionalism has been profoundly shaped by neoliberalism, which is the most doctrinaire expression of unfettered capitalism and absolute markets in politics and ideology. The British people have had the misfortune of encountering a global pandemic under the sovereignty of a mode of state and governance that has been for decades almost completely absorbed by neoliberalism. The degree of this absorption is higher than in most of the other high-income countries. This partly explains the exceptionalism.

Initial and then later resistance to lockdowns was consequently, animated by the imperative to keep Britain "open for business", even though and just as business was closing elsewhere. Incautious de-escalation of lockdown restrictions was, consequently animated by the imperative to restore as quickly as possible Britain's "openness" for profit-making; indeed, to ensure that business was restored faster than anywhere else that matters, so that there was no comparative competitive disadvantage for home-grown or home-based capitals *vis-à-vis* those of competitor countries. For exactly the same reasons, an aspect of the resolute defence of Britain's "openness for business" was also maintaining borders that were open to anyone and everyone who would bring commerce to these shores and who would convey it from these shores to elsewhere.

These are just the two most obvious manifestations of the phenomenon. These are also the actions of a ruling party that is fully integrated into the worlds of property and high commerce, so that the natural inclinations of its leaders are to prioritize private interests over public ones, commercial interests over matters of social welfare. These are traditional Conservative agendas, but they are radicalized by capitalist internationalization, since this has strengthened the grip of free-market fundamentalism (neoliberalism) on the politics of the party. What stands above all else in British exceptionalism, however, is the rejection of border-control policy. This more than anything else made the UK an outlier state in international relations in the pandemic world. A few more words on this is warranted.

I have argued throughout this book that the political, economic and ideological forms associated with neoliberal capitalism must play a key role in explaining the UK government's whole pattern of response to the pandemic. This is certainly germane when accounting for the initial policy inaction with regard to border defence. Neoliberalism, the policy-framing ideology of international corporate capitalism, is noisily insistent that economic disaster and social malaise must befall any state that is protectionist. Borders, according to neoliberalism, must be porous in the economic sense, so that the flow of income- and profit-generating transfers (whether tourists, guest workers, students, capital, goods and services, business practices, etc.) are unimpeded.

Since "globalization" is taken for granted by neoliberals, not simply as the source of all bountiful things, but as an irresistible force, this could support a disregard of border-control policy on the grounds that this would be futile in preventing importations of disease. Such an attitude may explain the failure of the UK government to enact border defence until it was too late. But, in any case, from the perspective of a neoliberal polity such as the UK's, even if such protective measures had radically suppressed the virus, there were economic consequences to think of. Success in defending public health would have been at the cost of obstructing the capacity of British corporations to operate on the global canvass. In this particular case of cost-benefit analysis, public health was the loser and boardroom bonuses and shareholder profits were the winners. But the Government got its sums wrong. The economic damage wrought by prolonged community lockdowns that were rendered almost inevitable by the lack of border protection, reckless re-openings, and subsequent lack of mass testing/contact tracing and quarantining, has been extensive and will be long-standing.

This explanation is along the right lines. But it does not appear fully satisfactory. This is simply because the UK was an international outlier in terms of eschewing border controls. Britain's state and government is certainly among the most neoliberalized in the world. But neoliberal governance is also an international phenomenon. Yet this did not stop other countries from implementing at-the-border policies in an attempt to curtail or slow the importation of COVID-19. In short, abstract neoliberalism does not alone explain the exceptionalism of the UK's lack of a border-defence policy.

The solution, I think, is to flesh out the above argument rather than to jettison it. The decision of the UK government not to attempt blocking the import of the virus doubtless reflects the particular status of British capitalism in world economy. Britain's capitals are among the world leaders in export business,[49] just as the largest British MNCs are in the front rank for global reach under the "transnationality index" – more so than those of the EU and USA.[50] Britain's economy is more export-oriented than those of the EU and its trade is more globally dispersed than is theirs. Moreover, the City of London is one of the world's biggest financial centres (vying with New York for first place), which is globally interlinked with all of the others.[51] Not only that, the interests of financial capital have been especially prioritized by governments in the UK *vis-à-vis* industrial capital over a long period of time,[52] and these financial services make a larger contribution to GDP than do those in virtually all other countries.[53] Indeed, it has been argued that this has been to the detriment of the country's "real" manufacturing economy which has largely been subordinated.[54] Today the British manufacturing sector contributes only 17 percent to GDP.[55]

Finally, the UK's tourist industry is among the world's biggest and most lucrative, and this also makes a significant contribution to GDP. Travel and tourism is an integral aspect of the UK mode of capitalism, which is heavily rooted in services rather than industry, with services making up 73 percent of GDP.[56] Travel and tourism contributed £237 billion to the economy in 2019 or approximately 9.3 percent of GDP.[57] A fundamental aspect of the tourist industry is of course international tourism. The UK is among the world's top ten countries for international arrivals, in fourth place internationally for expenditure on international tourism, and in fifth place for countries which are the most lucrative tourist destinations.[58]

In short, on the basis of a range of indicators, the British economy is more internationalized than most. Little wonder, then, that British political elites especially identify "British" (national) interests as those which are synonymous with economic "globalization". That is, as those which lie in promoting world trade and commerce and placing British capitalism at their centre. Since economic interests tend to be translated by their bearers into those which convey higher values, that is, as *moralized norms*, so it is also that neoliberal powerholders in the UK wish to invest in free international exchange the highest moral virtues: promotion of individualism (self-reliance), maximization of consumer freedom, redoubt against oppressive state authority, and so on. Seen in this context, the UK government's eschewal of border defence measures as a first line of defence against the novel coronavirus becomes comprehensible.

As for the rest of "exceptionalism", what did this consist of? Firstly, there was the radical under-resourcing of the public and welfare functions of the state that underscored the crisis of PPE and testing capacity that was discussed in Chapter 2. Secondly, there was the communicative ambivalence of the Government's pandemic messaging, which I addressed in Chapter 6. Thirdly, there was the test-and-trace debacle, also examined in Chapter 6. Finally, there was mask-scepticism, which was dealt with in Chapter 7. These phenomena too can be accommodated to the capitalistic and neoliberal explanatory framework.

Firstly, as I set out in Chapter 3, the crisis of welfare is the result of class warfare from above to shift resources out of public hands and into private ones. Austerity was initially a project to protect capital from the negative impacts of the Great Crash by shifting its costs onto taxpayers – most of whom are wage earners. Latterly, it has become a permanent policy of neoliberal states to redistribute income from workers and the social and welfare services they especially draw on to the big commercial enterprises in order to boost their international competitiveness.

Secondly, communicative ambivalence may be read as a strategy of neoliberal governance to either undermine physical distancing norms that could not be evaded, or to disincentivize the public from sticking to the practices these norms enforce once the norms are removed. This of course was in order to break down public resistance to full capitalist restoration or normalization. The attitude of Johnson, of other ministers, of Tory party members and government support staff workers towards mandatory physical distancing has been starkly exposed in recent months by the "Partygate" affair.[59] These people participated in a series of illegal social gatherings at No. 10 Downing Street, at the party's HQ, and other government premises, in 2020 and 2021, during periods where physical distancing rules were in force. Twelve of these parties have been subject to police investigation. Johnson's contempt for physical distancing norms of his own artifice is shown not simply by the fact that these were not to be permitted to prevent literal partying in the party. Additionally, this is confirmed by the fact that since Johnson and his chancellor Rishi Sunak were exposed over their own roles in the affair (and fined by the police for breaking the law), both have refused to be held accountable for their actions.

Thirdly, the test-and-trace debacle was a simple enough story of what is likely to happen where you hand over to your entrepreneurial friends matters of which they have no experience or aptitude to deliver and who are likely to milk the situation to line their own pockets rather than advance the public good. Neoliberals are not disposed to avoid these errors because for them capitalism and markets are simply virtuous ("dynamic", "innovative", enterprising", etc.) and must deliver everything more efficiently than the state.

Finally, as for mask-scepticism, this was a curiosity in that, unlike other aspects of exceptionalism, this hardly served the cause of unshackling capitalism from the constraints of physical distancing. Unlike physical distancing, mask-wearing has no impact on economic life. Not only that, mask-wearing, if legally mandated by government, is a strategy for trying to evade physical distancing controls, or even to release them, by way of providing an alternative to them. The mask scepticism of the UK government was not shared by other capitalism-friendly governments except Trump's in the USA. In that sense, it was an oddity. This manifests, from the standpoint of economic interests, as an irrationality. However, mask-scepticism in this case may be read as the expression of an economic liberalism and consumer libertarianism thwarted by physical distancing. This was perhaps a case of displacement.

This distils a general explanation of British exceptionalism. But there is, I think, more to be said about it. To conclude, what else might be said? At the start of the pandemic, British exceptionalism manifested simply as complacent inattention to the crisis. There was little evidence of advance preparations or scenario planning. The explanation for this, I think, lies simply in the interface between the dysfunctionality of Johnson's premiership, his wider government's and party's fervent Brexit nationalism, and its neoliberal internationalism. There are a number of factors that may be pertinent.

(1) There is, firstly, the "complex" personality of Boris Johnson. The present incumbent of No. 10 is not really a person who plans or reflects over much. He prides himself on his spontaneity and randomness, his "quirky" (as he sees them) departures from rules (as Partygate attests), his instincts, his laissez-faire attitude, his talent for dealing with stuff as it arises rather in advance, and his "bold" as he sees it risk-taking.[60] Johnson is no more renowned for his attention to detail than he is for allowing public service to deflect him from his enjoyment of life's pleasures. Johnson, as has been noted, neither "does weekends" nor "urgent crisis planning". He manifests as someone for whom being PM is more a diverting hobby than a serious endeavour. The period of time from winning the winter 2019 election up until the pandemic was for him a whirl of pregnancy (his partner's) and impending fatherhood, marital engagement (to his then-fiancée Carrie Symonds), divorce from his long-standing wife, and extended vacations – including in his country retreat and in the Caribbean.[61]

(2) Johnson's government in the few months since it was elected up until COVID-19 was not proactive in doing anything much (in terms of policy

initiatives), with one notable exception – Brexit. Johnson took the UK out of the EU on 31 January 2020, declaring a bright new dawn in which the full potential of the country would burst forth and the lives of all Britons would be improved. This was done with great fanfare and ceremony, including a national EU "Exit Day", along with street parties and the minting of a commemorative 50p coin. Post-election time generally was for the better part of three months a period of extended Brexit gloating and celebrating, littered with rousing patriotic speeches extolling the even-greater-than-previous-greatness of Great Britain that would now be unleashed on the world stage with the shattering of the chains of the European super-state. Aside from Brexit-mongering, the new government was preoccupied with cabinet reshuffles, feuding with the BBC, and browbeating senior civil servants. This was on exactly the same timescale as the WHO was red-flagging COVID-19 as an international public health emergency of the highest magnitude, owing to its tenacity, high transmission rate, and lack of a vaccine.[62]

(3) Perhaps related to the second point, the Government allowed itself in the crucial period from the emergence of the novel coronavirus in China up until the start of the British pandemic to be preoccupied by the (for it) overriding task of "getting Brexit done", to the detriment and neglect of all else. That is unsurprising since "getting Brexit done" and the trumpeting of this as the way to confirm Britain's greatness was the alpha and omega of the Conservative Party's election campaign and the sole active cause of its victory. Thus, governmental action post-election entailed renewed hostilities with the EU over the terms of separation, concerted efforts to establish a Canada-style trading relationship with former EU partner states, and renewed attempts to negotiate new trade deals with new international partners. In sharp contrast with the lack of COVID-19 planning, a Brexit taskforce, indeed department, was long established.

As late as 12 March (2020), just as the PM was announcing the start of physical distancing measures, and just as he was warning for the first time that people should prepare themselves for losing loved ones, his press officers were briefing the media that Brexit-severance talks with the EU would continue the following week as planned and that there was no change to the June deadline for concluding negotiations, whether or not a deal was reached.[63] This is indicative that, just as the WTO were insisting that governments everywhere must make *immediate* preparations – including for extensive testing, contact-tracing and quarantining – or else face appalling consequences, the attentions of Johnson's government were elsewhere, absorbed with Brexit euphoria, with spinning its post-Brexit free-trade mantra, and with its concerted efforts to re-situate British capitalism on the world stage post-EU.

(4) It is even possible that a nationalistic sentiment puffed up by Brexit success informed government inaction with regard to the impending pandemic. Thus, Britain, being of course *Great*, would simply not succumb to the virus, as lesser countries had. Somehow the British would muddle through, drawing

upon superior care and welfare services, and of course exceptional national character (bulldog spirit, etc.). Perhaps, genetically, Britons were seen as being made of sterner stuff, and so perhaps would have greater natural resistance to the disease than those unfortunates across the channel and in the distant places. This is speculative, of course, but it is not beyond the bounds of reason, not given the nationalist triumphalism of post-Brexit Toryism. Nor is it contradicted by Johnson's own behaviour on the dawn of the British pandemic. As the crisis spiralled out of control in Italy, what was he doing? He was attending a rugby international with his fiancée at Twickenham. He was also making it his business to engage in public handshaking,[64] even though a recent SAGE meeting had urged ministers to discourage any form of physical contact in public spaces. In the early days, Johnson reportedly described Covid as "kung-flu" and even invited Chris Whitty to inject him with the virus on national TV to prove that Britons had little to fear from it.[65]

(5)   Then there is the matter of "herd immunity". In Chapter 1, I discussed debates around whether or not the apparent complacency, inaction, tardiness, etc. of the Government with regard to the pandemic as it made its way towards these shores was simply a case of incompetence or negligence or could have been something else. Something else would be a policy of herd immunity through mass infection. When I originally discussed this issue – which was actually in the spring of 2020 – I concluded that the matter could not be settled. This is still the case. However, since then, several reports have come to light, to complement those back then, which strengthen the case in favour of the notion that Johnson may indeed have had a herd immunity policy in the run-up to the first lockdown. These are those which cite the PM as declaring that the lockdowns were misguided because "only" the elderly were being killed and that he would rather see "the bodies pile high" than take the country back into another lockdown, for example.[66]

(6)   Finally, there is the interface of Brexit nationalism and neoliberal internationalization that lies at the core of the Government's political vision of the world. Those capitalist interests to which public health needs were to be so disastrously subordinated were likely to have assumed a particular magnitude of importance in the eyes of ministers owing to the uncertainty of the post-Brexit economic situation. This uncertainty may indeed have swung policy in favour of herd immunity. The UK had finally exited the EU. But it had done so without having thrashed out a deal that would allow for new trade relations that would cancel out the deficits of formally leaving the single market and without setting up alternative or additional trading deals with the other Triad powerbroker states of North America and South Asia.[67] Yet a dazzling future of boundless national cultural and economic renewal was promised to the Brexit-voting electorate that now needed to be delivered on. As such, given this context, it was highly probable that Johnson and company were very eager indeed to send a message out to the world that Britain was indeed fully "open" for global business, and that nothing, not even a global pandemic, would obstruct that purpose.

Consequently, when delivering another of his trademark "Britain – champion of free trade" type speeches on 3 February 2020, Johnson even made a point of cautioning *against* taking any protectionist measures against COVID-19 that would obstruct the UK's mission of becoming a powerhouse of world trade liberalization. As he put it, "there is a risk that new diseases such as coronavirus will trigger . . . a desire for market segregation that go beyond what is medically rational to the point of doing real and unnecessary economic damage".[68]

The economic damage perpetrated on UK capitalism by Johnson's attempt to minimize it at the price of public health and human life is profound and will be long-lasting. This, alas, is history, but a history whose negative legacy will be with us for the foreseeable future.

22 June 2022

Notes

1 Worldometer (2022). *COVID-19 Coronavirus Pandemic: Cases and Deaths*. Worldometer (online). Available at: www.worldometers.info/coronavirus/. Accessed: 20/06/2022. The WHO estimates that the real numbers of people killed worldwide either directly by the virus or owing to reasons connected to the virus is likely double this number.

2 Worldometer (2022). *COVID-19 Coronavirus Pandemic: Reported Cases and Deaths by Country or Territory*. Worldometer (online). Available at: www.worldometers.info/coronavirus/#countries. Accessed: 20/06/2022.

3 HM Government (2022). *COVID-19 Response: Living with COVID-19*. (February), pp. 4–5. Available at: https://assets.publishing.service.gov.uk/government/uploads/system/uploads/attachment_data/file/1056229/COVID-19_Response_-_Living_with_COVID-19.pdf.

4 Mellor, S. (2022). 'From Scandinavia to Spain, Europe is unmasking and moving on from COVID. Here's who's relaxing restrictions'. *Fortune*. (11 February); Mellor, S. and McGregor, G. (2022). 'As Omicron gallops across the globe, some countries begin to ask the once unthinkable: should we just stop counting cases'? *Fortune*. (28 January).

5 Lovelace, B. Jr. (2021). 'WHO says Covid vaccines aren't "silver bullets" and relying entirely on them has hurt nations'. *CNBC*. (15 January).

6 Beaumont, P. (2021). 'WHO warns of "epidemiological stupidity" of early Covid reopening'. *Guardian*. (7 July); Boffey, D. (2021). 'Coronavirus: WHO warns against further lifting of lockdown in England'. *Guardian*. (15 June).

7 Mellor (2022); Mellor and McGregor (2022).

8 HM Government (2022), p. 5.

9 HM Government (2022), p. 5.

10 GOV.UK (2021). *Prime Minister Confirms Move to Plan B in England*. Press Release. GOV.UK. (8 December). Available at: www.gov.uk/government/news/prime-minister-confirms-move-to-plan-b-in-england.

11 Campbell, D. (2022). 'No 10 must implement plan B before hospitals fill up, NHS leaders warn'. *Guardian*. (1 December).

12 Hainey, F. (2021). 'Experts urge immediate "10 day lockdown" – but Omicron data "still lacking" as cases surge'. *MSN News*. (16 December).

13 Gregory, A. (2021). 'Covid news – live: get ready for plan B now, scientists urge as hospital admissions in England at a 8-month high'. *Newsbreak*. (22 October); Shearing, H. and Lee, J. (2021). 'Covid: bring back rules amid rising cases, urge NHS chiefs'. *BBC News*. (20 October); Sridha, D. (2021). 'Britain must control Covid now – or face a

winter lockdown'. *Guardian*. (22 October); Wylie, C. (2021). 'Covid case numbers are "unacceptable' as he warns of another lockdown Christmas – Nervtag adviser'. *Evening Standard*. (23 October).

14 GOV.UK (2022). *England to Return to Plan A Following the Success of the Booster Programme*. Press Release. (19 January). Available at: www.gov.uk/government/news/ england-to-return-to-plan-a-following-the-success-of-the-booster-programme.

15 GOV.UK (2022). *Coronavirus (COVID-10) in the UK: Healthcare in the United Kingdom: Patients Admitted to Hospital*. Available at: https://coronavirus.data.gov.uk/details/ healthcare. Accessed: 18/06/2022; GOV.UK (2022). *Coronavirus (COVID-10) in the UK: Healthcare in the United Kingdom: Cases in the United Kingdom*. Available at: https:// coronavirus.data.gov.uk/details/cases. Accessed: 18/06/2022.

16 Steerpike (2021). 'Five experts who predicted daily Covid cases would hit 100,000'. *Spectator*. (27 July).

17 Davis, N. (2021). 'UK Covid cases rise for second day running amid drop in testing'. *Guardian*. (29 July); Burke, D. (2021). 'UK Covid infections drop by 50% in just two weeks as 26,144 test positive'. *Mirror*. (31 July).

18 *ITV News* (2022). 'All coronavirus restrictions to lift in England – here's Boris Johnson's plan for living with Covid'. (22 February).

19 Merrick, J. (2022). 'How bad is the new Covid wave? Why the UK should be concerned about rising cases, but not alarmed'. *I-News*. (17 June).

20 GOV.UK (2022). *PM Statement on Living with COVID: 21 February 2022*. Oral Statement to Parliament. (21 February). Available at: www.gov.uk/government/speeches/pm-statement-on-living-with-covid-21-february-2022; GOV.UK (2022). *COVID-19 Response: Living with COVID-19*. Cabinet Office. Available at: www.gov.uk/government/publications/ covid-19-response-living-with-covid-19/covid-19-response-living-with-covid-19.

21 HM Government (2022), p. 5.

22 Morton, B. and Turner, L. (2021). 'Covid: amber list scrapped as travel rules simplified'. *BBC News*. (4 October).

23 DfT and DHSC (2021). *Travel Update: All Countries Removed from the UK's Red List*. GOV.UK (online). (28 October). Available at: www.gov.uk/government/news/ travel-update-all-countries-removed-from-the-uks-red-list.

24 Merrick, R. (2021). 'Omicron: passengers from South Africa were not tested and "got home in normal way"'. *Independent*. (28 November).

25 Calder, S. (2021). 'Red list update: six countries added as experts say new Covid variant is "worst we've seen so far"'. *Independent*. (26 November).

26 Quite aside from radically underselling Omicron, this dismissal of the new variant was blind to the far greater health risks posed by people contracting flu and COVID-19 together – which is a real danger for many during the flu season under circumstances where there is no social distancing. Research indicates that people infected by both experience especially radical health ill-effects. See Noble, K. (2022). *COVID-19 Mixed with Flu Increases Risk of Severe Illness and Death*. Imperial College London (online). (25 March). Available at: www.imperial.ac.uk/news/235116/covid-19-mixed-with-increases-risk-severe/#:~:text=The%20findings%2C%20from%20a%20study,likely%20 to%20require%20ventilation%20support.

27 Worldometer (2022). *Countries: United Kingdom: Total Coronavirus Deaths in the UK*. Available at: www.worldometers.info/coronavirus/country/uk/. Accessed: 25/06/2022.

28 Worldometer (2022). *Countries: United Kingdom: New Daily Deaths in the United Kingdom*. Available at: www.worldometers.info/coronavirus/country/uk/. Accessed: 25/06/2022.

29 GOV.UK (2022). *Coronavirus (COVID-19) in the UK: Deaths in the United Kingdom: Deaths Within 28 Days of Positive Test by Date of Death*. Available at: https://coronavirus. data.gov.uk/details/deaths. Accessed: 15/03/2022.

30 Worldometer (2022).

31 Worldometer (2022). *Countries: United Kingdom: Daily New Cases in the United Kingdom*. Available at: www.worldometers.info/coronavirus/country/uk/. Accessed: 25/06/2022.

32 GOV.UK (2022), Accessed: 28/04/2022.

33 GOV.UK (2022). *Deaths in the United Kingdom*. Available at: https://coronavirus.data. gov.uk/details/deaths. Accessed: 20/06/2022.
34 Merrick (2022). This reports epidemiologist Paul Hunter's judgement.
35 GOV.UK (2022). *Coronavirus (COVID-19) in the UK: Patients in Mechanical Ventilation Beds*. Available at: https://coronavirus.data.gov.uk/details/healthcare. Accessed: 28/04/22.
36 GOV.UK (2022). *Coronavirus (COVID-19) in the UK: Cases by Specimen Date*. GOV. UK (online). Available at: https://coronavirus.data.gov.uk/details/cases. Accessed: 22/05/2022; GOV.UK (2022), Accessed: 15/03/2022; GOV.UK (2022). *Coronavirus (COVID-19) in the UK: Patients Admitted to Hospital*. GOV.UK (online). Available at: https://coronavirus.data.gov.uk/details/healthcare.
37 *ITV News* (2022). 'Covid: England passes record for daily reported cases'. (1 January).
38 *ITV News* (2022). '38,409 more Covid cases recorded as coronavirus deaths rise by 15'. (21 February).
39 Pagel, C. (2022). 'The covid waves continue to come'. *British Medical Journal*, 377 (1504) (17 June), pp. 1–2. Available at: www.bmj.com/content/377/bmj.o1504.
40 Pagel (2022).
41 Altmann cited in Merrick (2022).
42 Ayoubkhani, D. and Munro, M. (2022). *Prevalence of Ongoing Symptoms Following Coronavirus (COVID-19) Infection in the UK: 6 May 2022*. ONS (online). (6 May). Available at: www.ons.gov.uk/peoplepopulationandcommunity/healthandsocialcare/conditionsanddiseases/bulletins/prevalenceofongoingsymptomsfollowingcoronaviruscovid19infectionintheuk/6may2022.
43 Burton cited in: Bawden, T. (2022). 'UK Covid cases double as Omicron BA.4 and BA.5 subvariants cause infections to rise by 105%'. *I-News*. (23 June).
44 Sato cited in *ITV News* (2022). 'Omicron subvariants may have evolved to target lungs, experts say as UK cases rise'. (21 June).
45 Pagel (2022).
46 British Medical Association (2022). *NHS Backlog Data Analysis*. BMS (online). (17 June). Available at: www.bma.org.uk/advice-and-support/nhs-delivery-and-workforce/pressures/nhs-backlog-data-analysis.
47 Ireland, B. (2022). *COVID: It Never Went Away*. British Medical Association (online). (19 May). Available at: www.bma.org.uk/news-and-opinion/covid-it-never-went-away.
48 Pagel (2022).
49 31.6 percent of UK GDP was for export in 2019. See: World Integrated Trade Solution (2020). *United Kingdom Trade Statistics: Exports, Imports, Products, Tariffs, GDP and Related Development Indicator*. World Bank (online). Available at: https://wits.worldbank.org/CountryProfile/en/GBR. This is far ahead of the USA's and Japan's output to export ratios (11.3 percent and 18.5 percent, respectively). See: Statista (2020). *Exports of Goods and Services from the United States from 1990 to 2019, as a Percentage of GDP*. Available at: www.statista.com/statistics/258779/us-exports-as-a-percentage-of-gdp/; Trading Economics (2019). *Japan: Export of Goods and Services (% of GDP)*. World Bank Development Indicators. Available at: https://tradingeconomics.com/japan/exports-of-goods-and-services-percent-of-gdp-wb-data.html The UK's proportion of exports to GDP is comparable to the large high-export economies of the EU – such as Germany and France – which are not typical worldwide. The bulk of Germany's and France's and the UK's export business is with the EU member states: 59 percent of Germany's were in 2018; 64 percent of France's; and 53 percent of the UK's were in 2019. See Federal Ministry for Economic Affairs and Energy (2019). *Facts About German Foreign Trade: Foreign Trade Figures in 2018*. Berlin: BMWi; Workman, D. (2020). *France's Top Trading Partners*. World's Top Exporters (online). Available at: www.worldstopexports.com/frances-top-import-partners/; Clark, D. (2021). *Brexit and EU Trade – Statistics & Facts*. Statista (online). (28 April). Available at: www.statista.com/topics/3126/brexit-and-eu-trade/#:~:text=EU%20still%20dominates%20UK%20trade,53%20percent%20of%20

its%20exports. The UK's trading dependence on the EU (which includes considerable food import dependency) is an obvious disadvantage in a post-Brexit and ex-single market context – and one that will not be resolved in the foreseeable future. This is because this will increase import and export costs for UK businesses owing to new tariffs, taxes, procedures, regulations, checks, and so on. The EU is also disadvantaged, for the same reasons, but much less so than the UK, because the GDP of the EU is much bigger than that of the UK, and the trading dependency between the two is asymmetric to the detriment of the latter. This is shown by the following statistics. Whereas 48 percent of UK exports went to the EU in 2017, 6.2 percent of EU exports went to the UK. Whereas 6 percent of the UK's GDP in 2017 was accounted for by exports to the EU, just over 2 percent of the EU's GDP was accounted for by exports to the UK. Germany and France, the EU's big players, are only fractionally more reliant on export trade with the UK than is the case for the EU as an aggregate. There was little prospect, then, during the negotiations around TCA, of the French or German governments feeling that their interests were better served by exerting pressure on the other member states to grant the UK special trading concessions. In the case of Germany, 6.6 percent of exports were to the UK in 2017, which is the equivalent of 2.6 percent of GDP. In the case of France, 6.7 percent of exports were to the UK in 2017, which is the equivalent of 1.4 percent of GDP. See Walker, A. (2018). 'Does the EU need us more than we need them'? *BBC News*. (23 December).

50 See Rugman, A. and Verbeke, A. (2003). 'Regional multinationals and triad strategy'. A. Rugman (Ed). *Leadership in International Business Education and Research – Research in Global Strategic Management*, vol. 8. Bingley: Emerald Group Publishing Limited, pp. 253–68. The "transnationality index" measures the supposed degree of globality of corporations in terms of the proportion of their sales, premises, properties, and investments that are outside their home country. In the early 2000s, the average transnationality rating of the top 100 UK MNCs was 69.2 percent. This compared to 45.8 percent for the USA's, 42.8 percent for Japan's, 59.5 percent for France's, and 49.0 percent for Germany's. There are, contrary to globalization theory, few firms that would even tenuously count as transnational corporations (TNCs), since most of their cross-border transfers are contained within a home region. Those MNCs that come closest to the ideal TNC are mostly from the smaller developed national economies than the bigger ones (e.g. of Switzerland, Finland, Sweden, Canada). These are more open to world commerce than the larger ones owing to the bigger limits on domestic sales. However, the UK economy is anomalous, in that it has a transnationality rating that is much closer to those of these smaller, more open national economies than those of its major larger competitors.

51 Financial Centre Futures (2016). *The Global Financial Centres Index*. China Development Institute (CDI) and Yen (online). (February). Available at: www.longfinance.net/publications/long-finance-reports/the-global-financial-centres-index-20/; *Financial Times* (2020). 'How London grew into a financial powerhouse'. (15 December).

52 Gamble, A. (1981). *Britain in Decline*. London: Macmillan.

53 Hutton, G. and Shalchi, A. (2020). *Financial Services: Contribution to the UK Economy*. London: House of Commons Library, p. 5. In 2020, the sector was the third largest in the OECD in terms of its contribution to GDP, earning the British economy £164.8 billion, or 8.6 percent of total GDP, with financial exports valued at £62 billion and with a trade surplus of £16 billion.

54 Gamble (1981).

55 O'Neill, A. (2022). 'Distribution of GDP across economic sectors in the United Kingdom 2020'. *Statista* (online). (15 February). Available at: www.statista.com/statistics/270372/distribution-of-gdp-across-economic-sectors-in-the-united-kingdom/#:~:text=In%20 2020%2C%20agriculture%20contributed%20around,percent%20from%20the%20services%20sector.&text=The%20vast%20majority%20of%20the,particular%20keeps%20 the%20economy%20going

56 O'Neill (2022).
57 *Statista* (2021). 'Travel and tourism in the United Kingdom – statistics & facts'. (26 August). Available at: www.statista.com/topics/3269/travel-and-tourism-in-the-united-kingdom-uk/#dossierKeyfigures.
58 UNWO (2020). *UNWTO World Tourism Barometer and Statistical Annex, December 2020.* (December). Available at: www.e-unwto.org/doi/abs/10.18111/wtobarometereng.2020.18.1.7.
59 Cavendish, C. (2022). 'Partygate lays bare the casual carelessness of Boris Johnson's ancien régime'. *Financial Times.* (15 April); Catterall, P. (2022). *Why Partygate has a Significance Beyond the Behaviour of an Individual Prime Minister.* LSE, British Politics and Policy. (20 April). Available at: https://blogs.lse.ac.uk/politicsandpolicy/why-partygate-matters/; Associated Press (2022). 'U.K. Covid "partygate" report blames culture of Boris Johnson's office'. *NBC News.* (25 May).
60 Bower, T. (2020). *Boris Johnson: The Gambler.* London: Random House.
61 Conn, D. et al. (2020). 'Revealed: the inside story of the UK's Covid-19 crisis'. *Guardian.* (29 April); Walker, P. (2020). 'Boris Johnson missed five coronavirus Cobra meetings, Michael Gove says'. *Guardian.* (19 April).
62 Conn et al. (2020); Helm, T., Graham-Harrison, E. and McKie, R. (2020). 'How did Britain get its coronavirus response so wrong'? *Guardian.* (19 April).
63 Conn et al. (2020).
64 Archer, B. (2020). 'Boris Johnson braves coronavirus outbreak with pregnant fiancée to support England'. *Express.* (8 March).
65 Cowburn, A. (2021). 'Boris Johnson offered to be injected with Covid on TV and called virus "kung flu", report suggests'. *Independent.* (26 May); Taylor, W. (2021). 'Cummings: officials feared PM would try to be injected with Covid on TV to stop "panic"'. *LBC News.* (26 May).
66 BBC News (2021). 'Covid: Boris Johnson resisted autumn lockdown as only over-80s dying – Dominic Cummings'. (20 July); Colson, T. (2021). 'Boris Johnson witnesses say they will swear on oath he said he'd "let the bodies pile high in their thousands"'. *Business Insider.* (27 April); Elgot, J. and Booth, R. (2021). 'Pressure mounts on Johnson over alleged "let the bodies pile high" remarks'. *Guardian.* (26 April); Ng, K. (2021). 'Boris Johnson said he "would rather let bodies pile high" than impose a third lockdown'. *Independent.* (26 April); *Reuters* (2021). 'UK PM's former adviser confirms Johnson said "let the bodies pile high"'. (26 May).
67 Conn et al. (2020).
68 GOV.UK (2020). *PM Speech in Greenwich: 3 February 2020.* Prime Minister's Office. (3 February). Available at: www.gov.uk/government/speeches/pm-speech-in-greenwich-3-february-2020.

INDEX

For Product Safety Concerns and Information please contact our EU
representative GPSR@taylorandfrancis.com
Taylor & Francis Verlag GmbH, Kaufingerstraße 24, 80331 München, Germany

www.ingramcontent.com/pod-product-compliance
Lightning Source LLC
Chambersburg PA
CBHW060248220326
41598CB00027B/4029